Advance Praise for *The Iberian Table*

"She may not like my saying this, but with *The Iberian Table*, Robin Keuneke has written a book that should appeal even to those food-lovers who don't care a fig about antioxidants, microbiomes, or fatty acids. I say that because I believe that one can probably eat better in Spain today than anywhere else in the Western world — from the most basic of foods (Catalonia's elemental *pa amb tomàquet*, the ubiquitous *espinacas con garbanzos*) to the most other-worldly innovations of modernist cuisine — and Keuneke has done a remarkably comprehensive job of telling us why and how. Her recipes are clearly written and seductive, and she eloquently evokes the soul and spirit of Spain — even those parts of it that are far from the Mediterranean — and, yeah, okay, all the health and nutrition stuff is pretty useful and informative as well, and only enhances the rest."

— Colman Andrews, author,
Catalan Cuisine: Europe's Last Great Culinary Secret and
Ferran: The Inside Story of El Bulli and the Man Who Reinvented Food

"Robin Keuneke has succeeded at a difficult task: writing about health statistics and recipes without becoming tedious. Most readers of such subjects eventually switch off. But Robin is a very fine, engaging writer. In addition, she is preserving in print, while it is still possible, an ancient way of life, now threatened by globalisation, commercialism, and climate change. For this, we should be grateful."

— Dr. Andreas Buttimer, Radiologist, Ireland

"*The Iberian Table* is many things—a story, a referenced text on health, a cookbook and a memoir helping us understand the Mediterranean diet on all levels. With thorough research and the voice of a seasoned storyteller, Robin Keuneke brings the Spanish Mediterranean diet to life."

– Isabel Bertomeu, formerly nutritionist-dietician
Mediterranean Diet Foundation, Barcelona

"Robin Keuneke uses her senses to bring a country, culture, its geography, food and people alive on inked pages. It is unusual for a writer to be so good at doing it."

– Udo Erasmus, Ph.D., Author of *Fats That Heal Fats That Kill*

"*The Iberian Table*, a fascinating road trip through the gastronomy of Spain, serves us on a plate the secrets of the Mediterranean diet. With two cups of grace and a pinch of passion, Robin Keuneke reveals the ancestral tradition of the Spanish people: that of simply eating our own landscape. Reading this book, you will discover that Spaniards have never been very impressed by Cordon Bleu recipes, but very attentive to fresh produce of the street markets; that a good fish doesn't need much more than a sprinkle of olive oil to be broiled to excellence. As you will find out in the fascinating interviews with chefs Arzak and Ruscalleda, eating in the Iberian Peninsula is not a refueling chore but a destination to an after-dinner conversation that can go on forever. So take a seat and enjoy!"

– Guillermo Fesser, journalist, writer,
filmmaker and creator of *Gomaespuma*

"*The Iberian Table* represents the wisdom of Mediterranean women in the development of culinary knowledge for a more delicious, sustainable, and healthy diet. A complete delight!"

– Alba Adat Caballero, formerly nutritionist-dietician
Alícia Foundation, Catalunya

"Robin Keuneke introduces us all to the unique and health-promoting 'Iberian Table.' It is filled with traditional, flavor-packed recipes that provide our hearts, minds and bodies with an array of phytonutrients sure to promote optimal health. Enjoy!"

– Donald R. Yance, MH, CN, master herbalist,
nutritionist, and author of *Herbal Medicine,
Healing & Cancer*, and *Adaptogens in Medical Herbalism*

"*The Iberian Table* whisks me away emotionally, historically and scientifically to incorporate this way of eating into my lifestyle. So simple and so much fun! With Robin's recipes I can visit Spain in my kitchen every night knowing that, in the process, I am promoting good health for my family."

– Sandy Gooch, author and natural foods retail pioneer

"A feast for the body, soul and spirit from wise woman Robin Keuneke, this book will delight your senses, and help you steer a clear path to health. Lots of Green Blessings here."

– Susun Weed, Author of *Abundantly Well: Seven Medicines*

THE
IBERIAN
TABLE

THE IBERIAN TABLE

Healthy Cooking Secrets from the Land of Longevity

Introduction to the
Spanish Mediterranean Diet

ROBIN KEUNEKE

BAY OF ROSES BOOKS

THE IBERIAN TABLE:
Healthy Cooking Secrets from the Land of Longevity—
Introduction to the Spanish Mediterranean Diet

Front cover photo: Eva Espinet and Olga Moya.
Book design: Vickie Swisher, Studio 20|20.

Publisher's Cataloging-in-Publication
(Provided by Cassidy Cataloguing Services, Inc.).

Names: Keuneke, Robin, author.

Title: The Iberian table : healthy cooking secrets from the land of longevity : introduction to the Spanish Mediterranean diet / Robin Keuneke.

Description: [Delray Beach, Florida] : Bay of Roses Books, [2024] | Includes bibliographical references and index.

Identifiers: ISBN: 978-0-692-98219-8 (softcover) | LCCN: 2024904041

Subjects: LCSH: Keuneke, Robin--Travel--Spain. | Cooking, Mediterranean--Health aspects. | Cooking, Spanish--Health aspects. | Diet--Spain. | LCGFT: Cookbooks. | BISAC: BIOGRAPHY & AUTOBIOGRAPHY / Culinary. | COOKING / Regional & Cultural / Spanish. | COOKING / Regional & Cultural / Mediterranean. | TRAVEL / Europe / Spain & Portugal.

Classification: LCC: TX725.M35 K48 2024 | DDC: 641.591822--dc23

permissions@iberiantable.com

This book is written in loving memory of my mother Nancy Grant
and
to my husband, Thomas, my confidante, my love
il miglior fabbro.

Excerpts

"That day, I was changed, too, for truly great cooking comes from a place deeper than the mind. It is a manifestation of all our experiences, but more than this, cooking is about how deeply we can feel and trust."

"Between forkfuls of delicious fried eggs and *jamón*, we spoke of ancient myths, pilgrimages, and invasions—of *la Reconquista*—and of a thwarted Charlemagne. We talked about the giant prehistoric creatures that once inhabited the outcrop of land that began the Pyrenees, and how the primordial mountains are older than the Alps."

"Our order is taken without fanfare by a serious, plump Catalan. The woman looks us up and down with piercing dark little eyes. Holding her pad with pen in hand, the server questions us—are we certain that we want *fideuá*? It's almost as though she will demand that we produce our passports. After a final severe glance, the woman shuffles away leaving a cloud of disgruntlement like bubbles trailing a displaced squid. We look at one another in suspense. What next?"

"Not to be taken lightly, good food marks an occasion. Aren't perfect summer berries a way to welcome this very special season—to memorialize a real moment, when morning sun pours through your kitchen window, heralding sybaritic weeks ahead, while you bask in it, allowing each berry to explode in your mouth in ravishing goodness? And finally, cooking as a way to explore other cultures somehow unites us all. Cooking has never mattered more."

"This land, where people have been cooking for a very long time, has yet to show me everything. Guided by rivers where lampreys have flourished since time immemorial, by tides of oceans and wind-swept seas, by berry-strewn paths winding through prehistoric mountains, by secrets revealed in ancient forests with tender plants that thrust through mossy soil every spring, I am still driven to know more. If you are like me, you will want to know it. As the artist-poet Juan Muñoz wrote, "'Our most beautiful days we have not yet seen.'"

CONTENTS

PART TWO

"On November 16th, 2010, the UNESCO intergovernmental committee for the safeguarding of Intangible Cultural Heritage at their meeting in Keyna agreed to include the Mediterranean Diet on the Representative List of Intangible Cultural Heritage of Humanity. The Mediterranean Diet is an immense and ancient cultural heritage that is in danger. Only the international recognition can result in the mobilisation necessary for its safeguarding."

– Fundación Dieta Mediterránea, Barcelona, Spain

As evocative as it is informative, *The Iberian Table* transmits the essence of the Mediterranean diet. We must keep in mind the origin of the word *diet*. The ancient Greek word *diaita* means balanced lifestyle, and this is exactly what the Mediterranean diet is. It is a lifestyle that combines ingredients from local agriculture, traditional recipes and cooking methods, shared meals and celebrations with family and friends, all in an active lifestyle that modern scientific research has proven to be in fact one of the healthiest lifestyles anywhere. Dr. Ancel Keys, thanks to his "Seven Countries Study," first described its health benefits in the 1960s, where he defines the role of this dietary pattern in heart disease. The dietary habits in the Mediterranean area drew attention because of Dr. Keys's finding that the incidence of coronary disease was significantly lower in Mediterranean countries than in others that did not follow the same lifestyle and eating habits.

The Mediterranean diet is a valuable cultural heritage that has been passed down from generation to generation over the centuries, evolving along with the history of the Mediterranean. It has been able to welcome new foods and techniques thanks to its strategic geographical position and its capacity to wisely incorporate them flawlessly. We can see a clear example of this with the discovery of the Americas. No one can imagine the Mediterranean diet without tomatoes, peppers, potatoes, etc. What would the Mediterranean diet be without these amazing contributions from the American continent? For one, Catalans would not have their iconic dish *pa amb tomàquet*. Something as simple but most treasured as a piece of bread rubbed with ripe tomatoes and a drizzle of olive oil would not exist. What a boring existence! We must also thank the Americas for "saving" one of the pillars of the Mediterranean diet triad of wine, bread, and olive oil. The phylloxera vine louse destroyed most of the vineyards for wine grapes in Europe in the late nineteenth century. After many years of trying to fight this blight, phylloxera insect-resistant vines from America were imported and used as root stock onto which European varieties were grafted, saving wine production in Spain and the rest of the continent.

The Iberian Table is many things: a story, a referenced text on health, a cookbook, and a memoir helping us understand the Mediterranean diet on all levels. With thorough research and the voice of a seasoned storyteller, Robin Keuneke brings the Spanish Mediterranean Diet to life with fresh and essential information that allows us to continue transmitting this cultural heritage down to our future generations. And she does so in a most practical manner as well as the best possible way, by spending time with our loved ones in the kitchen and around the table. Robin, the Mediterranean diet thanks you.

Isabel Bertomeu
Former Dietician-Nutritionist
Mediterranean Diet Foundation

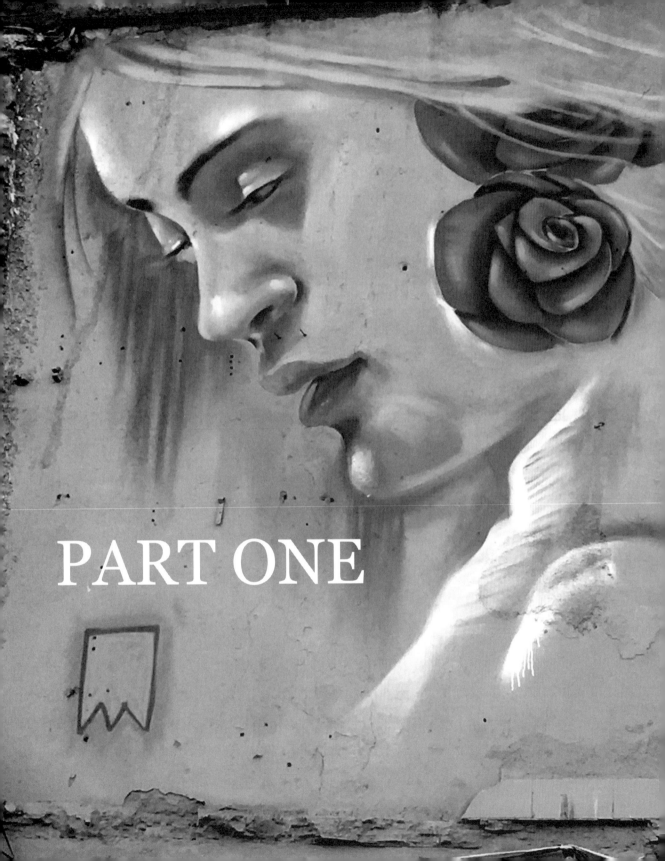

PART ONE

ACKNOWLEDGEMENTS

"The Mediterranean diet has consistently lowered cardiovascular events and mortality in numerous studies, and does not typically lower cholesterol levels."

— Donald R. Yance Jr., MH, CN, "What can Centenarians teach us about cholesterol levels and longevity—It isn't what you think" Blog post, donnieyance.com May 19, 2021

I could not have written *The Iberian Table: Healthy Cooking Secrets from the Land of Longevity—Introduction to the Spanish Mediterranean Diet* without the help of many people, but the chefs of Spain are first. The earth speaks to me through their cooking as if to say, "Let the flavors of nature reign."

Classes at New York's Macrobiotic Center in the 1980s propelled me into the world of natural foods cooking. I've always loved vegetables, so I attended the Center to learn more about preparing my favorite foods. I still treasure the ingredient-stained recipe pages from my classes there. The late founder of the center and my teacher, Shizuko Yamamoto, introduced many fine recipes, one of which was pickled daikon radish, prepared with a whisper of sea salt. In those days, nutrition science did not understand the crucial place gut microbiome held in human health, but Shizuko knew that if her pickles were eaten regularly, digestion would be revitalized, bettering health in countless ways. When the 2020 German study of European countries reported that for each gram per day increase in national consumption of pickled vegetables, the risk for Covid-19 mortality decreased nearly 36 percent, though Shizuko was no longer with us, admiration for my teacher grew.

Shizuko's contributions chronicle the development of natural foods healing and shiatsu worldwide. Along with her work in America, Shizuko launched workshops throughout Europe, starting coincidently in Barcelona, a setting for three chapters in this book. Born in Japan, young Shizuko studied with George and Lima Ohsawa, founders of macrobiotics.

Following my time at the Macrobiotic Center, I fell even more in love with the real and original way food tastes through my association with the Natural Gourmet Institute, also in New York. My thanks to the late founder, Anne Marie Colbin, Ph.D., author of natural foods cookbooks, and expert on the contributions of the Ohsawas as well as James Beard. I remain grateful to her Natural Gourmet program that lives on through the International Culinary Institute.

Surprisingly, a macrobiotic restaurant also set the course for this book. Though Souen closed in 2019, and owner Masaaki Yamaguchi, known as Yama, is no longer with us, I will never forget this fine man, or his light-filled SoHo restaurant, whose chefs cooked the splendid produce they purchased direct from Union Square farmer's market. Ingredients were always first-rate at Souen, whose Carrot Ginger Dressing was described by *New York Times* restaurant critic Mimi Sheraton in her 1981 review as "marvelous." In 2019, Souen was still on *The New York Times* radar with Christine Muhlke noting in her review that she "loved" Souen.

When traveling I searched for low-key, vegan-inspired places, always thinking of Souen. Trips overseas led to wonderful meals, but nothing compared to Souen. The same could be said about Norway, but there I sampled all kinds of herring. Clean, oily savors left me wanting more. As for Norway's ever-present pickled onions—thanks to Shizuko, I partook with gusto.

After the delicious herring of Norway, I longed for a gastronomy rich in healthy fats, which was met unexpectedly one night in a tiny, ramshackle gas station/restaurant in the Wadi Rum, some twenty miles outside Amman, Jordan, on the desert highway from Petra. As my husband Thomas and I entered, traces of wood-fire smoke wafted in from the stone oven out back. It was early evening, so the modest establishment seemed our own. Hummus, redolent with house-made tahini and olive oil was placed before us. The savory richness of the tahini was defining, and the olive oil, fresh. Next, a platter brimming with leaves of lettuce, scallions, sliced mild onion, and wedges of ripened tomato, all glistened with the promise of flavor. Of course there was rice. When the grilled chicken was served, scents of cumin, cinnamon, and garlic fluttered over the table like an exotic veil. The exterior of the chicken had just the right note of crispness, without being burned. Alongside the carafe of verdant olive oil were olives and yeasty, sweet-smelling pita, warm from the oven out back. The pita came in handy for mopping up every bit of that savory hummus, so freshly made it was slightly warm. A clay bowl filled with creamy yogurt beckoned. I tasted. It was house-made, too. Sensations of sweet, sour goodness flooded my soul.

A year or so later, when I made my way to Spain, I encountered a gastronomy that I loved even more. The spirit of Spain's plant-forward cooking, and quality of ingredients placed me on trajectory for this book. I learned that extra-virgin olive oil came in regional varietals of goodness and could impart bright lushness into all sorts of recipes. Flavors—sunny, full, and vivid—were extracted with little salt. Coaxed effortlessly, centuries of gastronomic expertise had been codified through the ages to showcase what Spanish chefs proudly called "raw materials." Exquisite products, prepared simply. Cold soups contained a variety of seasonal produce, and were blended with extra-virgin olive oil and almonds. There were so many ways to include nuts in one's diet. Who knew? Countless fish and seafood recipes helped me grasp that *more seafood, less meat* really could be put into practice. As for beans, I wasn't a fan, but it was the utter deliciousness of Spain's countless dishes that hooked me on this healthy food.

This special place intrigues me not just as a cook, but also as a health writer. The benefits of following Spain's traditional Mediterranean diet has been proven by the work of Dr. Ramón Estruch, leading researcher for the groundbreaking PREDIMED study. Conducted in Spain, PREDIMED clarified with peerless evidence that persons at high vascular risk for heart attack or stroke can reduce risk by as much as 30% by following Spain's traditional Mediterranean diet. The findings of PREDIMED were so dramatic it challenged the establishment. Some demanded the study must be reconfirmed. And it was. My appreciation goes to Dr. Estruch and all the researchers involved in PREDIMED for what may have seemed thankless work. Spain's traditional Mediterranean diet addresses a myriad of health problems. Heart health is but one.

Turning to the individuals whose help made this book possible, thanks first to my beloved husband, Thomas, whose enthusiasm for this project fueled me through years of writing and research. His appetite for adventure has taken us to disparate places, providing me with experiences in many traditional cooking cultures.

In addition, the following have my thanks:

Barcelonans Eva Espinet and Olga Moya styled and shot the photo for the cover of *The Iberian Table*. Their contributions also include photos of markets, as well as styling and photographing my recipes for this book. In addition, their tireless review of Catalan, Spanish, and Basque words and phrases were all executed with commitment and humor. Eva and Olga also contributed a recipe and coordinated the interview with chef Ruscalleda.

The Mediterranean Diet Foundation (Fundación Dieta Mediterránea) promotes investigation of the health, historical, cultural and gastronomic characteristics of the diet, as well as dissemination of scientific findings and health benefits among varied populations. The Foundation's Scientific Committee, consisting of recognized international experts, advises on scientific matters, edifying us all on matters integral to health. My appreciation for this organization would not be complete without acknowledging its successful initiative to preserve the Mediterranean diet and culture by bringing it to the attention of UNESCO, who then included the diet in the Representative List of the Intangible Cultural Heritage of Humanity.

In particular, Isabel Bertomeu, CN, previously nutritionist-dietician for the Mediterranean Diet Foundation, was part of the UNESCO initiative to gain special status for the diet. I wish to express appreciation to Isabel Bertomeu for this, and for her substantial contributions to this book, including her fine foreword, recipe and editing assistance. In addition, Isabel developed *The Iberian Table* website along with Albert Ariza, who hails from France. Presently, Ms. Bertomeu is Communications and Outreach Coordinator, Department of Epidemiology, Schulich School of Medicine and Dentistry, Western University in Ontario, Canada.

Chef Jaume Subirós somehow found the time to take an interest in this book. Before the appearance of nouvelle cuisine in 1961, the bellwether kitchen of his historic restaurant, El Motel, inspired a new generation of chefs, including Carme Ruscalleda and Elena Arzak, whom Chef Subirós kindly contacted on my behalf, opening the door to interviewing them for this book. In these interviews, Chefs Ruscalleda and Arzak bestow upon us a rare insider's look into their culinary habits. Monica Prensa coordinated the interview with Chef Arzak, and Mireia Bosch, Eva Espinet, and Olga Moya contributed translation assistance with Chef Ruscalleda's interview.

Chef María José San Román, lauded for her use of saffron and rice dishes, is a self-taught Michelin-starred expert on Valencian cooking. Her contribution of recipes to the book helped to extend *The Iberian Table* region south, reminding us that delicious, life-extending gastronomy occurs throughout all of Spain. Chef San Román's assistant, Julia Alonso, coordinated receipt of the recipes contributed to the book. Chef Xavier Arrey Vergés of Restaurant Indigo at Hotel Carlemany in Girona is praised for some of the best cooking in the region. His recipe for thyme soup can be found in appendix B.

Manu Manu's mural, *M'agraden les mares I dones del món sencer*, from the Sants neighborhood in Barcelona, graces the pages of the book. The artist, who has been profiled in *Graffitismo & Street Art* (Bellavite Editore, 2019), springs from a graffiti background, embracing crumbling urban context. His Sants neighborhood mural celebrates women of every age from across the globe.

The artist and photographer, Lourdes Solana, introduced to me by Eva Espinet and Olga Moya shared photos for this project including those of Manu Manu's mural which can be found in the opening of Parts One and Two, and in full among the color plates.

Alícia Trullén, an *aranesa* friend, has my thanks for her insights into the hearty and healthy cooking of her homeland.

Daniel A. Simon, Ph.D., poet, translator, journalist, and editor-in-chief of the diverse and globally-focused magazine *World Literature Today*, somehow found time to undertake copy editing for much of this book. To work with Daniel was an honor, for his own articles, editorials, poetry, and books remain some of the best contemporary writing published. Daniel's title observation moved me toward the final name for this book.

Master herbalist and nutritionist, Donald R. Yance Jr., MH, CN, RH, provided research and his time reading early manuscript drafts. Donnie, author of two books on herbs and healing, founded and operates Mederi Center, a thriving clinical practice, and Mederi Academy, having the purpose to provide online training to health care practitioners around the world. Donnie's insights helped us understand how thyme and rosemary, herbs central to the cooking of Spain, support the healing systems of the body. These herbs are so protective that new research findings are published about their benefits regularly. I also wish to acknowledge his wife, Jennifer, for her co-stewardship of Mederi Academy and Mederi Center, organizations dedicated to improving the health of people everywhere.

Udo Erasmus, Ph.D., author, teacher/philosopher, speaker, and blogger, wrote the seminal work *Fats That Heal, Fats That Kill*, which opened the door to a crucial nutrition story, previously overlooked. Udo's work increased my understanding of why Spain's olive oil-rich Mediterranean diet is so very protective. In total, his books have sold over 250,000 copies. Udo, who gave generously of his time reading early drafts of the book, remains a force in my life.

As with Udo, I became acquainted with Sandy Gooch and Niqi Cindric when writing my first book on health. I am grateful for their friendship, support, and inspiration.

Spain's diversity of language made writing *The Iberian Table* a challenge. Feedback was especially helpful during the early manuscript stage from Gerry Dawes, described by Chef José Andrés as the "first to really tell the story of Spain." Gerry, expert on wine and gastronomy, has lived in Spain and traveled the country for decades, providing context and insights that gave this project added texture. In addition, my thanks to Gerry for his contribution on sherry, for permission to reprint two photos, and for arranging my introduction to Chef María José San Román.

Talented Vickie Swisher, book designer for *The Iberian Table*, handled the project with clarity, good cheer and resourcefulness. Vickie is accommodating to work with, and her positive attitude meant much.

The resourceful Jane Plass is an editor, indexer, and general expert on assembling books. Jane assisted with copy editing, and she created *The Iberian Table*'s index. In addition, she solved an early problem related to the editing program that no one else could decode.

Designer/artist Rafael Sánchez's interest in this project provided inspiration on every level. My friend's love for literature, Spanish history, culture, and gastronomy was nourishing to this hungry writer's heart.

Thanks to Liz Stell who shared her late mother's recipe; to Jordi Mas, Don Harris (1936–2024), Jonathan Harris, Pere Selles, and Christine Weiss for providing support and inspiration. I also wish to thank Emily Labes and Emily Natsios.

Sara Baer-Sinnot of Oldways, offered constructive criticism early on. Jadranka Vrsalovic Carevic of The Institut Ramon Llull, New York City, provided the catalog *We Are What We Eat (Som el que mengem in Catalan): A Literary Evening* (2009). David Crumm and Ignacio Taboada, Spanish Vice Consul in Atlanta were a source of support during the early stage of writing this book. Ignacio's own work into the history of Spain's support of the United States during the Revolutionary War is fascinating.

Alba Adot Caballero, nutritionist-dietician, Alícia Foundation, Udo Erasmus, Donnie Yance, Guillermo Fesser, Gerry Kerkhof, Elias Gonzalez, and Susun S. Weed, all provided advance praise.

My friend and fellow author, Neenyah Ostrom, kindly helped proofread the final manuscript.

Loving gratitude to Edith and Maurice Rottner, my maternal grandparents who I lost years ago. Nanny and Poppy gave me so much. My Grandmother was an excellent cook. Summers at their beach cottage on the shore of Long Island Sound, was a budding nature writer's dream. My childhood, filled with their love, brimmed with splendors of the shore. The many passages with nature writing in *The Iberian Table*, sprang from life with them.

Coming into the home stretch, I wish to thank Dr. Andreas Buttimer and Colman Andrews for their support.

These acknowledgements would not be complete without a tribute to my beloved mother, Nancy Grant, who died in 2022. Her appreciation of all of my endeavors, whether painting, writing, or cooking, meant everything to me. She turned her remarkable ability with color and design into successful businesses and was an inspiration to me. Making everything seem easy, mother's free-wheeling, full-flavored recipes possessed a culinary freedom that I fall back upon to this day.

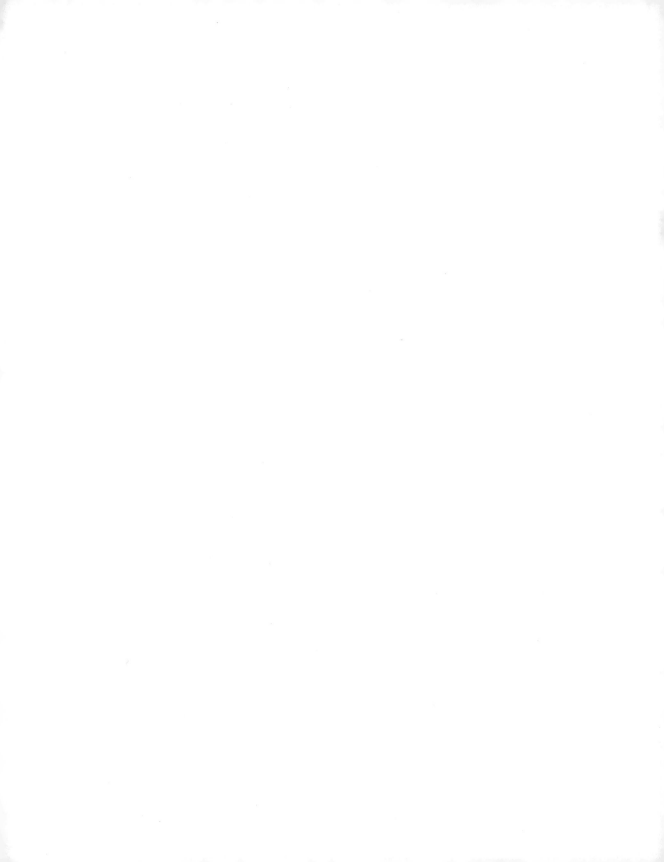

Some places remain with us long after we leave. Think of favored destinations one seeks as a child. In my own experience, nothing compared to Salt Island, part of the barrier islands off the coast of Westbrook, Connecticut, five hundred feet from the beach where I lived with my grandmother and grandfather each summer. When tide was low, the island was close enough to shore for even very young children to reach by foot, sometimes unaccompanied by adults. But only if we returned before the tide came in, else we would be marooned on the island with no dinner.

Part huge, shelf-like prehistoric boulders, embedded in the front of the island where water meets stone with three sand shark fossils, the island was half vegetation with reeds and wildflowers. But the large expanse of boulders took center stage. During low tide, when we could see the fossils, shallow, swirling, transparent tidal flats formed during the last ice age waved with eelgrass, revealing burrowing clams, scuttling crabs, assorted mollusks, and horseshoe crabs with spears! We stepped smartly.

In certain places the rock formations molded by incoming tides over untold years formed ridges so sharp the youngest were reminded to take care when touching them. There were scurrying hermit crabs of varying sizes with hairs on their outer skeleton, often battling each other, and losing a leg here or there. Horrified, we marveled at their spryness.

Periwinkles shined through low tides with glistening shells in shades of lavender. To this splendor, at higher points of the island, add white Queen Anne's Lace, with long, pliable stems to fashion into garlands to wear in our hair like crowns.

But for me, the highest point of Salt Island, a refuge to nesting seabirds and accessible only by scaling a narrow cliff, was the spot I remember most. The glistening waters of Long Island Sound beckoned below. As a child, I only saw this magic place, guided by my mother, who scaled the cliff with ease, for she had grown up there spending summers walking to the island. I held her hand, and once at the top, the wind whipped our hair. Wild roses appeared in tangled profusion at this high point along with Queen Anne's Lace, scenting the salty air, mingling into a perfume that I have never smelled before or since. With gulls cawing overhead, mother and I looked down over the expanse of water, sparkling in sunlight. The glory of the Sound would never be forgotten.

Life unfolds. Years pass. My grandparents died. As adults we find ourselves contemplating mortality, which for me, led to protecting my health, a journey that brought me to Spain and *The Iberian Table*. My mother died during the writing of the final chapters, but through this grief, as I finish, this book still feels shiny and new, just as Salt Island felt every time I walked there with her as a child.

Spain's Mediterranean diet was a story I had to tell. This book put many people on my path. Without you, colleagues, well-wishers, and especially you, dear reader, all sharing in my journey, *The Iberian Table* would not be the banquet that it has become for me.

"The food in Spain is based on the Mediterranean diet—lots of olive oil, wine, garlic, peppers, tomatoes, and grains—not so very different from Italian cooking except Spain has its own special ways of combining ingredients to make them taste outstanding."

– Penelope Casas, author of *The Foods and Wines of Spain*

"While seemingly every culinary corner of France and Italy has been explored under a microscope, Spain remains El Dorado with an immense untapped wealth of the kind of unfussy, elegant and alluring Mediterranean flavors we all swoon for these days."

– Anya von Bremzen, author of *The New Spanish Table*

Essentially, *The Iberian Table* is a continuation of my interest in writing about the health benefits of food, this time with focus on Spain, particularly the North. To Anya von Bremzen's celebration of flavor, I would add that the Spanish Mediterranean diet offers untapped nutritional wisdom that everyone will want to know.

My intention is to keep *The Iberian Table* packed with new findings and information not reported in my first book, *Total Breast Health: Power Foods for Protection and Wellness* (Kensington, 1998). My second, *The Detox Revolution: A Powerful New Program for Boosting Your Body's Ability to Fight Cancer and Other Diseases* (McGraw Hill, 2003), written with Thomas J. Slaga, Ph.D. the former scientific director of The AMC Cancer Research Center, examines which foods really enhance the body's ability to cleanse itself of toxins. Many foods the Spanish eat do just that.

This, my third book, conveys an excitement in discovering a way to eat that, as Peter S. Feibleman, author of *The Cooking of Spain and Portugal* said, "I would want to be close to for the rest of my life." Not only is Spanish gastronomy rife with fresh flavors, it offers the promise of health. Bloomberg's 2019 Healthiest Country Index and Money UK's 2021 index confirm that Spain is ranked number one in terms of longevity.

As a natural foods cook, the North of Spain intrigues me. I have come to realize that the region's cooking is the most naturally delicious that I had ever encountered. I had no idea these realizations would become the subject of a book, until I began researching an update to *Total Breast Health*. The story I had to write was already in front of me.

And so, anchored by years of travel, this book also honors people I have met along the way, who have spoken to me of their culinary habits, family recipes, and traditions. Some have become friends. I had the opportunity to meet and speak with many chefs. The interviews with Carme Ruscalleda and Elena Arzak add an exciting element to this book that for me makes it complete.

Admittedly, *The Iberian Table* suggests an area larger than northern Spain, and it is undeniable that the whole of Iberia including Portugal is *la buena mesa*. But when I read about the long-lived people in the North (including Andorra), in a 2016 report published in *The British Medical Journal of Epidemiology and Community Health*, regarding work led by Dr. Ana Ribeiro at the University of Porto, it grabbed me. Dr. Ribeiro's study identifies Mediterranean dietary patterns of eating as fundamental in making their conclusion.

But time marches on, and for some in Spain, the Mediterranean diet has been left in the past. With the globalization of diet, many young people have abandoned healthful eating, replacing it with fast foods high in harmful ingredients such as emulsifiers, calories and salt. This way of eating is also unhealthy because it is deficient in nutrients and beneficial plant compounds found in fresh vegetables and fruit. And so, obesity among the children of Spain is now a concern. Cases of breast cancer are increasing, too, especially among the young.

Just as alarming, since the early 1940s researchers have seen a steady increase in smoking among the women of Spain and what some call an epidemic of lung cancer. In terms of developing cancer, poor nutrition and exposure to toxins is a collision of great storms. As I examined with Dr. Slaga in *The Detox Revolution*, inadequate nutrition can lead to poor performance of detoxification genes, which in turn diminishes detoxification enzyme activity, so crucial to the body's ability to eliminate such pollutants as tobacco smoke.

Returning to good news, a recent report by the global organization NPD Group states that young adults up to thirty-seven years of age are driving a trend toward fresh and organic produce, full-fat butter and yogurt, and meat from free-range animals.

It is my hope that *The Iberian Table* and the many studies in the bibliography, which include a 2016 report about the prevalence of the toxic chemical bisphenol A (BPA) found in 67 percent of nearly two hundred food cans tested, should compel people to *want* to cook more! In case you did not know, BPA is linked to infertility as well as cancer. Another 2016 study shows many of these canned and processed foods contain "emulsifiers" that initiate inflammation in the gut, which in turn can trigger bowel cancer, as reported in the peer-reviewed medical journal *Cancer Research*.

Even when packaged foods are labeled "free from" adverse ingredients, they still lack life-extending extra-virgin olive oil, and are typically high in calories and salt. The prevention of heart disease, too, must be addressed with healthy diet. Also in 2016, scientists at the world's largest conference on cardiovascular disease hosted by the European Society of Cardiology reported that the new findings discussed at the conference and characterized as "extraordinary," show that following a Mediterranean diet is "more powerful than any drug, including statins" in the prevention of heart disease.

As pointed out, *The Iberian Table* expresses my own feelings about discovering the foodscape of northern Spain, a land of disparate, culturally-rich regions, each with its own version of the Mediterranean diet. The late Penelope Cassas wrote in her book *The Foods and Wines of Spain*, "While eating habits and hours are more or less uniform throughout Spain, cooking can be quite different."

So throughout this book, we move among Basque, Castilian, Galician, Navarrese, and Catalan in referring to recipes, foods, and places. In general, usage is dictated by the region in which I am writing. For example, the small city San Sebastián is called Donosti, or Donostia/San Sebastián by the Basques, who know their land as *Euskal Herria*. The Catalans spell their region *Catalunya*, and to the Spanish, well, it is *Cataluña*. Likewise, *Empordà* (Catalan) is known as *Ampurdán* in Spanish. And so on. It fascinates me that the cooking in this diverse land, with its own culinary rigor, is so healthy. This primal instinct— connecting wholesome, fresh food with life—has kept the distinct cultures alive in all of Spain through times of war and peace, since time immemorial.

I want to say a word about the recipes in this book. In Part One, with the exception of *sofrito*, I have presented recipes that illustrate Spain's incredible contributions to healthy eating. I have not done so with sofrito. Because it is such a fundamentally protective food, I urge exploration of its many uses, such as including it with ingredients for American style meatloaf.

Not surprisingly, many *cocina de vanguardia* chefs are interested in health. The Alícia Foundation, forty-five minutes from Barcelona, in Catalunya, under the strategic leadership of Ferran Adrià, explores technical innovation in food but also is dedicated to bettering nutrition for everyone. For example, one of their programs develops menus for persons with cancer.

Basque superstar chef Martín Berasategui, who happens to have eight Michelin stars, more than any other chef in Spain, released his cookbook, *Salsa Para tu Coco*, or "brain food." Berasategui's father-in-law was diagnosed with Alzheimer's, so the chef sought out foods he hoped would slow the progression of the disease. Healthy food can heal us. Cooking gives us hope.

And finally, regarding the literary passages. Just like the gastronomy, the dramatic topography of Spain inspires me, so I wish to convey these feelings to you, the reader. Let us drink from this fountain together. Because of this desire, much of what I have written is meant to feel spontaneous. I imagine you at my side. When we visit Altamira cave, for example, unspoken are the hours spent researching anthropology, prehistoric art, or time spent at the Altamira Museum.

I cannot wait to share *The Iberian Table* with you. The experiences I write about offer context for a way of eating that I hope you, too, will want to remain close to for the rest of your life.

"Every era of history modifies the stove,
and every nation eats according to its soul,
perhaps before its stomach."

— Emilia Pardo Bazán, 1851–1921,
Galician novelist, journalist, critic, and scholar

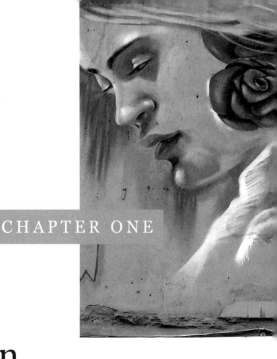

CHAPTER ONE

The Call for Prevention, Yet Again

"People in Spain are predicted to have the longest life expectancy in the world by 2040—beating Japan into second place—and much of the reason is to do with the way they eat, according to the authors of the most comprehensive study of the global burden of disease."

— Sarah Boseley, *The Guardian*, 2018

Well intentioned as it is to run a race to fund a cure for cancer, why is there no determined effort to prevent it? Should we not do everything we can to avoid this disease in the first place and, while we're at it, do the same to prevent heart disease, that other killer? Let me be clear. We cannot just rely on medical science to prevent disease. Consider an October 2022 report on a gold-standard trial that found colonoscopies did not help to reduce deaths from colon cancer. This does not go unnoticed.

Certainly, I am not discouraging diagnostics, but whether you agree or not, we must finally accept that diet really does play a role in the prevention of disease.

This connection first entered public consciousness with Dr. Ancel Key's introduction of the Mediterranean diet over fifty years ago. Since then, our understanding has evolved, and now we know that extra-virgin olive oil is fundamental in the ability of the diet to prevent disease. To prove this, in 2013 research led by Ramón Estruch, Ph.D. demonstrated that the olive-oil-rich diet is much more protective against heart attack and stroke than the low-fat American Heart Association diet.

Dr. Estruch's study, known as PREDIMED, the first clinical trial to specifically measure the effects of the Mediterranean diet on heart health, found that the benefit to the group using the most extra-virgin olive oil was so compelling that it would be "unethical" to prevent the other two groups from consuming more of it.

The Mediterranean Diet Beneficially Changes Gut Microbiome A 2020 study of elderly people published in the *British Medical Journal* found that following the Mediterranean diet for one year could beneficially transform gut microbiome leading to improved cognitive function, reduced inflammation and fragility. Microbiome is the term used to describe the collective genetic components of the microbial cells in our body.

PREDIMED also found that the olive oil in the diet is protective against breast cancer. According to Dr. Estruch, just four spoonfuls a day reduces the risk for breast cancer by almost 70 percent. Dr. Estruch's study was so persuasive that the story was picked up by international publications including *Time* magazine and the *New York Times*.

Gina Kolata reported on the PREDIMED study in the *New York Times* in February 2013 adding that "low-fat diets have not been shown in any rigorous way to be helpful, and they are also very hard for patients to maintain."

In 2016, *The Guardian* covered a report issued by the United Kingdom's Public Obesity Forum and the Public Health Collaborative that "the low-fat diet and advice to lower cholesterol have been wrong."

For those who still argue that what we eat cannot have a physiological effect on our health, consider that recently in China, scientists found diet so powerful that it altered the sex of unborn bees. And in the field of epigenetics, scientists found that tumor-suppressor genes can be ignited by good nutrition and exercise.

Isn't it empowering to know that even when cancer is encoded into our DNA, it need not be destiny? This book expands upon the discussion by focusing not only on the Spanish Mediterranean diet, but by embracing the way Spanish people eat from a region that many may not be familiar with. It is a land renowned for world-class cooking that we will explore in this book.

Though we know it is essential to eat vegetables and fruits every day, and the best way to eat from this so-called rainbow is to cook at home, in the United States the miles of take-out joints that line our highways, and the expanding processed and frozen-food sections in our supermarkets, and even so-called healthy snacks like kale chips, make it easy to grab food on the go. A June 2022 report from three prospective US cohort studies confirmed an association between ultraprocessed foods and risk of colorectal cancer in men and women.

It is tragic that we have strayed from the unprocessed foods that we are meant to eat. Yes, by now most of us have rejected margarine and found our way back to butter, but it is not enough.

What is enough?

For the answer, we look to Spain. People there boast one of the longest life expectancies in the world. We gain insight by examining their pattern of eating. After all, according to a December 2016 report by Reuters, there are over 17,000 people in Spain over the age of one hundred. Moreover, Spanish women have the lowest mortality rates from breast cancer in Europe—even lower than the women of Greece.

Though the consumption of processed food has tripled in the Mediterranean region in the past decade, many Spanish still follow a Mediterranean pattern of eating. Their diet is based on vegetables, fish—often for lunch and dinner—as well as nuts, fruits, grains, and olive oil, with little red meat. A 2024 *JAMA* study found that in a "cohort study of 25,315 women followed up for 25 years, higher adherence to the Mediterranean diet was associated with a 23% reduced risk of all-cause mortality." Results were even more dramatic, reported in *The American*

Journal of Clinical Nutrition, 2017, following this type of diet results in a 56 percent reduction of all causes of mortality.

Perhaps you think you know the Mediterranean diet. The recipes of Greece, southern France, the west coast of Italy, all the way down to Lebanon have been brought to light. Americans are familiar with ratatouille; we are accustomed to pasta with white beans, falafel, and chicken skewers with yogurt sauce; and we know gnocchi and lamb tangines.

However, the Spanish Mediterranean diet is relatively unknown, which is surprising, especially since *Lancet Medical Journal* pointed out in 2013 that Spain's version is the healthiest. *Lancet* knew this in 1998, when they published "Spanish Live Long and Healthy Lives."

Dishes are purposely simple so local product can be showcased. People are very proud of good farming there. Southern Navarra, or *Reino de Navarra*, is renowned for exquisite produce. What's more, many gardens in the northern regions are organic. El Mareseme, northeast of Barcelona, is such as place as is Delta del Llobregat. Because of the proximity of the sea, there is a humid saline atmosphere perfect for farming. Vegetables and fruits grown there are exceptional.

Cooking During Medieval Times
Baby aubergines stuffed with herby goat cheese is an old Catalan recipe that continues to be prepared in this region today. The dish is so ancient it is noted in the *Llibre de Sent Soví*, a cookbook written by an anonymous Catalan author in the fourteenth century. Because history of this cooking culture shows the evolution of Spain's Mediterranean diet, I speak of *Llibre de Sent Soví* many times throughout this book.

Chefs are inspired by these offerings and work closely with farmers. Peas are so outstanding that they give rise to recipes. Sisters Paquita and Lolita Reixach prepare these local peas with homemade *botifarra* sausage in their restaurant Hispània in Catalunya's Arenys de Mar.

It is not only peas that are excellent. The region's artichokes are considered some of the best in Spain.

Galician products are also highly regarded. Cabbage, turnip greens, potatoes and bread are outstanding, and beef from the native breed *Rubia Gallega* is recognized as the best in Spain. Galician seafood is prized, too. So is Galician seaweed, which is beginning to be available more widely.

No matter where you are in Spain, exceptional foods known as "raw materials" grace center stage. It's impossible to explore the North without marveling at this bounty. Dairy products from Cantabria and Asturias are the best in Spain—Asturian cheese is known throughout the world. In Aragón, where cooking is hearty and simple, produce is so revered that there is a festival for local peaches—velvety, plush, and juicy—and for turnips in *la* Cerdanya, the mountainous region of northern Catalunya that stretches across the Pyrenees between France and Spain.

Claudia Roden points out that there are more wild mushrooms in Catalunya than anywhere in Spain. And given the research showing Spain to be the sixth largest producer of mushrooms in the world, this amounts to a lot of fungi.

More on mushrooms later.

By the thirteenth century, Barcelona had become a major Mediterranean port, helping the city become a center for trade and through time, this melding of cultures made Catalan gastronomy and products the most diverse not just in the Mediterranean basin, but all of Spain. Keep in mind that Barcelona always had close access to farms, so fresh produce defines her gastronomy. During the seventeenth century, Catalan chefs were known to be the best in Europe.

Make no mistake, the Basques have their own distinguished heritage, reaching back earlier than anywhere in Europe. San Sebastián is a place celebrated for the strong food movement of the North. Here can be found gastronomy clubs called *sociedades gastronómicas* where home cooks and star chefs join forces to cook and feast. It is no exaggeration to say that every social relationship in the Basque region is centered around great food and cooking. As noted, the Basques bring to light some of the most trailblazing cooking in the world.

In this region, cooking is so defining that young people dream of becoming chefs. Basque millennials have formed a club devoted to gastronomy called *SUKATALDE.*

To the west, the young Cantabrian chef Ricardo González Sotres prepares lobster with cream and cauliflower and seaweed.

And in neighboring Asturias, chef Nacho Manzano renews tradition.

One of his creations, crunchy *pancetta* with *fabada* vinagrette, is inspired by the signature recipe of his land, *fabada asturiana*, which we will talk about in the next chapter.

Innovation can also be found in Galicia, where cuisine is inspired by a Celtic heritage and their Atlantic seafood. Michelin-starred chef José González-Solla, a member of *Grupo Nove,* a highly regarded gastronomic movement made up of local Galician chefs, draws flavors from his past while creating dishes that are at the forefront of cuisine, such as bread pudding with mango and coconut flan. Pepe, as he is called, is self-taught and began cooking in his family restaurant known for its traditional menu.

Many of Spain's most iconic recipes were developed by generations of women who cooked for their families or ran their own restaurants like Pepe Solla's mother. Professional chefs have high regard for the contributions of these women, and when cooking in the new style, may express homey old recipes in new ways.

We examine the work of these chefs not for prestige, but because their passion for cooking reminds us that we, too, can keep the act of cooking fresh.

What's more, chefs who cook in the new style called cocina de vanguardia, embrace sustainable and organic farming. Catalan chef Carme Ruscalleda, with her seven Michelin stars—more than any woman chef in the world and more than most men—was born into a family of farmers. She understands that sustainability must be supported. Terroir must be healthy.

It seems tough to find a bad meal in the North. Even truck stops offer good buffets with fresh salads, tasty fresh vegetable sides such as stewed zucchini with peppers, and homespun entrees like cod and garbanzo beans or garlicky roasted lamb, even offering little plastic tubs of real extra-virgin olive oil to anoint bread. Try finding that in an American truck stop.

This region is also a place where animals are generally not confined to small quarters nor given antibiotics and hormones; where cattle ranching translates into healthier meats and what I believe to be Europe's greatest cheese.

Because all of Spain is a mosaic based upon unique gastronomic cultures expressing their own versions of the Spanish Mediterranean diet, for brevity, we look to the North of Spain, where one gains insight just by observing. Again, consider Barcelona. Although there are thirty-nine municipal food markets throughout the city, distinguishing it as having the largest such network in Europe, for our purposes a tour of *Mercat de Sant Josep de la* Boqueria will help us appreciate what the Spanish Mediterranean diet actually is.

In *la* Boqueria, we discover that the Mediterranean pattern of eating is born from the farm. Tomatoes glow with the promise of flavor, and are so tasty that everyone eats them in abundance. Rubbed on toasted bread for breakfast and the base for gazpacho, tomatoes are also basic to *sofrito*, which begins countless recipes. Salads with tomatoes are ubiquitous.

I had never encountered a cuisine with so many tomatoes.

Tomatoes contain the antioxidant lycopene, which helps prevent prostate and breast cancers. Not only does consumption of tomatoes help prevent cancer, but a tomato rich diet also strengthens bones and protects hearts. And when the Spanish eat tomatoes with extra-virgin olive oil, which they do, lycopene becomes even more protective.

Consider that there are 120 varieties of tomatoes in Spain, with additional "lost" heirloom varieties rediscovered every year to be logged in the seed bank outside of Barcelona. Imagine the many plant chemicals with benefits to human health in these heirlooms yet to be discovered.

While Spanish researchers treasure heirloom seeds, in our country scientists are busy breeding nutrients out of our foods in favor of longer shelf life.

Dr. Donald R. Davis published a study in 2009 reporting that nutrients in vegetables and fruits plummet when plant breeders develop high-yield crops meant to sit on grocery store shelves for long periods of time. Dr. Davis learned that although we pay more for heirloom varieties, we are gaining in nutrition over common supermarket fruits and vegetables. Mineral content of vegetables and fruits declines, too, when phosphorous fertilizers and pesticides are used.

When I consider what is missing from our food supply, to say I am sad is understatement. Our lives depend upon buying and cooking the very best food we can find.

As the *British Journal of Cancer* advised in a 2014 article, "Spanish Mediterranean Diet and Other Dietary Patterns and Breast Cancer Risk," "when you plan your menus around a variety of vegetables, fruits, legumes, pulses, and monounsaturated rich foods such as nuts, avocados, and olive oil, you reduce the risk of breast cancer."

Flavonoid-Rich Foods Extend Longevity in Spain In 2016, nutrition scientists studied the diets of the longest-living people in Spain and reported that they ate many fruits and vegetables; the scientists concluded that the flavonoids in the foods are responsible for extending life. Researchers have known for many years that flavonoids, with their antioxidant properties, help protect against cancer. In another 2016 study, scientists reported that flavonoid-rich foods such as apples and green peppers may help prevent long-term weight gain.

In addition to containing monounsaturated fat, as pointed out, extra-virgin olive oil helps the body absorb antioxidant plant compounds such as lycopene, so when tomatoes are cooked in it, the oil provides a natural carrier for this anti-cancer compound.

Spanish people consume life-extending fats from many foods including nuts—all types, used in countless recipes—and they eat fatty-rich fish. What's more, desire for these foods begins early, even for olives, for which many Americans never develop a taste.

The Spanish also prevent disease by what they are *not* eating, beginning with commercial grade cooking oils, commonplace in American kitchens and restaurants. As explained by expert Udo Erasmus, Ph.D., in his groundbreaking *Fats That Heal, Fats That Kill*, these oils are treated with chemicals and often stored for indeterminate lengths of time on warehouse shelves, forming substances through use and reuse that are harmful to human health. By consuming health-bashing fats like this, people are not getting the nutrients and plant compounds needed from the vegetables they eat! Only healthy fats act as carriers for nutrients and plant compounds (not just lycopene), making these antioxidant substances accessible to our organs, tissues, and even our protective DNA. Not incidentally, we all have DNA programmed for health and programmed for disease. A healthy diet activates DNA meant for detoxification of harmful substances such as steroidal hormones.

In addition, damaging lifestyle habits also trigger disease. The American Institute for Cancer Research (AICR) reported in December 2015 that poor diet, inactivity, drinking, and smoking "cause up to 90 percent of cancers" and that the majority of cancers are "caused by lifestyle and not bad luck."

The AICR projected thousands of cases of breast cancer in the United States could have been prevented had women not been overweight and had eaten a better diet. And in 2021, two new studies partially funded by AICR suggest a better diet can help breast cancer survivors live longer.

The Spanish Mediterranean diet is the better diet. Cooking is simple. Sauces are minimal. Fresh produce defines. Flavors are fresh, big and satisfying. The diet is so satisfying that our pattern of eating stabilizes.

Through this normalization of blood sugar our instinct for well-being understands that health is on our path.

So we are motivated to develop our pantry. We explore. The ages-old smoky flavor of *pimentón* makes briny seafood shine. Saffron threads crinkle in our fingers, releasing perfume; and *sofrito* fills the kitchen with the rich fragrance of melding onions, tomatoes, and garlic, sautéing in extra-virgin olive oil. It becomes exquisite marmalade. As for the taste of roasted Marcona almonds, when crushed, well, another intoxicating perfume is released. There is incomparable *queso*, and honey to spill over the rustic cheese. And *turrón*, candy made from almonds and honey, is gently sweetened like a kiss.

And through this way of eating we sense when a dish is ready to be covered or uncovered, or when the fire under the soup must be turned down to simmer merrily away on the stove, filling our kitchen with delight. We discover the exact moment when peppers are roasted to perfection; when the darkened skin can be pulled away, as though revealing a rare jewel.

Not to be taken lightly, good food marks an occasion. Aren't perfect summer berries a way to welcome this very special season—to memorialize a real moment, when morning sun pours through your kitchen window, heralding sybaritic weeks ahead, while you bask in it, allowing each berry to explode in your mouth in ravishing goodness?

And finally, cooking as a way to explore other cultures somehow unites us all. Cooking has never mattered more.

Perhaps you ask, "I know cooking is important to my health, but who has the time?"

If this is how you feel, I urge you to talk to someone who has a terminal disease. Wishing we had taken better care *after* we lose our health should not be an option. Frida, a trim, vibrant woman of a certain age who I met at my fitness club—a survivor of wars—understands this and more. When Frida is chided for spending time in her kitchen, she retorts, "I'd rather spend my time cooking than waiting in doctors' offices for appointments."

As an advocate for real food, I believe there is much we can learn from Frida. Embracing her enthusiasm for cooking might just save your life.

The most important aspect of remaining free from disease—scientists are in assent here—is to have a strong immune system. After years of research for three books, I offer you no greater truth. For a strong immune system, we must eat whole, unprocessed foods.

Even if you've received a diagnosis of cancer, do not despair. Improve your pattern of eating. As the Spanish know, food is meant to be shared. Connect with family and friends. Spend time in sunlight and fresh air. There is much you can do to extend and improve your life.

Reduce portion sizes, for compelling studies show that when we eat less, dormant DNA programmed to heal is initiated, and DNA programmed for disease is silenced.

And so, for the rest of your hopefully long and fulfilling life, embrace everything that you can do and learn to create better health.

We will be learning together.

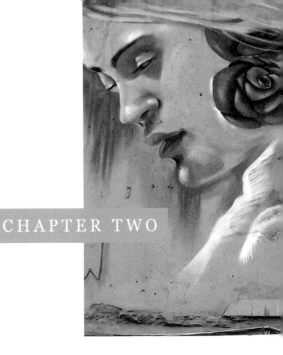

CHAPTER TWO

Inspiration Born

"The duende ... where is the duende? Through the empty archway a wind of the spirit enters, blowing insistently over the heads of the dead, in search of new landscapes and unknown accents, a wind with the odour of a child's saliva, crushed grass, and Medusa's veil, announcing the endless baptism of freshly created things."

– Federico García Lorca, *Theory and Play of Duende*, 1933

"This great calm, this silence everywhere, this untouchable tranquility in the air, a stillness of light and shade, makes me feel as if time has stopped its race through the centuries for just one moment of reflection, of waiting, or perhaps to look with melancholy to the past, to what has come before races or religion."

– Basque writer Pierre Loti, *Echoes of Jaizkibel*, 1916

My love for Spain began soon after I met my husband, Thomas. Each of us had just moved to San Francisco, and one night as part of a group, we went to a neighborhood Basque restaurant—cozy and informal, with communal tables large enough to seat twenty.

We were living in a Pacific Heights boarding house called the Pink Palace, a grand four-story shocking-pink Victorian mansion with turrets and spires and secret rooms clinging to a steep hill among palm trees and flowers. The San Francisco Bay and Golden Gate Bridges could be seen from the Victorian's many windows. Rose, the manager of the boarding house, was a snide, portly gourmet familiar with the city's many splendid restaurants and possessive of her favorite boarder, Thomas.

Rose was the kind of person you could dislike but not shake off because she was entertaining. Her remarks about the boarders were uncensored and, well, when she got your attention she kept it. One could never guess who might receive her merciless ire. Revealing secrets was Rose's specialty, so if you were a fool, you told her things; if you were not, you kept her around for laughs.

And so we tolerated her. Despite Rose's advice that all relationships were doomed—she was a real optimist—Thomas and I had been getting closer, so it came as no surprise that we found ourselves seated next to each other at the large plank table of the Basque restaurant that Rose had selected for a dinner party.

As usual, Rose organized everything, and this evening was no exception, handpicking favored boarders to join her with a seating arrangement that had Thomas at her side at one end, and me at the other end. But to my delight, Thomas had his own ideas.

It was easy to forget that anyone else was present because we had found our world. The simple Basque food was like nothing I had ever experienced either. There were many courses, and each was memorable. Dinner began with a roasted red, orange and yellow pepper dish that had been prepared with extra-virgin olive oil and garlic. Flavors were deep and colors vivid, just like my life was to be with Thomas.

Rainbow-colored vegetables, rich in anticancer carotenoids, encompass the energy of life, especially when cooked with olive oil—a caveat that I am certain did not enter the mind of the Basque chef who prepared our meal that foggy night in San Francisco.

We married, and years later found ourselves traveling by car through the Pyrenees on a journey from Nice to Madrid. Thomas and I were living in New York City, where I was painting. During this time, I began studying at the now closed historic Macrobiotic Center in SoHo and at the Anne Marie Colbin Natural Gourmet School.

For those who may not know, to follow macrobiotics means seeking health through a diet founded in whole seasonal foods of the utmost quality, simply cooked and presented. I frequented Manhattan's greenmarkets, where I learned to appreciate newly harvested foods with joy. I began to see my personality develop my cooking, too. In the fall, the sweetness of kabocha squash was elixir, and come early spring, tender fiddlehead ferns reminded me of woodland creatures from time immemorial. Summer inspired idiosyncratic salads such as juicy peaches joined with butter lettuce and dill. Winter was memorable, and chestnuts too. The shortest days of the year meant silence and snow falling over Manhattan rooftops, with the smell of brown basmati rice mingling with that of oil paint.

As my canvases sprang to life, I came to know that the changing seasons meant more to me than I ever dreamed, even among the concrete towers of New York.

During this time, I began creating recipes with macrobiotic foods such as tempeh and seasonal produce. I came to understand bean cookery, and how to make seaweed taste delicious. Whole grains fascinated. Pressing salads from raw vegetables to keep digestion vital was exciting too. So was miso, a fortifying condiment used for flavoring soups.

These experiences translated into better health, so I began to understand the direct correlation that real food had on well-being. No more headaches, allergies or anxiety. Focusing on so-called natural foods fostered a kind of elegant restraint, which manifested in a newly found passion for cooking I did not know I possessed.

For New Yorkers who loved to cook, the timing could not have been better. Manhattan was a gastronomic haven. Some chefs were beginning to fuse Japanese macrobiotic ingredients with French, and greenmarkets were exploding throughout the city. My favorite was at Union Square. I seldom missed a weekend.

It was meaningful to become acquainted with the hardworking New York and New Jersey farmers who grew the vegetables I so loved. They spoke to me about their work; about the generosity of the soil and their struggle to improve it; the impact heirlooms have on flavor; and their foraging discoveries such as a cache of rare wild mushrooms. Sometimes the farmers even shared recipes, too.

Those moments are imprinted on my soul. Don't laugh. Though I am no longer macrobiotic, I learned many things during this time, and how to really cook was only the beginning. I began to understand that devotion from farmers and chefs is a life force that can pass into the food, giving it energy. When one eats food grown and cooked with care, one can feel and taste the difference.

Unlike Manhattan, the Pyrenees is a place where time seems to stand still. My first trip there began on the French side, where Thomas and I attended a macrobiotic conference in Saint-Gaudens, packed with staunch devotees from all over Europe.

I read about wild mountain herbs and plants such as cardoons and borage and such, so I could not wait. What's more, I was in Europe where cooking is supposed to be spectacular, right?

And so, after arriving at the retreat, I expected a fine spread of vegetable dishes, and maybe some wild mushrooms, but after our initial meal of overcooked carrots and soggy brown rice, I realized that Thomas and I were in for a long weekend.

Following that dinner, when the highly touted lecture by the French macrobiotic expert got under way, I realized just how long the weekend promised to be. In the international language of English, the humorless, gaunt gentleman who looked like the "before" picture from a bodybuilder's magazine, spent the first hour extolling the virtues of rice cakes with his audience hanging on every word.

Delivered in droning monotone, I learned that dried brown rice was a philter against all ills. Wherever had I been? What's more, I had never seen so many Birkenstocks in my life. The room was packed, but not a whisper could be heard. The suspense was as thick as amasake pudding.

Walking the full length of the lecture hall, clutching a rice cake high for everyone to see, the scrawny Frenchman lectured in a scolding tone.

Suddenly I felt as though I had been called into the principal's office for talking during study hall. With my fanny beginning to feel as though it had been glued to the bridge chair for all of eternity, I listened up.

After a protracted pause—with drama rivaling Brando's performance in *A Streetcar Named Desire*—the macrobiotic expert cited a disease and then, still holding the rice cake high for all to see, made a hurling motion toward us, his faithful audience, in fiery admonishment.

Perhaps he pictured each of us slobbering down greasy burgers and fries?

All of this had been going on for about an hour, which for me seemed an eternity. And this was *not* what I meant about time standing still in the Pyrenees.

Finally, Thomas whispered, "Let's leave."

Giving no argument, we fled, taking care not to step on toes as we walked shamefully through the audience toward liberty.

Immediately upon returning to our spartan-like room, we packed our suitcases and placed them beside the door. Before sunrise the next day, we left the retreat as though escaping a gulag in Siberia.

I can't say we were unhappy, but I will say we were quiet. It was still dark when we backed out of the parking lot. The tires of our car against the gravel sounded as smooth as a silkworm on Michio Kushi's kimono.

Soon we were driving toward the Spanish side of the Pyrenees, somewhere near the border of northern Navarra. The wildness of the Spanish terrain was like nothing I had ever seen or imagined. It was rugged and beautiful, but also a bit threatening.

We drove for long stretches with no signs of civilization, drifting in and out of fog on remote cliff roads cut into mountains of stone. In the purple-gray distance, I glimpsed peaks that seemed to float against the horizon on air.

Snow. Big, fat flakes melted against our windshield.

Though it was cold, I opened my window, and suddenly the car was filled with the fragrance of newly fallen snow. We passed streams, reflecting patches of autumn sky. With Thomas beside me, it seemed that all rushed in that I'd ever loved. I watched mountains of granite turn to crystal when lit by the darting sun, and I saw age-old forests of emerald-green pines.

We were still climbing very high.

Then dusk.

Everything was wrapped in shadow.

We found an inn and stayed the night. Awakening early the next morning with my coat wrapped over my nightgown, I rushed outdoors. Mountain air warned of encroaching winter, and as the sun made its appearance, it is hard to describe what I saw.

In silence, as I watched the fog giving way to a plummeting valley surrounded by more astonishing mountains stretching and shaking into a horizon that was an inconceivable distance away, I saw a Pyrenees sunrise.

Pastures gleamed green amidst rocky cliffs of stone. Somewhere goats bleated. Smelling wild thyme, I watched red fall leaves blaze against cold blue sky. White snowcaps startled in the distance, and hemlocks and pines released elixirs older than humankind.

I looked up. Cries of carnivorous birds—perhaps vultures—shrieked. They were watchful, circling the very mountain we were on. Perhaps some animal had been wounded and lay dying. Maybe a young chamois had lost its way?

It was death, but it was also life. In the Pyrenees, the chain goes on.

Suddenly my neurosis, my human failings, and my dreams all became mere blips in the incomprehensibly long march of never-ending time. Just at that moment, I felt a sense of oneness with the sun, the mountains, and even with the fierce, hungry birds.

Then I wanted breakfast.

Thomas and I eagerly ate a wonderful one in the sunlit dining room of the old inn, overlooking a yard burnished golden by autumn. While savoring slices of toasted country-style bread that we dipped into good Spanish olive oil, beyond the yard we saw mountains surrounding the great valley below, which was filled with what reminded me of Washington Irving's "ocean of clouds."

Between forkfuls of delicious fried eggs and *jamón*, we spoke of ancient myths, pilgrimages, and invasions—of *la Reconquista*—and of a thwarted Charlemagne. We talked about the giant prehistoric creatures that once inhabited the outcrop of land that began the Pyrenees, and how the primordial mountains are older than the Alps.

There was cheese, too, with a smoky flavor that was the earthiest I had ever eaten. Between idyllic bites, we spoke of the Stone Age people that lived in the mountains we were in.

I peeled a clementina as we spoke of Europe's early sheepherders that made humankind's first cheese and about the pre-Christian moon goddess *Mari*, who when night falls as the Basques say, sometimes can be seen leaping from mountain to mountain, leaving flames across the sky.

Vowing to return, we remained at the table drinking good dark coffee with hot milk for a very long time. And return we did, many years and many trips later, traveling from the Atlantic Ocean to the Mediterranean Sea, getting to know the Basque region from coastal Bilbao and Donostia/San Sebastián in the foothills of the Pyrenees, to Basque-French Biarritz, across the border in France.

But more than this, our travels led us to Asturias, Cantabria, Galicia, Aragón, Navarra, and throughout Catalunya's Pyrenees to the coast—each region with its own distinctive culture and recipes. These discoveries changed the way I looked at life, and the way I cooked. I found myself immersed in the truest food culture on the planet.

The story of these people so profoundly connected to the earth begins with the Basques, the oldest inhabitants of Iberia, a race of people that came before nations or religion, and that during its beginnings in *Euskal Herria*, worshiped nature.

This comes as no surprise, for theirs is a land of astonishing coasts and mountains; of rushing trout-filled rivers; of valleys and pastures; of ancient fern forests and caves; and spectacular waterfalls that cut through gorges with vengeance. A rocky, radiant land that through a character in his novel, *The Garden of Eden* (published after his death), Hemingway described as "so beautiful that it makes one hungry to paint or write."

The mystery that surrounds the origins of the Basques makes it hard to understand just how long they have lived in their land, so beautiful that it created a hunger in Hemingway to write.

Anthropologists once thought that Basques migrated to Iberia but now believe they have always lived in the region despite a legend that claims Tubal, the grandson of Noah, escaped the great flood and arrived in northern Iberia right after. As the story goes, Tubal settled first in the high Pyrenees, eventually moving to lower Navarra, and the Basques are his descendants.

Scholars such as Ptolemy, Pliny, and Caro Baroja may split hairs about the origins of the Basques, but they agree that this northern region shaped the history of Iberia.

The Basque language, *euskara*, is the oldest in Europe and unrelated to any other, even Latin. Records show *euskara* has been spoken for over ten thousand years. The earliest cave paintings in Europe can be found here: *Altxerri* cave goes back 39,000 years. Clearly this northern territory is one of the oldest inhabited places on earth.

To put things in perspective, someone once said that cheese was made in this region before the earliest parmesan or brie.

A Cro-Magnon skull found in the Urtiaga Valley at the Basque Cantabrian border is believed by anthropologists to closely resemble the modern Basque skull. Images of sea bream—a fish still revered by Basques today—are found on cave walls throughout their land. The late Basque gastronomic historian, José María Busca Isusi, believed that the Basques still prepare bream today much like they did during ancient times.

Recipes in Catalunya date back to the Roman occupation. Colman Andrews, author of *Catalan Cuisine: Europe's Last Great Culinary Secret*, believes Catalan gastronomy offers a greater variety of foods over any other culture. In *The Foods and Wines of Spain*, author Penelope Casas wrote that Catalunya "is the most gastronomically oriented and exciting region of Spain."

To this land, Romans brought cuttings from olive trees, beans such as *fava* (*haba* in Spanish) and garbanzo, and the art of leavening bread. Visigoths arrived in Barcelona after sacking Rome and stayed without shaping Catalan gastronomy as did the Romans or the Moors who appeared later in the eighth century.

During the centuries that followed, Barcelona's position as an international port further exposed Catalunya to cultures from the Levant, North Africa, Greece, France, Italy, and Turkey, broadening the palette of flavors even more.

On the far western side of northern Iberia, Galicia and Asturias have an ancient gastronomy shaped by green terrain and a misty climate. Though seafood is ever present, Galicia's gastronomy, rooted in her early Celtic culture, offers olden dishes such as meat and seafood pies, and rural-style breads, some made from corn and rye. Cantabria and Asturias share the same coastline, with culinary treasures from the sea. The great stretch of soaring limestone mountains called the Picos de Europas, is known for a staggering variety of flora and fauna, and has what are thought to be the largest caves in the western world. Many of Europe's best cheeses are ripened in these caves. Asturian *Afuega'l Pitu*, the oldest cheese in Spain, is creamy and unctuous, and reminds that this region has its own ancient cuisine, which we will talk about throughout this book.

The evolution of cooking in the north shaped a varied and vivid gastronomy. In 2014, food writer Vernon Grant interviewed Luis Benavides-Barajas, author of numerous books on Spanish gastronomy. In this interview, Benavides-Barajas says that people in the north of Spain are the most "gastro-oriented" in the country and that cooking there is "the best in the land." Judging by the number of stars, the *Michelin Guide* seems to agree because no city in the world has more stars per capita than modest-sized San Sebastián.

One trip to northern Spain was planned to experience the full length of the Pyrenees and points west through Basque country, Cantabria, and Asturias. This led Thomas and me to the ancient town of Jaca, in Huesca, a province in Aragón where France and Spain meet and one of Spain's earliest Christian shrines, *Monasterio de San Juan de la Peña*, erected on a mountaintop in the tenth century AD.

As with our first trip, it was fall but early in the season, so instead of fog, the day was drenched in sun. It was arid and bright, and the smell was pure Spain—thyme, oaks and hawthorns, great pines and laurel. A mixture of dried leaves with something primordial was also in the air.

I yearned to identify every sight, sound, and fragrance for I knew this was to be my secret cache of impressions I would draw upon throughout my life. It was to be my sensory meditation about the earth, or the way I want to remember it.

When the world is too full to talk about, the silence between Thomas and me is a kind of promise. So we rode lost in thoughts that we knew we would share with each other later.

Through the grass that lined the road, I saw bees and wildflowers and beyond, rising cliffs of stone. There were tracks, too, of animals leading into the forest.

We were in the high Pyrenees of Huesca; almost touching heaven we rode, arriving at the tiny stone monasterio in late morning. Beneath an endless canopy of autumn sky, we could see for miles across mountains to a distant horizon of more rising mountains—some so high they were topped by eternal snow.

In the midst of these imperial mountains perched on one of its own, the classically proportioned little stone monasterio managed at once to be both bold and delicate. Monasterio de San Juan de la Peña, 920 AD, was carved from the mountain she was part of, as though the earth herself had birthed this tribute to humankind. I knew that inside the mountain was Monte Pano cave, where Christ's Holy Grail was believed to be secreted during the time of invading Moors. Adding more mystery, the little stone structure was constructed right at the forest's edge, over the remains of an ancient mosque.

Struck by this history, I could not help but sense the presence of others—for lack of a better word, feel free to call them spirits. Don't get me wrong. Psychic phenomenon and such strike me as hokum, but at that moment I felt communication perhaps from souls in the forest, or inside Monte Pano cave.

Wind rustled through the trees, but what I heard was "Remember us, for we are here."

When we finally left the monasterio and her ghosts behind, I felt a sense of longing for what I did not know, maybe for stories never told, or ones forgotten.

Being close to the border of France, I was reminded that cultures coalesce over food. What I mean to say is that, although Spain finally drove her invaders out, her gastronomy shows an embracing of Arab influence—such as the use of saffron and the tastes of sweet and sour, so I wondered if local cooking would reflect that of her northern neighbor?

Driving west, we selected a stone inn for lunch. The short menu offered a dish that reminded me of *gabure*, one of the oldest recipes in France.

It was a thick soup made with fall vegetables and tender lamb, and it had been cooked in a kettle over a fire, perhaps through the night. There were noodles in the soup, too. Though it had been cooked for a very long time, flavors were still bright, and the noodles gave it silkiness. A bowl of autumn sun.

I guessed the vegetables had been grown by the chef herself, whom we could see working in her kitchen. Aragón is a land with fifteen hundred acres of organic farms, and as we arrived we saw a garden behind the inn with fall vegetables, stone fruit trees, and sunflowers.

The taste of the hearty soup with its many vegetables and bits of meat that had unfolded from the bone mingling with whispers of thyme and laurel, was, in a sense, savoring the past. The soup would leave an imprint upon my culinary subconscious, meaning my approach to cooking would be forever changed.

That day, I was changed, too, for truly great cooking comes from a place deeper than the mind. It is a manifestation of all experiences, but more than this, cooking is about how deeply we can feel and trust.

And so, in complete satisfaction, we continued driving northwest toward the Basque country.

We began to see whitewashed stone houses, called *baserri*, that according to Basques are more than just structures. To the Basques, a house is a living entity whose inhabitants merely "pass through" to preserve it for future generations. This means that the solid mountain houses we were looking at had remained in families for centuries.

It wasn't long until we descended the Pyrenees and began entering her foothills. Through these low hills, I saw rivers leading to the sea, and then I saw the sea itself.

As we began to make our way along the coast, my musings turned to whales. I knew that some as long as thirty feet once swam along the Basque-Cantabrian coast that we were following. Though the great creatures are long gone, they will always be remembered in these parts as *balena Biscayenis* or Biscay whales.

Make no mistake, whale hunting was a risky business. For one thing, those Biscay whales weighed tons. Many men had lost their lives in the sea shimmering before me. But this bucolic-looking sea is known to be treacherous and deceivingly deep. What's more, Basque whaling excursions usually happened during winter at night, since this was when whales would venture near the coast. One whack of a whale's tail could capsize a small boat and throw eight men into a freezing midnight sea.

Then the old Basque saying sprang to mind: "The one who fears getting wet will never catch a fish." From the ridiculous to the sublime, I began to think about sardines. Perhaps it was because the Cantabrian Sea is known to have some of the best in Spain. The Cantabrian is colder than the Mediterranean, so sardines and anchovies from these waters have more fat, which makes them extremely flavorful. I knew that women known as *sardineras* used to walk from town to town, selling sardines from baskets on their heads. I am sure they had beautiful, strong legs and called everyone by name.

We turned off the Cantabrian coastal highway toward Santander, and caught the road to Altamira. We were in low Cantabrian hills that descended to the sea, now a couple of miles away. It was an unobstructed view of hills and sea, and it seemed undiscovered wilderness. Arriving at Altamira, I could see the sea in the distance. I knew that I was in a place where everything was as it has been since time immemorial.

When I got out of the car, I was surrounded by meadows of waving sea grass that when lifted by breeze, shimmered silver. It was quiet, except for the curious hum of bees. Since the meadows were filled with wildflowers, there were of course many. The low hills seemed to go on forever, so the buzzing was amplified against their silence.

Gulls swooped overhead, taking the peacefulness of their kingdom for granted. Occasionally one would cry out, and the sounds seemed brutal against the peace.

With the taste of salt in my mouth, I stood before Altamira cave—the same sacred place where Western civilization's first artists stood. The sky, reflected in the shimmering blueness of the sea, produced a kind of radiance. And through this light, the vividness of what lay before me made it easy to imagine life in these parts a very long time ago.

Suddenly, I saw myself inside the dark chambers of the cave painting on stone. It was cool and mossy, and the sound of my own breathing was all that I heard. Little ceramic lamps with burning animal fat sputtered away as I painted. Flames flickered against the walls of the cave, matching the cadence of my breath.

As I worked, an image of a bison began to spring from the stone. There was an inevitability to my creation, as if the creature had been lying there waiting for me. As though guided by hidden powers, the modeling of muscles formed the animal. They were graceful and anatomically accurate, showing years of drawing practice executed on skin or wood—materials that did not withstand the course of time. No one needed to find this evidence, for there was no question of my ability. Something powerful was happening.

When I finished, I slapped my hand against the stone: A woman was here. It was then I realized that after working all day, the artists of Altamira must have been hungry. For them to create life on cold, gray stone made them shamans to me, but even shamans must eat.

What did prehistoric people eat? I asked Thomas.

We agreed that though anthropologists theorized early people in Spain ate uncooked roots, certain herbs, mushrooms, eggs, fruit, honey, pine nuts and, when they could, fish and game, Altamira's artists must have known how to cook. Life in Altamira cave spanned many generations, but perhaps even her earliest artists—because of their sublime inventiveness—knew how to make fire?

It was not easy leaving this sacred ground that ruled centuries of artistic invention and still holds reign, for great art uses virtuosity to give meaning to the inexpressible. That is, although the Altamira artists discovered the principles of painting and drawing, the spirit of their work goes deeper. Picasso understood. Indeed, one cannot forget that the master said, "After Altamira, all art is decadent."

Though part of me remained at Altamira, Thomas and I left, continuing west.

Soon, dusk.

While we drove, rosada-colored light peeked through clouds bathing cliffs and olive groves, apple orchards and cattle, grazing on land bordered by sea. A land of mountains, caves, and sea, with a shoreline so beautiful it is said to be the loveliest in all of Europe.

Thomas and I spoke about Cantabria and Asturias—how they are separate regions but share the same sea and rivers, so meat, seafood, dairy, and crops have much in common.

Then silence.

As Josep Pla wrote, "The only sound was the breathing sea."

Now nightfall.

When we reached Oviedo, the capital of Asturias, we were tired, but a slightly alcoholic and effervescent apple cider called *sidra* was rejuvenating. Rich in healthful enzymes, it has been made in the region for so many years that the Greek geographer Strabos wrote of sidra during the first century BC, calling it *zythos*.

Altamira Cave, Discovered by an Eight-Year-Old Girl Through eons of time, local hunters had to have been aware of the cave's opening, but it took the persistence of eight-year-old María Sanz de Sautuola to explore the cave, which led her to discovering the paintings of Altamira. *Finding Altamira*, a docudrama set in 1800's Spain starring Antonio Banderas, tells this story in a researched but natural way. While the film unfolds, you will feel transported to Altamira, Santander, and Santillana del Mar, the town Jean Paul Sartre described as being "the most beautiful in all of Europe."

The waiter poured the sidra as it must be, holding the pitcher high; something about releasing the bubbles. During the pouring, one smells fresh red apples and something simple but precious. Perhaps really good soil, moist from morning rainfall? Bright, tart, and dry, after just one glass—even if you have a headache—one is restored.

As always in Spain, dinner was late but worth the wait. We ordered *fabada asturiana*, a defining dish of the region that varies from family to family, but always includes *fabes de la Granja*, beans so large they stand up to dishes that must be cooked for a very long time.

Fabada asturiana, with its huge buttery beans that compose most of the recipe, is usually cooked with sausages and a pork knuckle. It has been described by Peter S. Feibleman, author of *The Cooking of Spain and Portugal*, as the most "solid" dish in all of Spain, and is just the type of recipe that grandmothers still teach their families to cook.

We tasted. With the passing of generations, adjustments were made, perfecting the recipe we were savoring.

As with other great dishes of Spain, fabada achieves true flavor with few ingredients, but they must be first-rate. Then the recipe can be cooked slowly so that when it is finished, as you ladle it bubbling from the casserole into shallow bowls, vapors mist your face like dew. The ancient Iberian perfume of laurel, olive oil, and thyme, reach the deepest part of you, connecting you to the past, while anchoring you in the moment all at once. The taste of fabada is a culinary truth that for me means, after one bite, you will understand cooking in a deeper way.

Fabada, known as "survival food," has been cooked through times of war and peace, since time immemorial. The greatest of human spirit is behind the unpretentious old dish, composed of simple yet noble foods, cooked with heart in the humblest of kitchens.

This nourishing recipe, feeding families during wars and famine, is why Spanish chefs strive to keep traditions alive. With pride they call these dishes *cocina de la abuela* and don't want anyone to forget how defining these recipes are to their culture, and their hearts.

For the chefs know the embracing of simple sustenance and the dignity that lies therein, is the soul of Spain's greatest cooking. Peter S. Feibleman said about the cooking of Spain that "there is something more solid, sturdier and at the same time brighter and more wholly satisfying than the cooking of any other people."

Yet the cooking of Spain embodies more. Whether an informal beach bar in Galicia where one can have grilled octopus with pimentón, or a rickety roadside stand deep in the Pyrenees where the roasted herbed chicken is world class, or a tiny *pintxos* bar in Basque Hondarribia where young chefs surpass each other's rampant inventiveness while struggling to pay rent, chefs care.

One feels this heart, too, in Catalunya, even in the plainest of restaurants with paper tablecloths, while eating toasted bread that has been rubbed with tomato and garlic and finished with olive oil and salt.

It is a victory that this direct connection with nourishment lives on.

In November 2013, the online newsletter *This Week in Barcelona* reported that young people of Catalunya are continuing the work of their parents. I am grateful that the young are interested in the pressing of olives and the production of artisanal cheese, and the growing of grapes for wine. Despite the passing of time—and time feels so vast in Spain—the passion for excellence lives on.

Celebrate this, for to care is life force. Without it, we shall lose our way. Call me a romantic, but we desperately need connection to nourishment in our own lives, for it is primal.

Begin by frequenting your local farmer's markets as I learned in Manhattan. Get to know the people who grow and produce your food, for you will find that they care. As a cook, everything is possible when you select the freshest and best ingredients you can find.

And remember, like the Spanish, cook from your heart.

UPDATES FROM AUTHOR:

In July 2022, it was announced by archaeologists at the University of Zaragoza that Huesca, at the southern slope of the Pyrennes—the area we explored in this chapter—was once part of a huge urban complex "of monumental proportions" believed to have been built by the Romans between the first century BC and second century AD. Interestingly, this city whose name remains unknown, had to exist during the time that, according to legend, the Holy Grail was secreted to the Monasterio San Juan de la Peña.

In February 2023, it was reported that Neanderthals prepared seafood meals of roasted crabs, barnacles and so on, organizing these feasts to make rather sophisticated dinner parties with other groups of Neanderthals. *El Pais* headlined this news later by describing Neanderthals as "gourmet." This speaks to my musings earlier in this chapter about meal preparation at Altamira.

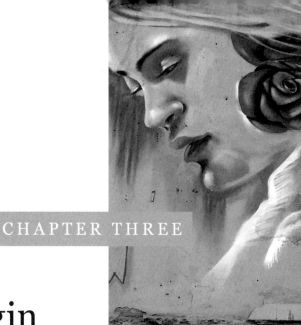

CHAPTER THREE

Spanish Extra-Virgin Olive Oil and the Benefits of Gentle Cooking

"When a diet low in all fats is adopted, the body consequently increases the consumption of carbohydrates (sugars), and we now know that an excess of carbohydrates are [*sic*] damaging to health ... Olive oil should be the main source of fat, but it is much better if it is extra virgin. Extra-virgin oils, as well as providing oleic acid, contain a large amount of polyphenols. These bioactive compounds are synthesized by plants to counteract physical threats, such as the sun, and to combat disease. When humans eat them, we acquire some of these same protective effects they give plants."

— Dr. Ramón Estruch, Co-coordinator of Spain's national PREDIMED study,
Senior Consultant at the *Department of Internal Medicine at Barcelona Clinical Hospital*
and Associate Professor at the *University of Barcelona Medical School*

O live oil from the first pressing, which is what extra-virgin means, stunts the growth of breast, prostate and other cancers, protects DNA, decreases the risk of coronary artery and cardiovascular diseases and stroke, increases circulation in the extremities, and lowers blood sugar, which means diabetics who consume plenty of extra-virgin olive oil will require less insulin.

The consumption of extra-virgin olive oil (EVOO) can reduce the risk of invasive breast cancer up to 68 percent. This is because the oil is high in monounsaturated fatty (oleic) acid and includes breast-protective antioxidants such as polyphenols, and vitamin E. In addition, research shows that EVOO aids in the absorption of calcium and other minerals, helping to prevent osteoporosis.

The Spanish Trade Commission's *Foods & Wines from Spain* tells us that there was a time when small family presses could be found throughout Iberia. Today, Catalunya produces some of the finest olive oils in Spain, many from trees as old as a thousand years.

Catalunya's Alt Empordà, which shares a border with France in the northeast corner of Spain, is dotted with villages that have oil mills. There, oils mostly from *arbequina* olives are pressed and sold in local cooperatives.

In fact, first-rate EVOO is pressed and bottled all over Spain and exported throughout the world where Spain is the biggest producer.

Many years ago, during the evolving days of nutritional awareness, nutritionists mistakenly believed that the Mediterranean diet was protective because it was low in fat. There was even a time when corn and cottonseed oils were recommended over EVOO.

Thanks to some scientists, especially Dr. Ramón Estruch (whose work I highlighted in Chapter One and will continue to discuss throughout this book), the benefits of EVOO have been brought to light, and today there is consensus that we should be consuming an abundance of it.

Since my first trip to Spain thirty years ago, I have been cooking with Spanish EVOO. As life unfolded, I learned that the olive oil from Spain usually places first in international awards, so my decision was a good one. In addition, the quality and taste are hard to match, and I knew it was authentic.

It also impresses me that Spanish olive oil was used in Dr. Estruch's PREDIMED study.

According to Dr. Estruch, following are the benefits of consuming extra-virgin olive oil as part of the Mediterranean diet:

Quoting Dr. Ramón Estruch, the national coordinator of Spain's PREDIMED study, "It is important to embrace the concept that healthy fats, such as extra-virgin olive oil, should be higher than 40 percent of total energy intake, and intake should be high, too, of grains, better if unrefined. Moderate to high consumption of fish, high intake of vegetables, legumes, and dried fruits, moderate consumption of white meats such as chicken and rabbit, and low consumption of red meat."

- Reduces the risk of cardiac problems by up to 30 percent.
- Reduces likelihood of developing coronary artery disease by 37 percent by consuming just two tablespoons a day.
- Contains oleocanthal, a substance that inhibits the proliferation of cancer cells, and when part of a Mediterranean diet, EVOO can reduce the incidence of invasive breast cancer up to 68 percent.
- Contains luteolin, the source of yellow coloring in EVOO and a component that inhibits the proliferation of human breast cancer cell lines and new blood vessels from forming malignancies.
- Aids in preventing osteoporosis by encouraging the absorption of calcium and other minerals into bones.
- Improves stomach function and reduces heartburn by acting as an anti-inflammatory.
- Assists the liver and gall bladder by aiding it in the digestion of fats.
- Reduces the incidence of gallstones and decreases hepatic excretion of cholesterol, thereby reducing its levels in the blood.
- Reduces risk of circulation problems in the extremities up to 66 percent.
- Helps lower blood sugar levels, which for diabetics means less insulin is needed.
- Contains a nontoxic chemical compound, DMB, that prevents gut bacteria from converting certain nutrients that can harm heart and brain health.

- Lowers blood pressure when eaten with vegetables such as spinach, celery, and carrots, resulting in the formation of nitro fatty acids, which help keep blood pressure from spiking.
- Helps to stabilize blood pressure and keep it normal.

Research on olive oil is ongoing with benefits being reported continuously including the 2024 *JAMA* study "Consumption of Olive Oil and Diet Quality and Risk of Dementia-Related Death": "In a prospective cohort study of 92,383 adults observed over 28 years, the consumption of more than 7 g/d of olive oil was associated with a 28% lower risk of dementia-related death compared with never or rarely consuming olive oil, irrespective of diet quality." A 2023 study published by Harvard T. H. Chan School of Public Health indicates "opting for olive oil instead of fats such as margarine and commercial mayonnaise...may reduce the risk of fatal dementia." And, according to *The American Journal of Clinical Nutrition*, in 2017, such a diet results in "a 56 percent reduction of all causes of mortality."

> TIP: **Extra-Virgin Olive Oil Spray**
> Fill a spray bottle with two-thirds EVOO and one-third water or vermouth. You are ready to mist seafood, fish, and more before cooking.
>
> Vegetables sautéed in EVOO are intrinsic to the Spanish kitchen. A 2016 study from Granada found that when sautéing potatoes, eggplant, tomatoes, pumpkins or hard squash in EVOO, phenols from the olive oil transfer antioxidants during the cooking process into the vegetables, acting as a carrier for the oil-soluble nutrients in the vegetables to be efficiently absorbed.

EVOO can taste pleasantly bitter, buttery, fruity, herby and peppery. Those oils with the strongest taste, and darkest green color, are highest in polyphenols meaning they are richest in antioxidants. The anticancer polyphenols in olive oil are terpenes, flavonols, phenols, flavones, lignans, and anthocyanins.

The variables that go into the making of olive oil produce differences in color, fragrance, and taste. Colors include yellow, yellowish green, dark yellowish green, delicate green and dark green.

In my household for basics, I make sure my EVOO is from Spain. For finishing oils, I look to Spanish food importers to collect fresh pressings of varietal oils.

In Chapter One, I wrote about Dr. Ramón Estruch's PREDIMED study in which he found that the Mediterranean diet, with four or five tablespoons of EVOO a day, offers almost a 70 percent chance of lowering the risk for invasive breast cancer, compared to a diet low in fat. In a study reported in the *Daily Mail* in July 2010, scientists discovered that "olive oil thwarts a gene that drives the growth of breast tumors" and "also switched off proteins that cancer cells rely on to stay alive." In 2010, researchers from Milan discovered that when women who routinely consumed EVOO were compared with women eating diets high in saturated fat, especially butter, the breast-protective benefits of the extra-virgin oil users far exceeded those of other women.

Thyme and EVOO, when cooked together as is common in the Spanish kitchen, show enhanced health benefits, and now we are beginning to understand why. A 2016 study by researchers in Tarragona shows that the combination of EVOO and thyme protects DNA.

Because research about EVOO is so compelling, I have been using much more of it myself. Recently, I made turkey meatballs, adding olive oil to the chopped meat as I folded in thyme, shallots, ground pepper, garlic, and breadcrumbs. The oil gave the recipe a richness that it needed.

In order to obtain the generous daily amount of EVOO as recommended by Dr. Estruch, begin by making your own vinaigrette, or as the Spanish call it, *vinagreta*. Commercial dressings rarely contain olive oil because of the expense and the fact that it solidifies at refrigerator temperatures. Besides, homemade vinagreta tastes so much better than bottled dressing.

Thomas and I make vinagreta a couple of times a week and it's not a difficult habit to establish. Once you discover how tasty homemade vinagreta is—not just over salads with leafy greens, but also with salmon burgers, cooked asparagus, etc.—nothing else will do.

> TIP: When we steam or sauté vegetables with EVOO, the antioxidant activity of the vegetables and olive oil increases by being cooked together, helping to prevent cancer, diabetes, and macular degeneration.

Here is my "go-to" recipe, however, you will find other vinagretas throughout this book. Over time, tweak the vinagreta to make it your own. Do you prefer shallots instead of garlic? How about a touch of honey? Change the recipe according to your taste.

A Su Gusto Vinagreta

INGREDIENTS: 1 cup extra-virgin olive oil, ½ cup aged Spanish Sherry Vinegar, 1 tablespoon Dijon mustard, 1 tablespoon country-style or grainy mustard, a small clove of minced garlic, a dusting of salt, ground black pepper to taste, and a pinch or two of cayenne.

THE METHOD: In a small, serrated ceramic bowl or a mortar, grind the garlic with a pestle together with a pinch of salt. Add mustard and slowly mix in the oil until blended. Using a small whisk ensures a creamy texture. While mixing, add the vinegar, pepper, and cayenne. Taste. If needed, adjust the salt and vinegar. Set aside for at least an hour, allowing flavors to meld.

When Cooking, a Knowledgeable Approach Can Extend Life

Whether grilling, frying, roasting, poaching, sautéing or using a *cazuela*, cooking is a gentle art. For instance, cocina de vanguardia chefs know that the best-tasting fish and seafood are cooked until just done, or as the Spanish say, *al punto*. Ferran Adrià, the Catalan chef, places clams and mussels into a strainer to dip them into boiling water for no longer than five seconds.

In 2010, scientists from Barcelona found that extra-virgin olive oil protects against breast cancer by launching "multiple attacks against tumors" and helps reduce mammographic breast density, one of the main risk factors for breast cancer.

Though studies have shown that overheating oil results in free radicals that have been tied to cancer, EVOO can stand up to pretty high temperatures relative to most other oils. In 2020, University of Barcelona conducted a study on the effects of heating EVOO and found that although beneficial polyphenols were diminished at temperatures common for frying and baking, they were still healthful. Nevertheless, the best practice for obtaining the oil's benefits is to avoid heating it to the smoking point or to use EVOO unheated as with vinagretas.

Oliago Soup with Fresh Figs

Oliago, which means olive oil and water, is a traditional soup that originated in Minorca. Colman Andrews describes it as a "sort of hot gazpacho." Classic oliago includes garlic, red peppers, onions, parsley, and olive oil. It is never allowed to boil, which helps retain the soup's health benefits. Chop equal amounts of onions, red and green bell peppers, parsley, and ripe tomatoes. Mince scallions and several cloves of garlic. Heat a pot with plenty of EVOO and add the chopped vegetables and garlic. The technique is "poaching" the vegetables and garlic in heated EVOO for 5-6 minutes, so do not cook on high. Then use a wooden spoon and press down on the tomatoes, breaking them into the mixture, and season with salt and pepper.

A 2012 study from Spain published in the *British Medical Journal* revealed there is no adverse association between foods fried in olive oil and heart disease, stroke, or death. This is because olive oil is one of the only oils that can stand up to high temperatures without breaking down, and still maintain its antioxidant properties.

Sauté for 5 minutes more. Then pour simmering water over the poached vegetables, mix together, and simmer for 30 minutes on low to medium heat, taking care not to boil. Toward the end of cooking, adjust salt and pepper. Finally, add the scallions to the soup and continue to cook for a couple of minutes more. Serve oliago with fresh ripe figs.

Burned Meats: A Concern

A recent study completed at the University of Minnesota reported that women who ate overcooked hamburger had a 50 percent higher risk for breast cancer than women who ate it rare or medium. And similar conclusions were reached in the famous Iowa Women's Health Study that found women who regularly ate well-done steak, burgers, and bacon had a higher risk for breast cancer than women who consumed these foods cooked medium or rare.

Cancer Encoded DNA is Initiated When We Consume Burned Foods
Nutrition scientists in the new field of epigenetics discovered that issues related to our environment, such as reducing or eliminating exposure to substances in burned foods called heterocyclic amines, or HCAs, can halt expression of genes programmed for cancer. There is a great body of research over many years showing that cancer can be initiated by HCAs.

Charred meat contains the toxic substances heterocyclic amines or HCAs. Researchers have known for decades that HCAs are linked to cancer.

However, charred fish and chicken are also damaging to our health. Though the strongest correlation was with red meat, the *Journal Toxicology Letters* reported in May 2014 that well-done fish and meat contain carcinogens with estrogenic effects, too.

TIP: Cancer researchers recommend removing not only the charred parts of meat before eating but the pan drippings too, because such substances are also high in HCAs.

Vegetables Help Protect

A recent study conducted by nutrition scientist Sabrina Trudo at the University of Minnesota reported that compounds in vegetables shield against the HCAs in burned meat. So when you are invited to a barbeque, discard the charred pieces, and eat the rest of your steak with vegetables.

Instead of grilling, the following lamb recipe inspired by Ash Mair, from his *My Basque Cuisine; A Love Affair with Spanish Cooking*, is roasted slowly:

Slow-Roasted Lamb Shoulder

Preheat oven to 275°F. Peel 2 pounds of purple onions and cut into chunks. In a heated sauté pan, add a glug of EVOO and several cloves of crushed garlic. Add onions and several pinches of salt. Sauté until golden, then remove onions to a large baking dish along with several sprigs of thyme. In the same pan place a 2–3 pound boneless lamb shoulder, seasoned with salt into a heated pan with EVOO, and gently brown on all sides. After lamb is cool enough to handle, rub with plenty of crushed garlic, rosemary, and more olive oil. Then place meat on top of onions skin side down and add a pint of organic chicken stock around the periphery. Cover tightly with foil and slow roast for 4 hours, removing foil to roast uncovered for 20 minutes more. Remove lamb from pot and place on serving dish. Allow to rest before slicing.

———•———

Something special happens when we cook with care. Consider sofrito. I can't wait to tell you about it, for this exceedingly rich and savory concoction offers tremendous benefits for health.

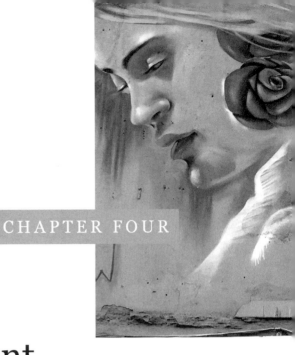

CHAPTER FOUR

Sofrito: The Madly Delicious Antioxidant Powerhouse

"We all cherish the memory of a tomato and garlic sauce at the hermitage and rosé wine sparkling in our eyes. And the last thing we shall see when we die, what our dead always see, is the prow of the hermitage, hanging between the sea and sky in a void of fabulous oblivion."

– Catalan writer Josep Pla, *The Gray Notebook*

Sofrito, that irresistible and shielding preparation of tomatoes, onions, and garlic, sautéed in extra-virgin olive oil, is the tag of Spanish Mediterranean cooking. Savory, mellow, piquant, and slightly sweet, this ancient culinary tradition began in Catalunya and is ubiquitous in the Spanish kitchen.

Research from the University of Barcelona, published in 2014 in the journal *Food Chemistry,* confirms that the combination of tomato, olive oil, garlic, and onion in sofrito, through the process of sautéing, increases the protective activity of the antioxidant plant chemicals in the foods. Tomatoes contain anticancer, antioxidant-rich polyphenols, carotenoids including lycopene, and vitamins A and C. Onions offer anticancer compounds known as flavonoles. Garlic contains the anticancer compound sulfur, and extra-virgin olive oil has monounsaturated acids, polyphenols, and vitamin E, all strong anticancer substances. Onions are especially important since they boost the shielding substances in tomatoes.

The earliest written reference to this mixture is found in *Llibre de Sent Sovi,* circa 1324. There, it is called *sofregit,* meaning to lightly fry.

While cooking, sofrito fills the kitchen with aromas so tempting they will even awaken an older sleeping dog, if she is anything like my Yorkie, Milly.

I don't mind giving sofrito the time it needs to build richness for I know that slow cooking increases benefits to health.

Besides, it's gratifying to watch the separate ingredients combine and bond with olive oil. And I love the intensifying aromas as sofrito reaches conclusion. The point at which the onions, garlic, and tomatoes explode to collapse into marmalade-like splendor, makes this medieval classic worth the wait.

Sofrito can begin a recipe, or added during cooking to boost flavor. If you want to use it as a sauce, this works, too. For a smooth consistency, simply sieve or blend and spoon over fish, chicken, etc.; however, I never get that far. Sofrito, rustic style, is just too irresistible.

Discover riffs on sofrito. Make it your own. Sometimes a little jamón or panceta can be added, or a touch of cumin. Or pimentón.

Catalan cooking is described as being *'barroc i saborós'* meaning rich and tasty. Many recipes begin with sofregit. No matter what you call it, sofrito is the secret for cooking recipes that offer rich, unexpected taste.

Author Colman Andrews observed that "Sofrito is the basis for things to come." I agree. Sometimes I use the mixture in ordinary ways, for example, to begin meatloaf, or Polish cabbage soup. Sofrito gives the soup unexpected depth that inspired even my Polish friend, Lena, to pronounce it wonderful.

Sofrito works in fusion cooking, too, including as a base for Asian short rib vegetable soup before adding lemongrass, five-spice powder and ginger. When finished, the flavor is bright. Because of the inherent sweetness of sofrito, this Asian soup needs no sugar.

Sofrito is not only sensuously flavorful, but it is a nutritional treasure when we cook it for at least an hour, as a May 2017 study published in the journal *Food Research International* from the University of Barcelona reported. Rosa Maria Lamela Raventós, who led the research, remarked that the cooking time and onions were key. Onions activate anti-cancer lycopene.

Research shows there are roughly forty different types of antioxidant-rich polyphenols and carotenoids in one cup of sofrito. This means protection against cardiovascular disease, hypertension, diabetes, and certain cancers.

I have already written of Dr. Ramón Estruch's work regarding extra-virgin olive oil, but he also has much to say about sofrito, since he led the University of Barcelona's team. Dr. Estruch and his colleagues found that sautéing in plenty of EVOO releases bioactive antioxidants in the tomatoes, onions, and garlic, making them more potent. Dr. Estruch recommends a cup of sofrito daily, but if you can't meet his goal, remember to eat this mixture often.

Still another nutritional plus for tomatoes cooked in EVOO comes from the American Institute for Cancer Research in a 2013 report that cooking tomatoes this way activates lycopene activity—lycopene being the plant chemical in tomatoes that helps prevent breast and prostate cancer.

My Basic Sofrito

6 medium tomatoes
EVOO
3 medium yellow onions, chopped
2 bay leaves
6 garlic cloves
Salt
Dried thyme
Dried rosemary
(Optional: crushed saffron threads or pimentón)

Cut tomatoes in half and, skin side out, grate using a coarse metal grater over a bowl to catch the pulp. Discard the skin, and set pulp aside. In a heated pan or cazuela, sauté onions lightly seasoned with salt in a glug of EVOO until they begin to caramelize, which will take about 25 minutes, stirring occasionally with a wooden spoon. Add the garlic—whole, chopped, or best of all, crushed, because studies show that crushing garlic and allowing it to stand for 10 minutes before cooking enhances anticancer properties. Add tomato pulp, another glug of EVOO, a touch more salt, 3 pinches of dried thyme, and 2 pinches of rosemary, stirring constantly. Continue to sauté until the tomatoes break down and meld with the onions, about 25-30 minutes. Adjust salt. A teaspoon of pimentón can also be added at this point. If you are saucing seafood, substitute crushed saffron threads for pimentón. Stir gently and cook a few minutes more. A good sofrito takes about an hour, which activates the protective synergy of the antioxidant foods in the mixture.

Chicken Casserole with Sofrito

Do you have leftover roasted chicken, still succulent and flavorful? Marinate it for a couple of hours in a dash of pimentón, a few pinches of dried thyme, rosemary powder, and a drizzle of extra-virgin olive oil. Begin sofrito, and as it cooks prepare quinoa. Place cooked quinoa in a casserole dish, cover with clean dish towel to absorb residual liquid. Using a wooden spoon, gently mix the sofrito with the chicken, and layer it on top of the cooked quinoa. Cover loosely with foil. Place casserole in a preheated 350°F oven for 10 minutes. Serve with trimmed scallions, and olives.

Baked Kabocha Squash Topped with Sofrito

During my macrobiotic studies, I learned to look for red kabocha since it is known to be consistently sweet; however, green kabocha is delightful, too. Cut squash in half, deseed, and cut into ¼-inch slices. Drizzle with a dash of olive oil. Season with fresh ground nutmeg, salt, and white pepper. Place slices on a parchment-lined baking dish that you first prepare with a thin coating of olive oil and bake in a 450°F oven for 25-30 minutes, turning once. Top with sofrito and serve.

———•———

All chefs know that a tasty recipe must begin with a flavorful cooking base. It is my opinion that Spanish sofrito offers more flavor than Italian *soffritto*, which uses chopped carrots and celery. It is also my opinion that sofrito has deeper flavor than French *mirepoix*, made from sautéed onions, celery, and carrots, cooked in butter. But, of course, I am partial.

Sofrito is so adaptable that when I became familiar with the practice of making it and exploring usage in recipes, it was as though I discovered a treasure chest filled with culinary secrets.

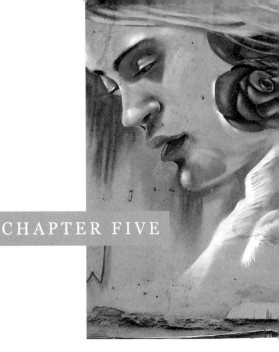

CHAPTER FIVE

¡Oye! la Boqueria:
The Ultimate
Natural Pantry

"The range of fresh fish and shellfish from the waters of two seas and one ocean is more inclusive, more spectacular throughout Iberia than anywhere else in the world."

– Peter S. Feibleman, *The Cooking of Spain and Portugal*

"I came to realize how extraordinary raw materials were in this part of Spain, and just how appealing—how varied, how (pardon the expression) 'world-class'—Catalan cooking could be."

– Colman Andrews, *My Usual Table, A Life in Restaurants*

There is a long-standing tradition of destination greenmarkets throughout Spain and Portugal—all fascinating to explore, but *la* Boqueria, Europe's oldest and most beautiful, is iconic. Manuel

Vázquez Montalbán, critic, journalist, and gastronome, described *la* Boqueria as "the cathedral of the senses."

When one enters the ineffable market, aromas of olives, oranges, and jamón intoxicate. They are dreamt-of tastes. There are sounds too, of bartering and of laughter. But what especially amazes are the seemingly endless narrow lanes, packed cheek to jowl with stalls offering astonishing foods arranged as a movie set, depicting the spoils of Eden.

But *la* Boqueria is real.

Although a market has existed in the area since 1217, around the time when Barcelona was becoming established as a major seaport, the so-called "modern" era of the Boqueria did not begin until the 1830s when traders selling their wares on *Les Rambles* were displaced and obliged to move to the present-day location built over the church of *Sant Josep* and the site of a convent. After the sale of the lands, the church and convent were demolished. Columns in the neoclassical style marked the new square, as did the metal modernist-style roof proclaiming "*St Josep, La Boqueria.*"

Despite the almost forty other greenmarkets in Barcelona, visitors to the city are drawn to *la* Boqueria. Perhaps they sense the history.

Writer Toni Monné brings us back to this world in her book *Barcelona, Gastronomy and Cuisine*. Monné points out that at the beginning of the nineteenth century, granddaughters and daughters of farmers from Baix Llobregat sold in the area in open-air stalls. These were hard-working farm women who unloaded wagons and piled up boxes of produce to table their scales.

Behind boxes of artichokes, broad beans, and cabbage were heroic acts—grueling labor often before dawn, bumpy rides in uncomfortable wagons along unpaved roads from farm to market, and then the weighing of fruits and vegetables sometimes in hard winds and rain, or under glaring sun.

Today, the vendors of *la* Boqueria remain the heart of the old market. Standing with dignity, faces express pride. Their expectation that vegetables and fruits are sold within a day or two of harvest is still fundamental.

But sadly, things are changing in Spain.

Until the mid-twentieth century, 80 percent of the population worked the land. Now at least 80 percent live in cities, so cooking habits are moving from tradition. Perhaps it is no small irony that a Dunkin' Donuts sits adjacent to the entrance of the market? An enemy at the gate so to speak, but as a Barcelona friend told me, this donut shop is for tourists.

Despite this, *la* Boqueria stands unfaltering, housing vendors whose grandparents taught them to walk forest trails in the mountains to forage wild mushrooms or to raise doves. Though much has been written about *la* Boqueria, nothing has been mentioned about how the foods of the great market protect health—an omission to me, since there is much we can learn just by observing. After all, *la* Boqueria is the embodiment of the Spanish Mediterranean diet.

Wouldn't it be great if you and I could tour *la* Boqueria together? Through the magic of imagination, we can, and what's more, we can leave now. You won't have to pack, but do grab your sunglasses—Barcelona can be a very sunny place.

Okay. At this moment, make yourself ready.

I am serious. Be still.

Close your eyes.

¡*Ahora*!

¡*Abre los ojos*!

Come on!

It is a vivid, Mediterranean morning—a spectacular Barcelona day!

Spain is the southernmost part of Europe, so it is not your imagination that it seems tropical here.

Some of the vegetation we stroll by, such as palm trees and yuccas, proves this so.

Though we are in the heart of a city, the presence of nature is obvious. The taste of salt is in the air because the wide avenue we are on, *Les Rambles*, leads to the sea.

Making our way down the broad tree-lined avenue, now we walk in shade. Branches of the plane trees above our heads spread and reach for the sky, showing they have been fused to the earth far longer than any of us strolling beneath them. But these trees are not as old as the convents that once stood along the dried stream bed on which *Les Rambles* was built.

We won't have to walk far before arriving at *la* Boqueria, and if you look over there, you'll see the stylish metal roof of the market that resembles a nineteenth-century train station. The sun, glinting on the metal, is a reminder that it is almost noon.

Pausing for a moment, we look down to admire a work of art at our feet. Many pass by lost in thought, but we cannot.

The large, colorful mosaic face seems as though it was created by a child, perhaps because of the broad smile, which verges on laughter, but, no, the master Joan Miró was the artist. The art form of using colored shattered pottery and enameled glass to create an image or a form is known as *trencadís*, and its origin means fragments, or to break, and this mosaic is a prime example.

la Boqueria is a labyrinth of stalls that line the aisles and crisscross the huge space. At last count three hundred booths make up the great market.

If Miró were here, and it was spring, he might shop the market to buy the ingredients for his favorite dish: *calçots*, a type of large, green scallion that grows in Catalunya that is roasted and dipped into an earthy, bold sauce, called *salsa de calçots*, made from crushed nuts, peppers, garlic, and olive oil. This dish is traditionally eaten outdoors with friends.

We cross the plaza and pass under the art nouveau metal entrance, but now we stop.

la Boqueria is crowded. What's more, everyone seems to rush about knowingly.

Everyone, that is except for us.

Peering in, remarkable displays of sparkling fresh foods astonish. It is harvest season. Summer produce is peaking, and autumn yields begin.

Vendors try to lure us with eye contact, but we hesitate. It is overwhelming.

See the grandmother walking toward us?

The dowager is stooped as she carries her string bag filled with items from the market. Notice that produce in her bag takes up most of the space, for this is how we should eat. See the onions, garlic, turnips, red potatoes, cabbage, and carrots? There is parsley, too, and garlic plus a few small, wrapped packages, probably meat—I imagine sausages, chicken, a beef, ham or lamb bone.

As she moves through the entrance towards the plaza, her sturdy black shoes clip-clop past us. Maybe she will cook a recipe from her girlhood, perhaps *escudella i carn d'olla*, a kind of homey stew made with nourishing broth, vegetables, chickpeas, and meat with a little pasta? Though the dowager's mother is long gone, the aroma of this dish while it cooks will remind her of her mother, for cooking awakens memory, you know. In my sensory imagination, I can smell the rich, deep broth made from chicken bones, collagen-rich feet, and garlic, along with vegetables and a lamb neck bone thrown in for good measure. These savory smells will meld with nutty-sweet garbanzos and the large meatball made from sausage. The unctuous, sustaining broth of this old-fashioned dish is meant to be eaten before the vegetables and meat. The meal will smell and taste just as it did when the old lady was a little girl, and ate with her mother at her side.

> Spain has 8,000 square miles of productive gray-green olive evergreens—the world's most extensive groves.

And for this, the old senyora still shops the great market, bunions, arthritis, and all.

Now our attention diverts right. A booth offering a fantastic display of olives begs to be explored.

The smell of brine intensifies upon our approach.

It is said there are as many as 250 varieties of olives in Spain, and it seems they are all before us now, glistening like primitive cabochon jewels. Recent studies show that olive consumption supports metabolic function, which helps people stay slim—a health caveat. Specific research shows that consumption of olives helps guard against cancer and strengthens bone mass.

I point out *gordales*, oval-shaped olives as large as quail eggs—fleshy and sweet, especially delicious when enhanced by spices. And these very small greenish ones are from the Ampurdán region a little north of here; and there are olives from Aragón, too. See the small grayish-brown ones? These are arbequinas—renowned but difficult to find outside of Catalunya. Oil made from these olives is know by chefs to be first rate.

American women rarely eat olives—a shame because olives contain a significant amount of antioxidant nutrients as well as plant chemicals and monounsaturated fat, which reduces the expression of a particular breast cancer gene by almost half. The *Journal of Agriculture Food Chemistry* reported in 2011 test tube studies that show pentacyclic triterpenes found in the skin of olives help human breast cancer cells to die. Other studies report that hydroxytyrosol, another plant chemical in olives, has been linked to cancer prevention.

As we make our way deeper into the crowded market, I don't want you to miss the large portrait showcased in a stall we almost pass.

Let's stop, for I know his story.

The picture is of a dapper fellow who dons a bow tie and bowler hat, sporting the most outrageous moustache ever. Meet Ramón Cabau, a respected restaurateur who owned and ran L'Agut d'Avignon, which many say influenced Ferran Adrià and chefs who followed. Cabau sold L'Agut in 1984 to become a farmer, growing hard-to-find specialty items such as flowering courgettes, and selling them at *la* Boqueria where he had many friends. But something in Cabau's life remained unsettled and one day, after giving each of his closest associates a rose, he took a capsule of poison and died here, in the market in a friend's arms.

We have been meandering along and now find ourselves at a tiny stall featuring premium extra-virgin olive oils.

The seller, an earnest young fellow dressed in a preppy way that underscores his boyish looks, is having a heated discussion with a dignified silver-haired gentleman, who looks like a professor or a researcher. Satisfied they are not going to come to blows, we begin examining the oils.

Notice the labels proclaiming *Denominaciones de Origen*, for they are a standard established by the Spanish government to ensure oils are from olives grown in a specific area and limited to the ones described on the label.

Don't miss this oil from Les Borges Blanques, or the one from Siurana, west of Tarragona. They are made from the arbequina olives we just saw, revered for their sweet, fruity taste. Arbequina oil is especially delicious when used to finish dishes.

Finishing oils bring to mind one of my favorite salads eaten by Majorcan farmers for breakfast early before they work in the fields. There are many variations, but here is a recipe for my favorite:

Majorcan Farmer's Breakfast Salad

Layer the following vegetables in a shallow bowl, sprinkling salt on each before adding the next: scallions cut on the diagonal, a thinly sliced fennel bulb, and 1 large sliced tomato. Top with slices of ripe pear, add a final sprinkling of salt, and drizzle everything with EVOO. Let rest for a few hours at room temperature before serving. Apples or peaches can be used in place of pears.

Denominaciones de Origen

Denominaciones de Origen is a government label that assures high standards for a variety of Spanish foods, not just extra-virgin olive. Products with this label are regulated and controlled by a council that confirms authenticity and characteristics, such as, in the case of olive oil, the variety of olives used, and that the oil is free of other substances that alter the product. In addition to extra-virgin olive oils, this council oversees condiments and spices, such as *Pimentón de la Vera*, as well as cheeses, cured hams, bread/crackers, rice, honey, candies and wines. For example, when regulating Pimentón de la Vera, the Denominaciones de Origen assures that the capsicum peppers are grown within the designated area, that they are picked when ripe, and that they do not contain artificial colorants or other substances that modify the spice. All of this is not to say that products without Denominaciones de Origen are somehow inferior, especially ones that do not neatly fit into the government's guidelines.

If you're interested in another version of this salad, check out Colman Andrew's *Catalan Cuisine; Europe's Last Great Culinary Secret.*

As we leave the little stall, the men are still in heated discussion, however the younger one looks up and smiles. Though we purchased nothing, he seems honored that we spent time admiring his oils.

At this moment, the seafood area we are entering is thick with shoppers, so we move toward the cases slowly.

The fish and shellfish are so fresh that it looks as though they were caught this very morning, which most likely is true.

> After Japan, Spain consumes more fish than any other country in the world, and nothing goes to waste.

Because seafood is so exceptional in the North, many times it is cooked simply, just with lemon and EVOO to showcase the purity of the product.

The variety of fish and shellfish before us is crushing. Examining what is known to be some of the best seafood in the world—even going back to the ancient Greek geographer Strabo, who praised the oysters of Barcelona—we see eels and all kinds of crabs, and many different types of fish, some so unusual that I have no earthly idea what they are.

Consider monkfish. These aggressive-looking creatures taste so good they are known as "poor man's lobster." Don't let these sea urchins fool you either. Those spiked, grisly-looking things are so tasty that there are festivals along the Costa Brava celebrating them.

That massive spider crab is a *centollo*. If you want to get cozy, we can find smaller spider crabs—see over there?

Vendors sense our interest, but since we carry no bags of food, they determine we are tourists and leave us to comment to each other in wonder.

We spot rockfish, admittedly not a pretty picture, and the even uglier *chocos* next to them.

These small cuttlefish disguise themselves in different patterns and colors to trick their prey. Farther down are *cigalas*, better known as langoustines in America.

How about these sluglike creatures? They used to be considered lowbrow fare, but now people pay more per pound for *espardenyes* than lobster.

Razor clams.

Don't they look just like their name? But don't let the menacing shapes deceive. Slightly chewy and subtly salty—these clams are so good they are habit-forming. And look: Galician sea scallops. See them in their pretty shells? And don't miss the sea bass, over there.

Whole Sea Bass Roasted over Potatoes

In Spain, when cooked with fish, potatoes are meant to be tender. Clean fish and set aside. After parboiling or steaming sliced potatoes until slightly firm, season with salt, pepper, and add a little EVOO. Place potatoes in a large baking dish. Tuck in sprigs of fresh thyme, and thinly sliced onions and tomatoes, along with cloves of slivered garlic. Place the sea bass over everything, and season with salt, black pepper, and EVOO. Cover and roast in 425°F oven for 25 minutes.

Look at the little darkish-red tentacle-covered creatures, for these are sea anemones, one of the most ancient predators on the planet. Called *ortigues*, they live amid green algae close to the surface of the water, in pools of sunlight, and come in all sizes, some even large enough to consume frightfully bigger ocean dwellers such as giant clams.

Sea anemones have a bright, concentrated, pure sea taste, and though the texture is somewhat slimy, Catalan chefs know how to cook them.

Anti-Breast Cancer Sea Anemones
Recent studies in Australia found sea anemones to contain a substance having anticancer benefits. The School of Medicine at Flanders University identified thirty-two species of sea anemones that can produce lethal cancer-killing peptides and proteins, causing apoptosis, or cell death. They found that "venom from these creatures has great potential to induce significant cell cycle arrest in lung and breast cancers."

I have to say a word about these silvery fish.

They are a delicate-tasting deep-water fish in the family of cod, called *merluza* by the Basques, who have been eating them some say since the beginning of time. In America this fish is known as hake.

Hake is sometimes prepared *a la plancha* style, meaning the filets are cooked on a hot flattop grill and served with just lemon, but more often it is cooked in a pan, then topped with salsa verde, a kind of very delicious Basque green sauce made from parsley and EVOO.

During ancient times, Basque fishermen developed recipes that define the region today. One is *marmitako*, a stew made from tuna of which, I see that this case has more than its share.

The same can be said of red mullet, turbot, trout, mackerel, megrim, whiting, cod, and bream. Sometimes a whole gilthead bream is roasted on a bed of thinly sliced potatoes, green peppers, and onions, with olives, and disks of botifarra, a sausage that is filled with flavor. The recipe, combining tastes of the sea and the earth, is emblematic of Catalan gastronomy.

Looking up from the case, we see salted dried cod, known as *bacalao* hanging from the top of many stalls. The old-world image seems a market scene from a Renaissance painting.

For over a millennium, salted cod has fed the masses throughout Europe, and it was popular during the Renaissance, but never truly celebrated until 2015, when it was deemed one of the top ten "new" gourmet trends of the world. Some say no culture cooks desalinated cod as knowingly as the Basques. Cod is primarily an Atlantic Ocean fish. The Basques had secret fishing grounds, which were as far away as North America where they were air- and sun-drying cod,

TIP: Ohio State researchers found that eating fatty fish and taking fish oil supplements increases the amount of omega-3 in the breast, which has been shown to reduce the chance of breast cancer. Women who do not have breast cancer have high amounts of omega-3 in their breast tissue.

Prehistoric paintings of merluza appear on cave walls throughout the Basque/Cantabrian region, and recipes for this fish can be found all the way back to the fourteenth century in *Llibre de Sent Soví*, and the sixteenth-century *Llibre del Coch*, both Catalan cookbooks, among the oldest recipe books in the world.

well before Columbus arrived, so they know a thing or two about cooking it.

Basque *bacalao al pil-pil* is one of the earliest known recipes in Europe. When cooked, the cod turns velvety and emits an unctuous fat that congeals with the olive oil and garlic. A single dried chili pepper adds dimension. The sauce gives an unexpected twist to the dish.

Still ogling the seafood case, now we see an array of gourmet-looking tinned and jarred seafood, all reflecting artisanal pricing. Products from Galicia, Cantabria, the Basque country, and the Costa Brava—regions known for exceptional sardines, baby eels, anchovies, tuna, white clams, and more—look intriguing. Containing protective vitamin D, and omega-3 fatty acids, these foods are also health boosters.

Cod as well as tuna, mackerel, salmon, sardines, anchovies, trout, hake, and halibut all contain omega-3 fats that slow or stop the development of breast cancer cells in laboratory studies with mice, and in test tube studies in which breast cancer cells are examined, as reported in 2014 by Ohio State University's Comprehensive Cancer Center.

TIP: **Anchovies Add Savory Punch** Crumble anchovies and put into a pot of simmering tomato sauce toward the end of cooking, mix through roasted garlicky vegetables before serving, or add to vinaigrette for salads.

Here are jarred Costa Brava L'Escala anchovies, packed in salt. They must be rinsed in milk or water before eating and are especially delicious as a topping for tomato garlic bread, pa amb tomàquet. The tinned anchovy filets over here are a traditional product of Cantabria. Anchovies provide umami flavor to dishes whether tossed with pasta, added to sauces, or as a garnish on salads.

Now, almost at the end of the aisle, our attention shifts to the ladies selling fish. They stand behind the counter, joking with customers, and some are what my grandfather Maurice used to describe as "lookers." The ladies are nicely coiffed and made up. Many wear sweaters with sparkly clips. After all, reaching into the icy case all day makes one wish for a sweater.

But don't let their stylish looks deceive, for these demure women know everything you ever wanted to know about gutting and cleaning fish.

Cocina Rápida

Garlic Prawns

Take 16–18 prawns, remove shells but leave tails intact, rinse, and season with salt. Heat a large, shallow pan, or a cazuela, coated with a little drizzle of EVOO. After oil heats, add 6 cloves of sliced garlic. When the garlic is fragrant, add the prawns along with ¾ teaspoon pimentón and 1 teaspoon medium-hot chili flakes. The moment the shrimp changes color, turn and cook until just opaque, taking care not to overcook. Remove shrimp from pan, put on a plate, and season with coarse salt, EVOO, chopped fresh parsley, and juice from ½ lemon.

———•———

As we stroll from the seafood aisle and make our way deeper into the market, a legend that has been told since the ninth century about St. James and the scallop shells comes to mind.

It has been said that every story enters one's mind exactly at the moment it must be told, so I will tell you this one now.

Hundreds of years ago in Galicia, a wedding was taking place on a beach when a storm developed. Lightning illuminated the sky and clouds opened, releasing a deluge. The waves grew violent. A ship careening toward the rocky coast faced certain destruction. But this was not just any ship. It was a special ship from Palestine and carried the remains of the apostle St. James!

Though the wedding party had no idea that the ship was carrying the apostle, without hesitation, the groom left the side of his bride and mounting his horse, urged it into the sea. Suddenly a huge wave pulled the groom and his frightened mare downward. Clinging to her neck, the young man prayed for help. Moments later, an unseen force transported him, his horse, the ship and all on board to the safety of a sandy inlet. When the groom and his shaking horse emerged from the sea, scallop shells covered their entire bodies.

This legend of St. James and the scallops is the reason why scallop shells mark the path to Santiago de Compostela in Galicia, known as the *Camino de Santiago*.

We have been moving through the crowded market talking.

Now we find ourselves pausing in front of a stall strewn with garlic and onions, shallots, and leeks. These foods are prebiotic, meaning they can influence digestive health in an immune enhancing way, even helping to prevent severity against Covid-19 and long Covid. In 2020, the journal *Cell Report* published a study showing that prebiotics boost gut microbiota, which can have antitumor protective effects related to the prevention of colon cancer and melanoma.

Known as aromatics, alliums ignite protective DNA, are anti-inflammatory, and contain compounds such as sulfur that support production of glutathione, a protector that helps the body to detoxify invaders such as pesticides.

On the virus prevention front, the biting fragrance surrounding us means these alliums are rich in sulfur and allicin, shielding compounds known to enhance immunity and fight infection. Alliums are also rich in quercetin, a star in the fight against Covid, as well as cancer.

All onions contain anticancer quercetin, but reds have the most. However, do not store any type of onion for more than a week, else they lose this shielding compound.

Alliums are ever present in the gastronomy of Spain.

Sofrito would not be a flavor star without onions, and no salad would be complete in Spain without them. Just ask the Andorrans, who love raw onions so much they have been eating them with honey in salads for over a millennium.

TIP: **Caramelized Onions Make a Base for Seafood** Roast cod, salmon, squid, or shrimp on a bed of sautéed onions. Sauté the onions in extra-virgin olive oil until they turn golden.

In Cantabria and Asturias, sautéed onions accompany sausages, and are used to make *porrusalda*, an old-fashioned style Basque leek and potato stew. In Valencia, home of *paella*, traditional *paella valenciana* is customarily served with fresh trimmed scallions instead of bread. Today, chef Pedro Subijana of Michelin-starred Akelarre in Donostia/

San Sebastián makes pasta from leeks. *Aioli*, an addictively delicious, garlicky condiment invented by the Catalans (*allioli*), graces noodle and rice dishes, asparagus, and more.

Ferran Adrià, who frequents Rafa's for lunch, adds scallions and chives to a potato salad recipe in his inspiring book, *The Family Meal*.

Okay, I know that onions are popular here, but the way people are grabbing them from that big bin is obsessive.

Now I see.

Figueres onions. Small, smooth, pink, and mild, they are one of Catalunya's most important crops, named after the town where they are grown. Figueres is in *Alt Empordà*, a region that extends from the mountainous French border in the North downward along the Mediterranean and inland toward Barcelona. The cooking there is highly praised.

Rafa's, the tiny, extraordinarily fresh seafood restaurant in Roses, serves a salad of sliced tomatoes and garnishes with raw leeks sliced paper-thin. Lemony vinagreta and large green olives finish this starkly simple salad.

TIP: Crushed garlic galvanizes the protective enzyme alliinase, which releases potent shielding plant chemicals. If you crush raw garlic and let stand for 15 minutes before cooking, benefits soar.

Look at this purple garlic known as *ajo morado* from Las Pedroñeras in the province of Cuenca, known for the best garlic in Spain. In all varieties, in addition to allicin, sulfur, and quercetin, garlic is rich in the anticancer mineral selenium and offers this important nutrient in a particularly absorbable form.

From a cook's point of view, depending upon how we use it, garlic can be sweet, sour, bitter, or hot. Chefs love garlic so much in Spain they even revere the shoots, called *ajos tiernos* which spring from the cloves and are added to salads and omelets. A dish encountered in the Basque country, *huevos revueltos con ajos tiernos*, combines the green garlic shoots with scrambled eggs. And garlic mousseline, a kind of soufflé topping made from garlic shoots that sauces fish, scallops, and more, is another Catalan invention. Garlic mousseline was created at the historic restaurant El Motel, in Figueres, which we will talk about again. Many traditional dishes were recast into new forms there, often intensifying flavors and, in every sense, modernizing cuisine. By the way, Salvador Dalí loved El Motel and ate there every week with his wife, Gala. The writer and gastronome, Josep Pla, was another regular at the restaurant.

About garlic, Pla said it is "the Genghis Khan of Catalan cuisine."

Raw, crushed garlic is combined with salt and extra-virgin olive oil to make aioli; however, some chefs roast the garlic to create a mellow version. In the Pyrenees, aioli thickened with honey and blended with apples, pears, or quince is often served with wild game.

I am missing *calçots*, but we can't expect to see them now because it is not spring.

As we leave the booth, the scent of alliums gives way to a fragrance that humankind has trailed and searched for, for hundreds of years.

In moments we are before a stall dedicated solely to mushrooms. There are so many varieties it looks like a display from the Museum of Natural History in New York. Baskets brimming with jumbled mushrooms are on the table before us.

Leaning in, the taste of forest is on my tongue.

With eyes of Argos, I see orange and red ones, and mushrooms that are almost black. There must be at least thirty varieties before us, and many I never dreamed existed.

I must tell you about Dr. Font i Quer, a naturalist who was crazy about mushrooms. During the 1930s, Font i Quer identified and cataloged 627 types. His findings were so remarkable that other mycologists jumped on Font i Quer's bandwagon, and the number of mushrooms the group identified exploded. Over the course of five years, more mycologists joined the original group, coming from France, England, and as far away as America, and together with Dr. Font i Quer at the helm, the group categorized over 1,500 types of mushrooms, all from Catalunya.

Don't miss those orange fall rovellons, the color of psychedelic tree fungus. With the mushrooms beside them in creams, dusky grays, and browns, the display makes an autumn tapestry.

Let's have a silent moment for these black mushrooms, for they are *trompetes de la mort.*

Here are wild *Boletus edulis*—with the fragrance of truffles—smell them? Mmmmm.

The Pyrenees are said to be the European center for wild mushrooms, so folks here know how to cook them. During autumn, everyone heads to forests and pastures with little baskets searching for wild mushrooms—like philosophers seeking the truth. Chef Reyes Gracia Pina, in her retaurant La Avenida located in the Pyrenees, prepares risotto of boletus with black truffles and rabbit with wild mushrooms, to name just two.

In Ganbara, a popular pintxos bar in Donostia/San Sebastián, I have seen mushrooms so large they were practically the size of footballs. The forager of these "Alice in Wonderland" beauties was an older guy wearing a neck scarf and hat, with the brim upturned. He stood with stylish nonchalance amidst a crowd of devotees, accepting congratulations as though he were a rock star.

Later I would discover that those giant mushrooms were *Boletus aereus*, and the caps sometimes reach a diameter of sixteen inches. They are highly prized, not just in Ganbara, but throughout the Basque country and Navarra.

No doubt many patrons of Ganbara did not know it, but global studies report that when we consume a variety of mushrooms, the spectrum of protective compounds increases even more.

A study done at the University of Western Australia in 2016 found that just a third of an ounce of common button mushrooms a day decreased breast cancer risk by 64 percent and, interestingly, if you regularly drink green tea, the risk reduces even more, to 89 percent. The City of Hope, a cancer research center in Duarte, California, also found that the consumption of mushrooms lowers breast cancer risk. Shiitake mushrooms, widely available in the United States, have been found by researchers to block tumor growth, so why not eat button mushrooms and shiitakes regularly?

Heading towards an open place where several aisles converge, I spot a tomato stand—but unlike any we have seen. As we approach, two nimble-

> Compounds in mushrooms increase immunity. In addition, certain phytochemicals in mushrooms are antiestrogenic while other compounds reduce COX-2 expression. And mushrooms contain vitamin D, conjugated linoleic acid, lectins, various B-glucans, selenium, and polysaccharides including lentinan, which is so powerful researchers have seen it literally destroy gastric cancer cells.

fingered ladies operating the stand weigh produce and ring up purchases, all the while joking with customers.

Another woman—a chef, I think—stands apart in contemplation. I am curious to observe her selections. She examines heirloom tomatoes with the scrutiny of a detective on a hot lead. Finally pointing out her choices to a young man hovering nearby—obviously her assistant—he completes the transaction deftly. We are onlookers, as they move on.

Consumption of tomatoes helps prevent heart disease, breast cancer, and osteoporosis, and aids in gene repair through stabilizing and reprogramming genes coded for cancer.

Tomatoes cooked in olive oil are especially protective.

There are people in Barcelona who may not know the health benefits of tomatoes, but they are beloved here no matter how you slice them. At Ca l'Isidre, a traditional restaurant in the Raval district of Barcelona, renowned for seasonal local products, one might be served tasty heirloom tomatoes with edible flowers.

Speaking of Ca l'Isidre, another story comes to mind.

This restaurant, for those in the "know," is acclaimed for traditional Catalan cooking. It is filled with original art, candlelight, and flowers, and the atmosphere is clubby. Intimate. The cuisine is known to be exceptional, however, as the

In 2017 scientists at the Mushroom Technological Research Center in La Rioja, Spain, reported that grilling or microwaving mushrooms releases the optimum antioxidant action of phytochemicals. They also recommend cooking mushrooms in olive oil for "improving the fatty acid composition" with "minimal increase in calories."

In addition to shielding lycopene, tomatoes also contain beta-carotene, photoene, and phytofluene, all cancer-fighting carotenoids, as well as the free-radical-fighting vitamin C.

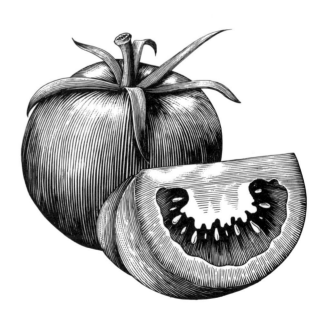

story was told to me some years ago, a young upstart from the Guide Michelin advised the proud owner, Isidre Gironés, "You serve excellent food but your restaurant is in need of updating." Unruffled, the elegant Catalan—and one of Barcelona's most respected chefs and restaurateurs—responded, "You stick to selling tires, and I will continue serving great food."

Now we see many varieties of tomatoes.

Red and green-veined Montserrat tomatoes; the small ones are Penedès, and these are bull's heart. And look—don't miss the pink tomatoes from Huesca.

There are about 120 known varieties of tomatoes identified in Spain, many native to a particular region, but agriculturists believe there are many more. Back in the 1960s, one could find innocuous-looking flatish heirloom tomatoes that were anything but bland. These *costolutos* could fit in the palm of one's hand but had an intensity of flavor that Nancy Harmon Jenkins found so delicious that it "was like no other" as she reported in *The Essential Mediterranean*.

Now I spot the freshest looking purple broccoli I have ever seen—and black turnips, and mounds of cauliflower!

All in this booth, right next door.

As we enter, an older woman—the vendor—senses my eagerness. Our eyes meet. A feeling that I've known her all my life washes over me. In broken English, with smiling eyes, "Vegetables, organic." Her face is webbed with wrinkles. The pride she shows in her work creates glory in her face, filling it with delight.

No doubt this woman knows many home-style dishes we would love to learn, including *menestra*. Originating in Navarra, this assortment of season-

Nutrition to the Max: Tomatoes Cooked in Extra-Virgin Olive Oil
Science shows that cooked tomatoes offer the most benefit, so for instance, a ½ cup of tomato sauce a day provides a significant boost of lycopene. What's more, since lycopene is fat soluble, the ultimate way to consume tomatoes is with EVOO as the Spanish do.

Heirloom Tomatoes, A Treasure
As the *New York Times* reported in a May 2013 article entitled "Nutritional Weaklings in the Supermarket," "heirloom and wild varieties of produce have been found in separate studies to outshine their cultivated cousins."

al vegetables might include asparagus, artichokes, lettuce hearts, carrots, peas, brussels sprouts, or cauliflower. Menestras are made by sautéing the vegetables separately before combining them, which assures they are cooked until just done, or al punto. No over cooking! Sometimes menestras are garnished with slivers of jamón.

Cabbage, brussels sprouts, cauliflower, and other crucifers such as turnips contain several highly protective compounds that help prevent breast cancer. Indole 3 carbinole converts cancer-promoting estrogens into shielding estrogens, and isothiocyanates help prevent cancerous substances from reaching their target.

In the Pyrenees of Vall d'Aran and Vall de Camprodon, there are festivals celebrating cabbage-potato cakes, cooked with a little bacon, called *trinxat*, another favorite of the long-living people of Andorra.

Increase the Efficacy of Sulforaphane A 2013 study reported frozen broccoli lacks sulforaphane, so be sure to buy fresh and eat in the same meal with arugula. A recent study reported that the plant compounds in the arugula support the bioavailability of sulforaphane.

Another plant chemical found in crucifers renowned for battling cancer is sulforaphane, especially abundant in broccoli. Studies also show that sulforaphane decreases certain enzymes that speed cartilage breakdown, something runners should keep in mind.

Exposure to environmental chemicals is cumulative as we age, so for those interested in cancer prevention, it is crucial to eat freshly cooked crucifers daily.

Galicians have been cooking turnip greens or *grelos* for centuries, and in Aragón, *Talltendre* turnips grown in the valley of Cerdanya are renowned. I'm not seeing it now, but salsify with its black exterior has been eaten in Europe since medieval times. But I do see turnips, which can be eaten raw and cooked.

Now cabbage. Green, red, Chinese, and curly.

Don't miss this fine-leafed curly *brotenera*. All types of cabbage are filled with plant compounds that break down harmful hormones, and curly leafed is known to be richest. Not incidentally, purple cabbage

TIP: Pound for pound, watercress packs
twice the vitamin C of oranges. The
CDC has pointed out that watercress is
the most nutrient-dense food we can
eat. Also, watercress has been found to
shield against free radicals.

contains shielding anthocyanins—more on these plant compounds in a moment.

Consider the many ways that the Spanish cook cabbage. They braise it with pork, sausages or ham, and use it to make *cocidos*, a national dish prepared with chickpeas, vegetables, stewed meats, and sausage. In the North, cabbage appears in countless soups and the leaves are used to wrap corn and rye bread before baking. And cabbage might be stuffed with deboned partridge, as was prepared for Josep Pla at El Motel Restaurant, after Pla lost his teeth.

Chef Carme Ruscalleda, who was a farmer before she was a chef, cooks with cabbage often. She prepares this humble vegetable raw for salads, boils it with potatoes, and drizzles EVOO over it to accompany meat or fish. The chef also combines leftover cooked cabbage with potatoes, and fries them together with a small piece of bacon to make *trinxat*.

Ruscalleda prepares turnips in many tasty ways, too. She peels, slices, and boils turnips for ten minutes in salted water. Then she sautés them in olive oil, and combines with apples and nuts to make salads.

Watercress contains erucin, a plant chemical that researchers found to inhibit hormone-receptor-positive breast cancer cells. Kale contains indoles and nitrogen compounds that may prevent certain lesions from converting to cancerous cells in estrogen-sensitive tissues.

Chard—we see mounds of it here—is sautéed with pine nuts, raisins, and garlic in Catalunya. Chard is also regular fare in Navarra and in Aragón, where it is believed by the older folks to support healthy digestion. Science has confirmed that chard supports the body's natural efforts to rid it of toxins and may help prevent cancer and heart disease due to the plant chemical it contains, kaempferol.

As we leave, the older lady is busy weighing produce but she finds a moment to glance our way bidding valediction.

"Until next time," her warm eyes say.

"Until we meet again," mine answer.

On our way, we admire the purple broccoli that drew us, reminding that purple vegetables and fruit are rich in anthocyanins, a plant chemical identified in 2010 as having exceedingly beneficial anticancer properties.

Now standing in the middle of the aisle, it's not easy to decide where to go next.

Let us not miss the large, orange hard squash in that booth nearby.

We stroll over.

Pumpkin and hard squash are important foods because they contain anticancer beta-carotene.

Janet Mendel points out in *Cooking in Spain* that the flesh of the pumpkin, or *calabaza*, ranges from pale yellow to bright orange and that "The bland slightly sweet flesh of the pumpkin can go sweet or savory, though in Spain it is most often used as a vegetable in hearty potages with beans and sausages."

Pumpkin is also stewed along with onions, tomatoes, and green peppers. And according to Mendel, hard skinned squash can be "baked, steamed or fried."

I must speak about Chef Ruscalleda again. In *Mediterranean Cuisine; 100 Easy Recipes*, she shares a pumpkin consomme recipe made with porcini mushrooms, courgettes, and brown rice.

Pumpkin seeds, a common snack in Spain, contain immune-enhancing nutrients such as zinc and plant sterols, which act as antioxidants, especially protective against prostate cancer.

Now we arrive at a large stall offering an extensive selection of seeds and nuts. It is one of the most crowded all day, a testament that this food is wildly popular here. Nuts, an important component

Huertos y Caza As explained to me by my Aragonese friend Alicia, older folks in her homeland eat as they did many years ago. "They eat *hortalizas*, meaning from the garden: figs, olives, almonds and other nuts, peaches, cherries, legumes, and many vegetables, especially chard, borage, cabbage, cauliflower, green beans, potatoes, etc. And they eat *caza*, meaning wild game from the hunt such as boar, partridge, deer, and hare, often if not always prepared with vegetables."

of the Mediterranean diet, are used in the cooking of Catalunya in endless ways.

We see a couple of teenagers sharing almonds from a small bag. I see they are Marcona almonds.

I must have some.

The flavor—rustic, oily, and sweet—leaves me wanting more.

Almonds are slivered and toasted for pilafs and pulverized to make sauces and cold soups; they are made into desserts such as *panellets*, a type of Catalan confection; almonds are used as thickeners for soups and to make *picada*, a flavor-packed thickener often used to finish stews.

Chocolate or Saffron Picada Made with Almonds

Using a mortar and pestle or a food processor, combine 1 handful of slivered, lightly toasted almonds, 1 clove of roasted garlic, 1 tablespoon EVOO, 2 tablespoons stock or water, 1 tablespoon roughly chopped flat-leafed parsley, salt, 1 thin slice day-old (or toasted) French or Italian bread lightly fried in olive oil, and a pinch of saffron or ½ ounce dark chocolate, broken into pieces.

———•———

When it comes to nuts, don't be overly concerned about counting calories, for researchers have recently determined that they are not as fattening as previously thought. We all can benefit by eating a moderate amount of this nutritious food every day.

Between delicious bites, I point out hazelnuts, pistachios, pine nuts, walnuts, peanuts, pumpkin seeds, and *chufas* or tiger nuts, a specialty of Valencia that is made into a chilled drink.

As the vendor weighs purchases as though he was competing in a category of the Olympics, laughingly, we move to the side and talk.

The mono and polyunsaturated fats in nuts are now understood to play a prominent role in protecting the heart, a significant element of the Mediterranean diet that in early days was not understood. Nuts contain plant chemicals called sterols that help reduce the absorption of cholesterol from one's diet.

Nuts also contain antioxidant plant chemicals, including flavonoids, phenols, and kaempferol, that suppress the growth of tumors. Evidence is building for a correlation between the consumption of nuts and long life. A 2014 study conducted among more than 200 thousand men and women in the United States and China, as reported in the *Journal of the American Medical Association*, found that the more nuts people consumed, the lower the death rate from all causes, especially from heart disease and stroke.

Consider walnuts. The omega-3 fatty acids in them help protect against cancer, particularly breast. A 2014 study reports that walnuts have the most benefits for breast cancer patients since they are richest in flavonoids, phenols, and antioxidants. And nuts are rich in vitamin E, important since researchers feel this nutrient is not absorbed efficiently from supplements and is best taken from foods that contain it.

Piñones, or pine nuts, are especially popular here. Catalans cook them in desserts, and in savory recipes, such as accompanying greens sautéed in garlic and as a garnish for vegetables. Pine nuts are pulverized to thicken sauces and used in making deserts.

We spoke about romesco sauce, one of the greatest sauces in Spain. Also a Catalan invention, it is made with crushed hazelnuts or almonds. Sometimes both.

Now, chestnuts.

Throughout the north, chestnuts appear in desserts, soups, vegetable dishes, and as stuffing for wild game. In the Pyrenees, lamb meatballs might have a chestnut in the center, and often in the winter, they are toasted over live coals by street vendors.

Walnuts Support Gut Micobiota
In 2019, researchers at Penn State University published a study that showed eating walnuts daily as part of a healthy diet improved gut function, thereby reducing the risk of heart disease.

Chestnuts simmered in milk to make a puree might accompany roasted meat or poultry. Comfort food to the max.

Perhaps you did not know that chestnuts are a remedy for keeping witches at bay?

It is said in Galicia that if you keep a chestnut in your pocket, witches leave you alone.

Results guaranteed.

Okay, there is no science proving that witches hate chestnuts, but there is showing that nuts in general shield against heart disease. This is due to the healthy fats I continue to speak of, so crucial to health. And isn't it comforting to know that nuts increase the activity of the hormone insulin, which keeps us from binging?

At this moment another booth beckons, but it's extensive. We decide to wait and explore it tomorrow.

And so, like the dowager earlier in the day, we become lost in the crowd moving away from the market to *Les Rambles*.

Strolling down the avenue we join old people, lovers, and children at play. Everyone seems at peace, and united in *la alegría de vivir*.

There are street artists in elaborate costumes and makeup. One young woman is wearing a white tulle ball gown. She is an unsmiling beauty with a chalky face, and powdery white rococo hair. Even her lips are white. She is an apparition, frozen in time, from days gone by.

Another artist transfixes, but we are not the only ones.

There is a group surrounding the creature. It, too, stands completely still, but this individual is costumed as an Antoni Gaudí lizard, in pastiched fabric of green, sewn together like a shattered *trencadís* from Parc Güell. The creature is convincing—even threatening—and

Pine Nuts in Medieval Spain Catalans invented the versatile nut sauce, picada, which means crush. Picada is an important element of Catalan cuisine used as a thickener and flavoring for sauces, soups, and stews. It is added moments before a recipe's completion, creating another layer of flavor. There are many versions of picada, some with saffron, others with chocolate.

Chestnuts are rich in anticancer B vitamins and folate, a substance that helps repair DNA and protect the heart.

suddenly breaks its lizard-like pose to terrorize a leashed dog that had been watching in bristly suspicion. The dog bares its teeth and barks with fervor. Together, with the dog's master, the three of us laugh, but the dog doesn't see the humor. What's more, the animal seems to take our laughter personally, which makes us laugh all the more.

In a recent study published in the *Journal of Nutrition*, researchers at Marshall University reported that eating just a few walnuts a day significantly lowers the risk of mammary cancer in mice. When walnuts are eaten raw, they contain the greatest amount of cancer-fighting substances over any other nut.

Finally, his barking stops. Our laughter dies.

We part in high spirits, and in the softness of late day sun, now I walk toward the hotel. The wide avenue narrows, and I walk on cobblestones, in shade. Elegant old coach lanterns line the street, and someone on a rooftop above, keeps doves. Now I think of the writer Mercè Rodoreda. As I make my way down the narrow street, the cooing of the doves seems to mark the passage of time.

A short time later, in my small one-window room, I lean back on pillows sipping Catalan *vi negre*. The full-bodied red wine smells like Mediterranean forests with a whisper of black olives, and tastes of wild berries.

The wine is velvet in my mouth.

It feels good to be alone. With curtains billowing at the open window, the only sound I hear now is the cooing of the doves.

I reach for my laptop and write.

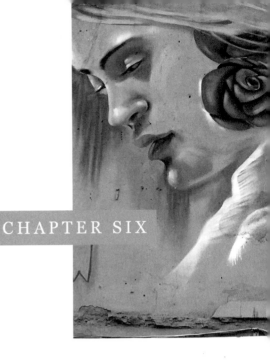

CHAPTER SIX

The Following Day, Our Return

"You must understand how serious we are about our vegetables . . . to give you an example, I have a friend who was going to build himself a new house a few years ago. He estimated that construction would take eight months. But the first thing he did, before beginning on the house, was to clear a garden and plant tomatoes."

　　　　　　– Colman Andrews, *Catalan Cuisine: Vivid Flavors from Spain's Mediterranean Coast*

"The art of cooking begins with selecting the produce, then you must treat it well, know how to store it, clean it, handle it and cook it."

　　　　　　– Chef Carme Ruscalleda, *CR20: 20 Years of the Sant Pau*, Mont-Ferrant

"There'd be lots of vegetables: petits pois, asparagus, kale, lots of greens, each prepared separately and cooked just right with olive oil."

　　　　　　– Chef Elena Arzak describing her final meal, *The Guardian*

Sunlight floods my little room, heralding the new day. With birds doing everything in their power to make sure I don't fall back into slumber, I am reminded that there is still much to explore at the great market and because time passes far too quickly in Barcelona, I resist bed gravity and call for *café con leche*, "*rápido, por favor.*"

The little restaurant where we plan to meet later in the day is near the market and makes no pretense toward decor. Often arguments can be overheard from the kitchen. The chef is known to have a temper.

But the little restaurant is also known for a dish that I love, and the strange little place does it well. Knowing this propels me as I walk from the hotel to the modest restaurant.

Soon I will be eating something shockingly delicious.

We meet, and enter. Looking about I see that the dozen or so tables are mostly occupied with locals quietly eating their afternoon meal.

Our order is taken without fanfare by a serious, plump Catalan. The woman looks us up and down with piercing dark little eyes.

Holding her pad with pen in hand, the server questions us—are we certain that we want *fideuá*?

It's almost as though she will demand that we produce our passports. After a final severe glance, the woman shuffles away leaving a cloud of disgruntlement like bubbles trailing a displaced squid.

We look at one another in suspense.

What next?

A short while later she serves our *fideuá negre* and allioli with a flourish, as though saying we will be taught a thing or two in her establishment. I nod in vigorous appreciation, but she gives me a withering look as if to say "Don't think I am not on to you," for the woman knows the funky black noodle dish is unlike anything else and suspects we might send it back.

But it would not be possible.

This *fideuá*, made with black squid ink, is a variation on the traditional way it is prepared in Valencia. Originating on the coast in Gandia, it began as the rice dish *arròs a banda*. What makes this fideuá so good are the noodles that Colman Andrews calls "Catalonia's own pasta."

The aroma is inviting but vaguely mysterious. As for the way it looks, well, remember thrift plays a role here. Fideuá was developed to use whatever is left at the bottom of the fishing net. We see broken squid tentacles, baby shrimp, etc., to which are added bits of sausage, caramelized onions, and slivers of sautéed green peppers.

Today there must be détente in the kitchen. We begin our meal in silence.

Essences spin in my mouth—they are so savory and pungent that the Japanese word *umami* comes to mind: exactly right for the moment, but impossible to describe.

Let me try.

Flavors are wonderfully old world and, as Catalans say, baroque, meaning for example that dozens of improbable ingredients are combined into one sensuously delicious dish. Fideuá, sweet, briny, and savory, is made distinctive by the black, unctuous sauce. But to the uninitiated, the concentrated umami and taste of the sea can startle.

Don't miss the the server watching us from the kitchen as we eat.

It is not until we finish the final delectable bites of the vermicelli-like noodles swathed in the bold, scrumptious sauce, every morsel of tender seafood and succulent pork, and every lush drop of garlicky allioli; and not until we leave the darkened restaurant to walk into the glaring sun—as we move down *Les Rambles* dodging text lemmings—do I explain there are many recipes for fideuá and the one we just finished was the black seafood version.

The cook began our dish with sofrito—made with diced green pepper—to which he added seafood except for the crustaceans and, blurring boundaries between land and sea, bits of sausage. When everything was cooking nicely, noodles were added, followed by saffron threads, cuttlefish ink, and heated seafood stock. The stock is slowly added, and the noodles are cooked until just tender. They should be glazed with the sauce and not overcooked.

TIP: Cuttlefish are larger, thick-fleshed relatives of squid. If you can't get cuttlefish (which is known as *sepia* in Catalunya), squid can be substituted. By the way, squid is known as *calamar* here.

Squid or Cuttlefish Ink Offers Tremendous Nutritional Benefit
Green foods such as wheatgrass have been on the radar of nutrition researchers for a long time, but more recently the focus has been on the benefits of black foods such as rice, and squid ink, a condiment rich in antioxidants and anthocyanins that has antitumor and antibacterial properties and protects immunity. In addition, squid ink contains protein, lipids, minerals, taurine, and dopamine, a neurotransmitter that encourages positive mental outlook.

Claudia Roden wrote, "The historical rice-growing regions where rice is a staple are the Mediterranean regions of Catalonia, Valencia and Murcia." Navarra is also a major rice-producing province. Interestingly, a porridge recipe from Navarra is documented in *Llibre de Sent Soví*, combining rice with the broth and meat of capons, or chicken. Then later, in the fifteenth century, *El Llibre del Coch* by Robert de Nola, refers to "stewed rice," bringing focus to the Catalan recipe of rice in beef broth, topped with egg yolks, and baked in the oven.

TIP: **Soupy Rice, known as *arroz caldoso*** Make soupy rice your own. Spanish people use whatever is in season and what the family can afford, and they don't worry about measuring. For soupy rice, short grain is best. These recipes are hearty, comforting, and warming during winter. Soupy rice can be "finished" in the oven while drier dishes such as paella are cooked over a flame.

Finally, a few clams or mussels are added, and after they open, it is then that one feasts. Wedges of citrusy lemon and garlicky allioli provide counterpoint.

Fighting carb overload, we make our way to the bustling market.

It's like entering another dimension. Wondering where to start, we decide on the ridiculously large stall we saw yesterday before parting.

Moments later, we find it.

Given that the proprietor is *guapo*, it isn't difficult to begin our investigations.

The cloth bag of rice you're admiring is from Pals, an ancient rice-growing region in Catalunya, and that *bomba 'La Perdiz'* by *Arcesa* you are holding is grown in Valencia. Both are exceptional. I explain that for paella, unwashed bomba rice rules.

The higher starch content of this medium-grain rice allows it to absorb a greater amount of stock while still remaining separate grains. Never wash rice for paella—it destroys the texture—and never use long-grain rice for paella or slow-cooked casseroles because it does not absorb adequate broth.

We see rice from the flatlands of the river Ebro in Navarra, and from Aragón.

Our conversation puzzles the handsome vendor who now looks our way. He reminds me of Martiño Rivas, the startlingly handsome star from the television series *El Internado*.

I am guessing that the guy wears his dark hair slicked back to show his profile, which he must know is remarkable. Like Rivas, he even has dimples.

Suddenly, I spot something I can't let you miss. Forget about Mr. Wonderful.

See this vegetable? It is called *borraja*, or borage, as we know it. Borage, which is extremely healthy, is prepared in soups and with clams and rice. The vegetable appears often in ancient cooking texts and is still treasured in Navarra, the Basque country, and Aragón, where borraja is gathered wild from the slopes of Moncayo Mountain to be cooked with boiled potatoes and good extra-virgin olive oil.

Researchers found that borage is a source of gamma linolenic acid, an omega-6 fatty acid derivative cytotoxic to tumors, meaning it has a weakening and in many cases, deadly effect on cancer cells. Moreover, GLA is vital to human health and plays an important role in restoring immunity and more.

Now stalky plants sidetrack. It's like they are on steroids.

These cartoonish looking things are cardoons, known as *cardos* here, another favorite of the people of the north who love this prickly vegetable so much that it is commonly cultivated in gardens. Cardoons grow wild throughout the Mediterranean and are so tasty they are cooked simply and dressed with just lemon, olive oil, and garlic.

The stalk is what is desired, and after trimming, cardoons are either cooked, which is the traditional way, or minced and served raw. Many so-called modern chefs in Navarra and elsewhere prepare cardoons to serve raw, as a salad.

Now I see sprouts.

Spain's modern chefs sometimes garnish with sprouts (symbolizing the freshness of the foods they cook and serve); however, the use of germinated

Consuming borage may help ward off stomach cancer and extend life. In 2013, Dr. Jose Miguel Sanz Anquela, a physician at the Hospital Universitario Principe de Asturias of Alcalá de Henares, noted that one dish of borage every three days has been correlated with these benefits. Cardoons contain plant chemicals that protect DNA: luteolin, silymarin, caffeic, ferulic, and dicaffeoylquinic acids. Cardoons are also a rich source of B vitamins and calcium.

As noted in the *Llibre de Sent Soví*, cardoons were popular in medieval Europe as were carrots, parsnips, cabbage, artichokes, Swiss chard, spinach, and leeks. *Llibre de Sent Soví* also notes early usage of wild plants such as dandelion, nettle, and chickweed.

seeds as food and medicine is said to be twice as old as the Great Wall of China. Sprouts are so high in nutrients that Vasco da Gama and Magellan grew them aboard ship to keep their men from dying of scurvy.

Sprouts contain live enzymes, minerals, and vitamins as well as chlorophyll and amino acids. All sprouts are healthy, but broccoli sprouts rule. Just one tablespoon a day offers protection. This is because sprouts contain concentrations of isothiocyanates, a life-saving plant chemical that sparks hundreds of beneficial genetic changes.

Now a classic. Potatoes.

The people of Spain cook them often and in surprising ways. Try roasting them on a bed of coarse salt. Just pierce your favorite large variety with a fork and roast on salt in a preheated 450°F oven for about an hour.

The Basques love potatoes slowly cooked casserole style in a gentle oven, sliced thinly with onions or chives and olive oil.

Ambrosia.

Patatas bravas is an icon in Barcelona's tapas bars. I will tell you about this recipe in a moment.

The George Mateljan Foundation reports that potatoes are loaded with vitamin B6, which is associated with lower rates of heart disease. Moreover, potatoes contain protective flavonoids, and are a source of vitamin C, potassium, and choline which is essential for healthy brain, nerves and muscles. Naturally gluten-free, cooling potatoes after cooking allows resistant starch to form, supporting the body in many ways including acting as a prebiotic.

Of the varieties before us, the small, elongated deep-purples have the highest nutrient value. Known by the French name, *vitelotte*, they are a favorite of mine. In America, purple potatoes are also called black, blues, violets, and truffled.

Whatever you want to call purples, they contain nearly four times the amount of nutrients and plant compounds such, as antioxidants, over common russets and more anthocyanins per spoonful than blueberries.

If this weren't enough, purples are lowest in starch over any other potato, meaning when we eat them blood glucose won't spike, which is important to keep in mind because a recent study found that cancer risk goes up 15 percent for every 50 units of glycemic load.

Basque chef Juan Marí Arzak serves wild duck with puréed purple potatoes, as described in *Arzak Secrets* (Grub Street Publishers).

Patatas Bravas

Throughout Spain, this spicy-hot, tomato-rich potato dish is often tapas. THE RECIPE: Make sofrito with 1 large chopped onion, several cloves of crushed garlic, 1 bay leaf, 14 ounces of chopped tomatoes, EVOO, salt and pepper to taste. After the sofrito cooks down, add ¼ cup of white wine, 1 tablespoon crushed red pepper flakes, 2 teaspoons vinegar, 2 teaspoons hot pimentón. Adjust salt and olive oil. Cook for 25 minutes or until sauce thickens. Meanwhile, wash and cut 2 pounds of potatoes. Leave skins on. Fry potatoes in EVOO for 20 minutes, until golden. Remove from pan, drain on paper towels, and season with salt. Transfer into a serving bowl, heat the sauce and serve on the side.

———•———

Now the herby, spicy smell of fennel.

The strong scent means this yield is rich in a type of anticancer oil.

On the culinary front, in Spain, fronds of fennel are sometimes tucked into fish before roasting, as with sea bass. Recently, I have been roasting fennel with lemon, garlic and olive oil as a side. And it is good raw, mixed with salad greens.

Herby Fennel Drizzle
to Serve with Roasted Pork or Seafood

Makes about 1½ cups of sauce. Take 2 cloves of garlic and crush with a pinch of sea salt in a mortar, until it forms a paste. Add 4 tablespoons chopped parsley, 5 tablespoons of EVOO and 1½ teaspoons fennel seeds. Pound the mixture and as it breaks down add the juice of ½ lemon, along with a few pinches more of salt and black pepper.

———◆———

Spinach.

During the eighth century, a Catalan chef had the idea to sauté spinach with toasted pine nuts, garlic and raisins. Ever since, they have been cooking *espinacas con pasas y piñones* here so you know it's good.

Spinach is loaded with nutrients. The body utilizes the antioxidants in it to make glutathione, that highly shielding substance I keep referring to, so crucial in supporting the ability to eliminate environmental toxins and steroidal hormones that trigger hormone-sensitive cancers.

All in for Spinach Take a clue from the Catalans and sauté spinach with pine nuts, which are loaded with fiber and offer potassium, phosphorus, and vitamin E. Pine nuts are also a good source of healthy fats, protein and zinc.

This mad profusion of chard shows us how popular the leafy green is here.

The long-lived mountain people of Aragón consider chard to be beneficial for the digestion. In Andorra, Aragón's neighbor, chard is also frequent fare.

The fact that chard is high in minerals such as potassium proves its place in Spain's long-life paradigm.

These turnip greens or *grelos* look like they were picked this morning. They are showcased in *caldo gallego*, a home-style soup made in Galicia with pork, pork bones and potatoes.

Turnip greens offer an abundance of the cruciferous plant chemicals that we continue to speak of, so helpful in the prevention of breast, uterine and prostate cancers.

Carrots. Talisman of chefs and home cooks alike.

Carrots are cooked in all sorts of ways here, and are included in everything from jellied meat pâtés to homestyle stews and more.

Regarding health, raw carrots are known by researchers to be abundant in anticancer falcarinol. In vitro studies show that exposing isolated cancer cells to falcarinol slows their growth. And carrots are especially shielding when eaten with eggplant, still another vegetable frequently on the menu here.

Here is common celery, but what it offers heart, bone, and breast health is

The strong sulfur smell of turnip greens and other crucifers such as broccoli and Brussels sprouts means that these vegetables help support the production of glutathione, the potent detoxifier.

The Iberian Table **Dynamo** Science shows the nutrients in carrots and eggplants galvanize when consumed together, meaning the vegetables become even more protective. In the North, carrots appear in soups, stews, salads, and terrines as part of a meal that frequently includes eggplant.

anything but common. Celery contains the anti-breast cancer compound apigenin as well as vitamin K, which helps prevent osteoporosis by transporting calcium into bones. Vitamin K also blocks excess calcium from gumming up blood vessels and supports normal blood coagulation. And celery does more by aiding in the assimilation of life-extending anticancer, antiviral vitamin D.

Before us, a huge display heaping with avocados stops us in our tracks. Avocados spill from half a dozen large baskets onto quite a long table. The Spanish have only been growing avocados commercially for the past few decades, so they are a modern addition to Spanish cuisine. You won't find traditional recipes with avocados here, as one finds with the cooking of Mexico.

Among many benefits to our health, avocados aid in the absorption of the important nutrient vitamin K, just mentioned when we spoke of celery.

Standing alongside her mother, who is choosing avocados with the focus of a chess player, we can't miss a *preciosa* girl. She looks to be about five. The *chiquita* has dark blond hair, and beribboned braids crown her lovely head.

Looking bored, the child clutches her mother's hand while gravely considering our admiration.

I can't help but think this little girl will be fortunate to grow up eating avocados for as she matures, nutrients and shielding fat from this food will help protect her from breast cancer. The monounsaturated fat in avocado will also help her avoid heart disease.

It is helpful to know that eating avocados keeps us slim. Nutrition scientists have discovered that when we eat avocados, the richness of this food promotes appetite satisfaction. A recent study reported that eating avocados with lunch, led on average to 83 percent fewer calories the rest of the day.

Nearby, these sweet potatoes are an excellent source of vitamin C and beta-carotene, nutrients that protect DNA from cancer-causing substances. Studies also show that sweets contain salicylic acid, a compound that specifically can help in the prevention of breast and prostate cancers.

> TIP: **Courgettes Protect** Courgettes or zucchini are also a source of salicylic acid, that anti-inflammatory plant chemical we just talked about, that lowers breast and prostate cancer risk. Other vegetables that contain salicylic acid include okra, cucumbers, green peppers, broccoli, and previously mentioned sweet potatoes.

At this moment, the adorable little girl follows her mother to the register. While waiting for *mamá* to pay, she sees us admiring her.

Now she sends us a kiss.

"*Besitos*," we say, laughing.

Her mother raises her eyebrows bewailing that her daughter loves the limelight. Some things are the same everywhere. Little girls just know they are charming.

Resuming our adventures, I zero in on zucchini, or *calabacín*, another vegetable endemic to Spanish Mediterranean cooking, also excellent for health.

Now moving to eggplant, the varied shapes and sizes are many—clearly another vegetable highly regarded here. In the North, cuisine reaches very far back indeed.

In Catalunya, it is common to roast eggplant with bell peppers at home in the fireplace, or outside, even on the beach. This is *escalivar*, which means to roast vegetables in the embers of a wood fire. The tradition likely began centuries ago, as did samfaina.

Escalivada Vegetables

Serves 6

Clean and dry 3 medium eggplants, 4 medium onions, and 4 red peppers. Rub vegetables with EVOO and place on a large baking dish drizzled with more oil. Roast in a preheated 375°F oven or grill for approximately 20 minutes. After vegetables cool, peel off blackened skin of eggplants, onions, and peppers and arrange on a platter rubbed with a clove of crushed garlic. Drizzle lightly with vinegar and EVOO, and season with salt and ground black pepper.

Samfaina, a boldly delicious sauce made from eggplant, is very similar to ratatouille. According to Colman Andrews, "to the Catalan mind, samfaina is the most important unique and incorruptible dish which the Catalan cuisine has brought to gastronomy" and because "the Catalans once held sway in that part of France ... who is to say that the Catalans didn't bring the dish to the French shores in the first place?"

Purple Foods Reign These "royal colored" foods contain an abundance of anticancer anthocyanins, so eat them often. Select from eggplant, onion, potatoes, berries, kidney beans, red grapes, pomegranates, pole beans, kohlrabi, broccoli, snap beans, açai, bilberry, chokeberries, and elderberries.

Eggplant also contains chlorogenic acid, which protects DNA from mutations, as well as nasunin, which shields cells from damage.

The George Mateljan Foundation's *World's Healthiest Foods* website reports that eggplants help lower LDL, or bad cholesterol, and that when laboratory animals were given extract of eggplant juice, the blood cholesterol in their artery walls and aortas was considerably lowered.

Samfaina with Anchovies

My version of this eggplant concoction contains anchovies. Use it to sauce fish, pasta, or chicken. Cut a large eggplant into approximately 1-inch cubes, salt lightly, and set aside for 30 minutes to remove bitterness. Discard liquid and pat the cubes dry with a clean towel. Set aside. Grate 2 pounds of tomatoes. See instructions for making sofrito in chapter 3. Deseed and chop 1 red bell pepper and peel and chop 1 pound of onions. Cut 2 medium-sized zucchinis into chunks. Peel and crush 6-8 cloves of garlic. Open a tin of tomato paste. Set aside. In a large pan, heat EVOO and sauté onions on high for 10 minutes, stirring. Salt the onions lightly and season with 3-4 pinches of dried thyme. Add 2 cloves of garlic. Continue sautéing for about 4 minutes to begin breaking the garlic down into the onions. Combine eggplant, red pepper, and zucchini with the onions, and sauté on medium-high for 20 minutes. Vegetables should be lightly caramel colored. While sautéing, season lightly with salt and ground pepper. Add tomatoes, a little more EVOO, 3 cloves of crushed garlic and lightly salt. Continue cooking on medium-high for 10 minutes, then add 2 pinches of dried thyme. Add ⅔ cup of water or chicken stock to the mixture and a little more EVOO. Along with remaining garlic, add ⅔ cup of tomato paste, season with ground pepper, a touch more salt, and a modicum of EVOO. Gently combine tomato paste into the mixture. Next, add ¼ to ⅓ cup of crumbled anchovies, which adds savoriness, and of course salt. Taste. Adjust salt. Simmer uncovered for 20 minutes more, or until vegetables are almost soft, occasionally stirring. Samfaina is meant to be soft but not mushy.

———•———

Resembling a giant beehive with thorns, a show-stopping display of artichokes beckon.

Artichokes have been eaten in these parts since early medieval times. They are mentioned frequently in *Llibre de Sent Soví*.

This brutish looking vegetable lowers harmful cholesterol and helps protect against cancer. A 2016 study found that the compound luteolin in artichokes has an inhibitory effect on the proliferation of human cancer cells and discourages the formation of new blood vessels that grow tumors. Nutrition scientists know that diets high in luteolin are linked to a reduced risk of breast cancer.

Don't miss these small purplish artichokes.

They are so tender that they are sometimes eaten raw in salads here. In early spring, even the stems of baby artichokes are especially delightful.

And here, bell peppers, a treasure of antioxidants and an icon of the Spanish Mediterranean diet.

Bells burst with nutrients, and no other Mediterranean culture cooks with green bell peppers as frequently or, I believe, with as much range as the Spanish.

Red, green, yellow, and orange bells gleam. A banner confirming life. Announcing a wealth of beta-carotene, antioxidants, and anticancer compounds, as reported by the American Institute for Cancer Research in 2016, bells are an excellent source of ascorbic acid—another name for vitamin C—which protects DNA from free radicals.

It's not just bells that protect. The Spanish cook with a variety of peppers, but if I were to talk about all of the peppers before us now, we would be here all night, so let me choose a few.

Reported in the *Journal of Pharmacological Science*, the artichoke compound silibinin promotes triple-negative and hormone-receptor positive (ER+/PR+) breast cancer cell death. And because of the bitter flavor, consumption of artichokes supports the liver, which means potentially dangerous sources of estrogen are detoxified.

Since discovering the cooking of Spain, I have become a pepper fangirl. But remember, the peppers used in Spanish gastronomy are a world apart from the hot ones of Mexico.

The many tastes of Spanish peppers can be likened to flamenco music. The range is sophisticated and can be seductively mellow, or bright and tangy, and sometimes harmoniously fruity. Some, like *ñoras*, are so old-world that you have no flavor to compare them to.

Spanish peppers offer up that critical, hard to find "missing taste." Let's dive in. I promise your palette will develop a taste for them all.

Peppers are so intrinsic to Spanish Mediterranean cooking that the Spanish have a favorite phrase, *me importa un pimento*, meaning it is as important as a pepper.

These dark-red dried burgundys are the *ñoras* I just spoke of. They are reconstituted in hot water and intrinsic in the making of romesco, *salmorreta*, and picada sauces, and are used in bean dishes and fish or meat stews.

Guindillas. These long, thin fresh peppers figure prominently in the Basque starters called pintxos. They are available in the US from some Spanish importers and are usually jarred.

Don't miss these small fresh green peppers, for they are Galician *pimientos de Padrón*, madly delicious when roasted, but once in a while a random one can be so hot it's like consuming fire. Russian roulette, Galician style.

Romesco Sauce for Vegetables, Roasted or Steamed, or to Sauce Poached Fish

Coat ½ of a deseeded red pepper with EVOO and roast in a 375°F oven until the skin slightly chars. Remove from oven. Place in a bowl with a lid until cool, which makes it easier to remove the skin. Reconstitute 1 small *ñora* in hot water. Remove stem and seeds. After the roasted red pepper cools, remove skin, cut into small pieces and combine with the reconstituted *ñora*, along with 3 cloves of minced garlic; ½ medium seeded tomato, peeled and grated; ¼ cup lightly roasted hazelnuts (or pine nuts, almonds, walnuts); 2 tablespoons red wine vinegar; ¼ cup olive oil; ¾ teaspoon salt; a few flakes dried hot chili pepper, and a splash of red wine. Use a large mortar with a pestle to combine ingredients into a sauce, or blend into a puree. Do not over blend. A slice of dried crumbled French-style crusty bread can be added for body.

———•———

We have been exploring the good-looking proprietor's stall quietly, but now a display of culinary herbs is so extensive my voice lilts in anticipation. The guapo looks our way, but when he sees it is only us—hardened "observers"—he quickly shifts his attention.

Two Herb Sauces to Energize
Poached Poultry, Fish, and Roasted Meats

Nuts and Herb Sauce: Combine parsley with mint and marjoram along with pounded hazelnuts and walnuts. Add a generous glug of EVOO and sweeten with a touch of honey.

Garlic, Oregano, and Parsley Sauce: Mix chopped garlic with chopped fresh parsley and oregano; add a dash of white wine vinegar and a generous drizzle of EVOO.

———•———

Ancient *monasterios* were renowned for having extensive herb gardens, and for offering some of the best cooking in Europe. Vestiges of these gardens can still be found today. In the fourteenth century, when monks were some of the most skillful cooks in Spain, sage, mint, laurel, cumin, parsley, and coriander were noted in the recipes of *Llibre de Sent Soví*.

These herbs and more are before us now, in this stand.

Flat-leaf parsley, another rich source of the breast protector apiginin, is pervasive in the cooking of Spain. Parsley's sharp, grassy flavor adds dimension to meatballs, stews, fish sauces, herbal sauces,

The Impressive Benefits of Culinary Herbs Herbs contain a spectrum of plant chemicals offering strong antioxidant actions. Common rosemary contains carsinol and rosmarinic, plant chemicals that inhibit the proliferation of various human cancer cell lines, including MCF-7, which is breast adenocarcinoma. Evidence also confirms that rosemary extracts can retard chemically induced cancers. Thyme has been found in recent studies to protect against mammary cancer. For more information on rosemary and thyme, see Appendix B.

TIP: Dry thyme is concentrated. Every tablespoon of fresh thyme equals the flavor of one half tablespoon of dried.

and marinades. In the Basque region, flat-leafed parsley was until recently so plentiful that butchers used to give it away for free with purchases of meat, and still today, across Spain, parsley is often added as a gift along with purchased vegetables.

Thyme has always been defining to the cooking of Spain. It makes repeated appearances in the recipes of *Llibre de Sent Soví*, circa 1324.

A 2016 study by the *Olive Oil Times* reported that "thyme-enriched olive oil prevents DNA damage," which means when we cook with thyme and extra-virgin olive oil, the phenolic compounds in each empower the other. A 2011 study found that compounds in thyme, ursolic and rosmarinic acid and luteolin, are associated with anticancer activity in animals, and a 2012 in vitro study concluded that wild thyme extract is effective in reducing human breast cancer cells.

Bay laurel is another herb that has a long history in Spain. With the passing of time, the nutritional benefits of laurel are becoming more known. Benefits include lowering blood sugar, reducing inflammation, and alleviating gastrointestinal and respiratory problems. Laurel also offers anticancer properties because it is an excellent source of the compound eugenol.

Eager to leave this booth in which we have lingered for probably an hour, I realize we overlooked asparagus.

Our handsome vendor looks up exactly at this moment—he sees us prepare to leave but then change our minds to stay.

His face is confounded—can't the poor man ever rid himself of us, two peculiar people who spend a great deal of time admiring his foods but purchase nothing?

The polite Catalan looks away.

Trying my best not to laugh, I explain that asparagus, or *espárrago*, is another vegetable valued throughout Spain. Both green and white are beloved here. White, which is revered, makes its appearance in early spring and has a gentle herby taste, with overtones of fresh peas. Navarra is known to grow the best white asparagus in Spain, and one can purchase it in the US through Spanish food importers.

Asparagus is Widely Popular in Spain and Everyone Benefits In 2013, the University of Hawaii Cancer Center in Honolulu published the results of a study showing that asparagus contains plant chemicals and nutrients that may help prevent breast cancer. In addition to a rich supply of antioxidants and protective B vitamins and folate, asparagus is a potent source of glutathione, the premiere cancer-shielding enzyme.

We finally take our leave, but this time the handsome vendor does not look our way.

After meandering through the bustling market, we find ourselves at a meticulous booth offering an extensive selection of dried beans and legumes. Everything has been arranged with so much thought it is as though we are in a library.

"*Bona tarda*," I say with my best Catalan accent.

A placid woman with horned-rim glasses and tied back tawny hair, nods welcome.

The showing in her booth is a bean nerd's dream.

Through cellophane, we see many types, and the impressive display pays tribute to the sophisticated bean cookery of the North. Some beans are so unusual I guess them to be heirloom. Some are in bins of water ready for customers to cook as soon as they arrive home. Others, like these, are named after the towns in which they were grown. Reds from Burgos and famed Tolosa blacks. Those tiny green ones over there, *verdinas*, were grown in Asturias, in Llanes.

The more I discover about the benefits of beans and legumes the more I cook and eat them. Recently, researchers reported that consuming as little as two tablespoons a day of beans can add years to one's life.

In Aragón, white beans are cooked with boiled potatoes and sautéed garlic, and black beans with wild greens in the dish *panicostra*. In Catalunya, *botifarra amb mongetes*, combining pork sausage with white beans, offers up a cozy meal.

Look—large beans for *fabes asturianes*—one of my favorite dishes of Spain. Also cooked in Cantabria, here are white beans. They are prepared with cabbage and pork in the rural dish, *cocido montañés*. Beans are so popular there, Santander has a covered food market with three stalls and beans are all they sell.

Beans with Clams

Rich in calcium, clams are bone-strengthening and when combined with fiber-rich beans, as is done in northern Spain, people obtain even greater benefits. Cover 24 small clams with salted water. Clams will purge. Meanwhile, in a large sauté pan, make about a cup of onion, tomato, and garlic sofrito. After prepared, stir in 1 cup cooked white beans, along with 1 cup of fish stock, 2 cloves of garlic, and a sprig of fresh rosemary. Cook for 12–14 minutes. Add several pinches of saffron powder in the final 2 minutes. Add clams and season with salt and pepper. After clams open, serve soupy, in shallow bowls, garnished with minced flat-leafed parsley.

Beans and legumes are loaded with lignans—the shielding compound I keep talking about. Women with low rates of breast cancer have high levels of lignans in their blood. Beans also contain antioxidant, anticancer phytochemicals, flavonoids, sterols, and protease inhibitors, as well as resistant starch, meaning they supply the colon with healthful bacteria that produce certain short-chain fatty acids, which shield colon cells.

Here are garbanzos, or chickpeas. And lentils. The humble quality of these nourishing foods must be respected.

The Cantabrian stew, *cocido lebaniego*, combines garbanzos with cabbage and pork, and in *espinacas con garbanzos* they are mashed and refried with sausage and spinach. Recently, I cooked garbanzos with grilled chopped portabellos in plenty of garlic.

Preparing garbanzos is little trouble—just make sure to use enough water—and the rewards are worth the two-hour cooking time. When made from scratch, the taste of chickpeas is nuttier and sweeter than what comes in a can.

Lentils are beloved and essential to the cooking of Spain. Like garbanzos, they are prepared often. Once again, Spanish people benefit, for lentils are effective in lowering harmful LDL cholesterol and rich in fiber. Lentils cook quickly, so there is no excuse not to make them.

Harvard's School of Public Health reported that women who consumed beans at least twice a week slashed breast cancer risk by 24 percent, and in 2014 *BMC Complementary and Alternative Medicine* showed that mung beans help halt a highly aggressive cancer cell cycle linked to cervical cancer.

Mediterranean Diet, Beans and Gut Bacteria Recently, nutrition scientists are focusing on healthful gut bacteria as central to the reason the Mediterranean diet is so protective, and consumption of beans has been found to play a major role.

Cocina Rápida

Basque Style Chickpeas and Sausage

Combine cooked chickpeas with cabbage, sautéed onions, leeks, and garlic. Season with bay leaves, salt and pepper. Add a glug of EVOO, and sausages from animals that were naturally raised (pork, chicken, or beef) and gently simmer on the stove top, covered, for 50-60 minutes.

—•—

Though having only scratched the surface of Spanish Mediterranean bean and legume cookery, we must leave the little booth and, as has become our habit, stroll through the humming market talking.

Basque *Alubias Rojas*

Rinse 2 cups red beans and set aside. Chop ½ reconstituted, deseeded, and destemmed ñora pepper, 1 onion, ½ red bell pepper, 1 tomato, ½ small leek and 3 cloves of garlic, and sauté in a cazuela or enamel baking dish with EVOO until just tender. Add the beans and two pinches of cayenne. Continue cooking for 30 minutes more. If you wish, add two sliced and fried sausages that have been drained of fat. Season with ground pepper and a splash of olive oil, and transfer, covered, to a 350°F oven for 20-30 minutes. If you don't have a ñora pepper, you can add a slightly bigger piece of red bell.

———•———

Now we find ourselves heading into carnivore central. Every animal imaginable—and unimaginable—behind the glass before us, now!

It turns out that chicken legs and thighs offer unique health benefits. This is because the dark meat contains fat soluble, menaquinone (vitamin K2), which is important for the brain, heart and bones. Research has shown K2 to have an inhibiting effect on colon and prostate tumor growth, hardening of the arteries due to plaque buildup and is important for proper blood clotting. Other foods commonly consumed in Spain that contain a meaningful amount of K2 include egg yolks and hard cheese such as Manchego.

See the furry haunches of wild boar hanging just above your head next to the wild hare?

Steel yourself. Pig trotters.

But now, our attention shifts.

Fixing our gaze upon chickens with strange pearly skin, I explain they are *pollo catalán and capón del Prat*, an old-fashioned breed known for its delicious sweetish meat, prepared for special occasions.

There was a time when the average Spanish ate any type of meat only on special occasions. The older generations probably remember eating chicken just two or three times a year.

Janet Mendel, the author of *Cooking in Spain*, says "a chunk of boiling meat, a quarter of a stewing hen, a piece of salt pork, a ham bone, a few pork ribs, and black pudding and red sausage ... all went into the cocido with garbanzos and vegetables and provided a nutritious and filling meal for a whole family."

One of Spain's most established nutritionists, the late Francisco Grande Covián, said "red meat is not essential, even though Western culture has made it an important feature of [its] diet."

When your diet is vegetable-centric, a little meat can be a healthy choice. In Spain, meat from a ranch where animals are allowed to roam, is called *cría ecológica*, and this is exactly the type of meat linked to promoting health.

Current research shows that saturated fat of any kind, meat or otherwise, may not be as unhealthy as we have been led to believe. As reported in the *New York Times* in 2014, Dr. Ronald Krauss, chairman of the American Heart Association, said that evidence connecting saturated fat to heart disease is lacking.

Eaten in Small Amounts, Red Meat Can Be a Healthy Choice Red meat contains cancer-fighting antioxidants including glutathione and superoxide dismutase. Red meat from grass-fed cattle is also a source of essential amino acids, vitamins A, B6, B12, D, and E, and omega-3 fat.

Proving this, despite the fact that the Spanish eat plenty of eggs and naturally cured pork, they live long lives, with low rates of cancer and heart disease. Incidentally, Japanese women, who have the longest life span and lowest rate of breast cancer, regularly eat Kobe beef, which is loaded with saturated fat.

Providing insight, Sarah Charles reports that "U.S. beef contains relatively high levels of estrogen compared to beef produced in other developed nations." And "the sources of estrogen in beef include soy-based feed and the use of growth promoters such as zeranol that are routinely administered to U.S. cattle."

I believe part of the reason Spanish—and Japanese—women live long lives is because they consume meat free of additives. But I also think it imperative that meat be consumed as part of a meal composed mostly of plant foods.

Let us consider the *Ibérico* pig, a direct descendant of the black-hoofed wild boar. Ham from Ibérico comes in different grades depending upon what the animal eats and how long the meat is cured. The ages-old Iberian process involves salt and air. And yes, the salt used in Spain for curing meat is natural.

The finest grade is *jamón ibérico de bellota*, from pigs eating a diet exclusively of acorns for all or part of their lives. A 2013 study shows ham from Iberian bellota hogs offers a high level of antioxidants. Meat from these animals is marbleized with fat rich with oleic acid similar to the fat in extra-virgin olive oil.

Lesser grades include *jamón ibérico de recebo*, from hogs fed a mixture of grain and acorns, and *jamón ibérico de cebo*, fed only grain.

Interestingly, 90 percent of all the hams produced in Spain come not from Ibérico but from Serrano, made from a more common breed of grain-fed white pigs, widely available in the states and much less expensive. Serrano ham, a delicious alternative to ibérico, on a toasted slice of country-style bread rubbed with tomato, fresh garlic and drizzled with olive oil, makes a quick breakfast for busy Catalans.

However, ibérico de bellota offers benefits.

According to the European Union, dried cured ham is a natural source of zinc, phosphorus, selenium, thiamine, riboflavin, niacin, and vitamins B6 and B12. B6 is more absorbable in cured ham than it is from plant foods because it is derived largely from tryptophan, an amino acid.

Though ham is produced in Italy and the south of France—two other

Mediterranean regions—Spain's ibérico is more revered for reasons having to do with flavor as well as health. It's not just the oleic acid, either. Vitamin B12 can only be found in meat, and jamón ibérico is the richest source. B12 as well as B6 and folates reduce homocysteine levels in

In 2015 the American Heart Association reported that Spanish women have one of the lowest death rates from cardiovascular disease of any in the world, surpassing even the women of Japan.

the body, significant in cardiovascular health. This is still another reason to celebrate the Spain's version of the Mediterranean diet.

Spain's specific artisanal methods for curing meat and fish have been honed for thousands of years. Prehistoric people used salt and air curing long before refrigeration.

Cerdo Ibérico de Bellota Steak

See Resource Guide to discover Spanish suppliers for this meat. Place 1½ pounds of *ibérico* pork steak in a shallow bowl. Grate 1 small clove of garlic over the meat, add a little EVOO and a couple of pinches of dried rosemary or half a fresh sprig. When in season, you can squeeze juice from ½ blood orange and add to the meat, garlic, EVOO, and herbs. Let meat marinate in this mixture, covered with a bamboo mat or plastic wrap before cooking, for no longer than 5 minutes. Do not refrigerate—you want the meat at room temperature before cooking. Roast in a 450°F oven or grill on open flame. Be sure not to overcook. Rare to medium is best. Allow meat to rest for ten minutes before slicing. Salt and serve.

Bones and collagen-rich feet from poultry have been cooked with soups and stews in Spain for countless years. Ham bones provide flavor for stock, soups, and beans; lamb bones are used to make sauces and cocidos; and beef shank bones are cooked with sausage and other meats with vegetables for stews.

Collagen Protects Health, and Nourishes Skin, Hair and Nails
As reported by the Weston Price Foundation, nutrients in bone broth produce amino acids glycine and collagen, which help prevent joint disorders and skin diseases, and support gastric acid secretion. Glycine is considered a "conditionally essential" amino acid, which means that it is helpful in producing other amino acids as well as bile salts, hemoglobin, and the nucleotides DNA and RNA. Glycine also helps produce the detoxifier glutathione. And gelatin has been reported to boost bone minerals and restore connective tissue, so it is excellent for those who suffer from arthritis, and helps keep skin, hair, and nails nourished.

Bone broth, a tradition based upon thrift, offers inherent nutritional wisdom. Certainly you have read about the benefits of bone broth. Studies confirm that it boosts immunity, and because of the collagen, the broth is a beauty secret. Use as a base for stews and soups, and watch your skin, nails, and hair thrive.

Incidentally, in ancient China, collagen-rich bone jelly was believed to be so healing it was considered medicine.

Still in the meat section, now we see duck, venison, thrush, quail, and red-legged partridge—all freshly killed. No doubt some of the wild game is farm raised, due to loss of habitat.

In the restaurant *Las Duelas* in Haro, La Rioja, chef Juan Nales prepares venison with steamed organic vegetables, quince, nuts, and berries. The meat, simply flavored with olive oil, salt, and pepper, is seared and served with fruit, nuts, and berries, surrounded with organic vegetables.

Regarding wild game, make no mistake, the fatty-acid profile of meat from animals that live in the wild is much higher in protective fats and lower in saturated fat over any other.

Oxtails.

Look at these big fat ones.

The people of Spain eat oxtails often. During winter, I braise *rabo de buey* in red wine for a couple of hours. The oxtail meat and softer collagen-rich bone tissue melds, becoming tender and rich with flavor.

Now a spectacle of liver and kidneys.

And more organ meats. Shocking.

Ears, brains, tongues, hooves!

Look. Something spongy.

Don't let them see you roll your eyes.

Even bull cojones are cooked here but, thankfully, I don't see them. Called *criadillas de toro* or from *toro de lidia*—from fighting bulls.

Which do *you* prefer?

Okay, perhaps not something your grandmother used to make.

But maybe she liked to cook gizzards?

My grandmother Nanny could make a fine meal in haste or cook for three days and make a feast. She knew that turkey giblets, along with alliums, bay laurel, and broth, made excellent gravy.

Catalans prepare wild game giblets with wine to make demi-glace. They also combine giblets with nuts, herbs, and garlic for picada. *Alta cocina* chefs sometimes use these bits mixed with sherry, caramelized onions, and such, as a pasta filling to accompany the roasted bird it came from.

The Long-Living Andorrans Break Nutritional Clichés The World Health Organization has identified the people of Andorra (the tiny snowcapped Pyrenean mountain principality we referred to throughout this book) as having the longest life expectancy in the world. They regularly eat bacon, sausages, and salamis—a diet that an Andorran chef referred to as a "mountain version of the Mediterranean diet." It is interesting that their diet is similar to the diet of the long-living people in Sardinia.

Spanish people derive nutritional benefits from tripe, a good source of anticancer selenium and immune enhancing zinc.

As a finale, the whitish, spongy substance we are standing before begs our examination.

Let's look.

This is beef tripe, the lining of the stomach of the cow, and the Spanish love it. Tripe happens to be very nutritious, so don't be put off.

Leaving carnivore central, I explain there is no one path to health. People can be healthy and eat meat, others unhealthy and not eat meat.

It is approaching time to make dinner, so now nearly everyone holds bags with long loaves of bread. It's challenging to walk and talk while dodging loaves, but we do.

And yes. Bread is a central food here, and it is delicious.

Hen's Eggs Offer Protective Nutrients Eggs contain carotenoids, choline, vitamins D and K, as well as phospholipids, which are extremely valuable fats located within the yolk. Eggs are also rich in shielding beta-carotene and vitamin D3, which have been found to influence cancer-related genes, as reported in the *Journal of Steroid Biochemistry and Molecular Biology.*

Nutritional Gold: A Raw Yolk in Your Breakfast Smoothie Scientists from the University of Alberta point out that two eggs in a raw state contain almost twice the antioxidant properties as an apple and that they shield against cancer as well as heart disease.

The implacable Spanish duo, eggs and potatoes, was first noted in the 1817 *Cortes de Navarra*, in a reference to *tortilla de patatas* where it is described as "the perfect dish for combating the hard conditions of the times."

Now we find ourselves standing in front of a tiny stall that looks like a country barnyard tricked out with every type of egg imaginable, all arranged fetchingly on real hay.

¡Dios! This is actually happening.

It seems as though every bird imaginable has partied here, including ostriches.

All the table space has been taken up with stacks of eggs in every size.

Looking above our heads, we admire gaily painted cut-outs, depicting cavorting hens and ducks. Now we see the vendor, but she is anything but cavorting.

The savvy Catalan has quickly assessed we have no bags, so she knows there will be no sale.

Without the slightest nod, the peckish-looking woman goes back to conversing with bona fide poachers, scramblers, boilers, and bakers. Though we won't be involved in those activities anytime soon, we stand as still as mice in a henhouse, taking in what can only be described as egg heaven.

Research shows that when hens are fed an organic diet, their eggs contain one-third less cholesterol and one-fourth less saturated fat. Organic eggs also offer two-thirds more vitamin A, twice the amount of essential fatty acids, three times more vitamin E, and seven times more beta-carotene.

Yolks are especially beneficial because they are rich in antioxidants and as mentioned, folate, which lowers the risk of heart disease. And yolks contain vitamin B12, which works together with folate to protect the heart. They also contain sulfur, helping to rid the body of toxins.

Which brings to mind Sra. Ana Vela Rubio, a Barcelonan, who at the time of her death in 2017 at the age of 116 was the oldest person in Europe. Ana attributed her longevity to eating two raw egg yolks every day.

Spanish chefs sauce mushrooms with yolks and stir them into all sorts of soups and sauces, including homemade mayonnaise and allioli. A poached or fried egg—always with a runny yolk—tops countless dishes.

Sometimes duck eggs are used.

Alta cocina chefs find new ways to cook eggs. Perhaps it is because eggs have always been a culinary touchstone of Spain, and gastronomy is about reinvention?

Besides, chefs love a challenge here.

Homage to the egg is paid at Girona's La Penyora, where the chef makes autumn pumpkin soup topped with a tower of meringue.

A lofty iceberg afloat on a pumpkin sea.

Somehow at Barcelona's Ca l'Isidre, desert chef Nuri Isidre makes warm chocolate egg custard in the shell itself. Presented in a perfectly cracked egg—halves seem like miniature porcelain bowls, broken by a boozy elf in her kitchen. Warm yolk joins melting chocolate as though destiny.

And now, as we leave the tiny booth, the vendor is still conversing with customers. The ladies seem to be in a discussion regarding the best diet for doves, so

Applause for Spain's National Dish: *Tortillas* Over time, nutrition research has increased our appreciation for the Mediterranean diet, including why Spain's egg-rich version may indeed be the most protective. Hugely popular in Spain, eggs are nutritional power-houses, but Ancel Keys apparently did not know that organic eggs can elevate the protective HDL cholesterol and lower the LDL cholesterol, or that the yolks are especially beneficial since they are rich in folate, which protects the heart. In *Eat Well, Stay Well* (1959) Key's twenty-eight-day menu plan only permitted two mornings when he allowed eggs for breakfast—and only one each day. He couldn't have known that eggs are heart-protective, with free-range eggs offering a highly absorbable form of lutein and zeaxanthin, both carotenoids that shield against free radicals and protect our eyes. He did not know that eggs help support brain function since they are a rich source of choline, and contain sphingolipids, a compound that has been shown to inhibit the formation of colon cancer.

we leave without interrupting.

Making our way back toward the entrance, I realize that I am on market overload.

It seems ironic to have spent so much time admiring food while forgetting our dinner, so we head out of the market on to the plaza.

Looking down, pigeons tutting at my feet seem dejected, as though they have gobbled every last crumb and every last nut.

But we have nothing to feed the greedy birds.

They flee as we turn and go our separate ways.

Spanish Egg Farmers Embrace Rigorous Self-Imposed Standards
In Spain, egg farms are cleaned every day and the farmers avoid toxic products. Regarding foods from Spain that include eggs, such as pastries, frozen tortillas, etc., you can be confident that you are receiving an excellent product. The article "How Spanish Eggs Have Avoided European Pesticide Crisis" in *El País*, August 2017, by Hugo Gutiérrez, reports that although seventeen European countries distributed eggs tainted with fipronil, and millions recalled, no tainted eggs were from Spain.

Now, heading toward my hotel, I continue down the darkening street. In the coolness of early evening, with blinking neon as background, I pass a chef scurrying to work and someone alone, perhaps trying to mend a broken heart.

Suddenly an emaciated cat slinks from a bed of yuccas.

His coat: knife-thin, deep auburn stripes slice into grimy, charcoal gray. The subterranean gray seems the closest color to black, without being black, that I have ever seen, and the knife-blade pattern is arcane, as though the cat has sprung from centuries of cats that spent their lives in the bowels of Barcelona.

A splash of moving soot with a truncated tail, the cat rudely swerves ahead of me, but does so with grace. I watch the animal raise what is left of his stubby tail with dignity as he sallies down the street.

Moving swiftly through the night, the animal is a poem.

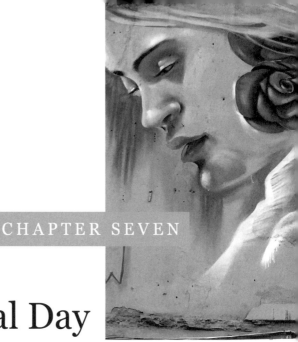

CHAPTER SEVEN

Our Third and Final Day

"Nothing is invented, for it's written in nature first."
– Antoni Gaudí

What a strange night.
I had a dream so vivid and mysterious, that when I awoke I was almost confused as to what century I was in.

Rushing to dress, and then a short time later, we meet at the entrance of *la* Boqueria and make our way in.

As we enter, I recount my dream.

Antoni Gaudí cooked for me.

The same genius responsible for the creation of *Sagrada Familia*, and other Modernism masterpieces that define this magnificent city, cooked … for me.

First, Gaudí and I met in a museum. Each with our own sketch books, we talked. Then we strolled through Barcelona drawing palm leaves and when we could, insects and birds. I struggled over a drawing of a dragonfly. The wings seemed impossible. It wasn't until Antoni explained that they were concave instead of flat, that my dragonfly sprang to life.

To celebrate the success of my drawing, we went back to Antoni's flat to cook. He told me he was a vegetarian and knew some very fine recipes.

A follower of the Kneipp health movement that was spreading through Europe, Antoni lived and ate simply. Sometimes just leaves of lettuce dipped into a bowl of milk was his lunch, "eaten at my desk while I worked," he confessed.

But I assure you, that night he prepared something far more interesting.

Antoni decided upon wild mushrooms. As he shook the cazuela, aromas sprang from a culinary well so deep that the associations had no time or place.

Were the aromas of cooking medieval? Perhaps. Maybe even earlier, going back to the time when cave dwellers roasted mushrooms over fire.

Antoni was an artist, so he knew to honor the natural taste of food. I watched while he cooked with olive oil, garlic, salt, only shaking the cazuela instead of stirring.

After the mushrooms were ready, Antoni held the pan out for me to admire. I could not help but notice his eyes, which were the truest blue I had ever seen. His mood was somber.

Then Antoni extinguished the candles and drew the curtains closed, making the room pitch-black.

What next?

Sitting there in the dark, trying not to spill anything on the bodice of my taffeta gown—I told you this was the nineteenth century—I reached back to rearrange my bustle.

Then navigating the fork to my mouth, I tasted. Forest. Earth. I lost myself in the tastes that humankind has guarded and searched for, for thousands of years.

And though he did not partake, Antoni served *Codorníu*, a sparkling dry white wine that was the newest thing.

We ate and talked throughout the night with abandon.

Antoni confided childhood health problems, which included a kind of arthritis. Herbs, homeopathy and a vegetarian diet helped him. Antoni was committed to using nature as medicine ever since.

And he spoke of a woman who broke his heart.

Endure, abstain. Antoni's maxim.

Towards morning, my host opened the curtains with a flourish, as though we were about to watch a play. Since his garret was on the highest floor—all those steps—Antoni paid little in rent but he did not mind.

Day broke. It was then I realized why he loved his garret. The view was breathtaking. Elaborate black spires and turrets of Victorian rooftops looked surreal against the morning sky, which was splashed with the colors of gladioli.

It was hard to wake up.

We find ourselves standing before a booth with cutouts of gaily painted wooden silhouettes. The images are engaging.

Taking in cartoon cows, sheep, and wedges of smiling cheese, we notice the engaging proprietor. He looks like Javier Cámara, a film star who happens to be bald and a bit chubby, but possesses a certain droll charm that some men have who just know they are funny.

Maybe you saw Cámara in the classic *Torremolinos 73*?

The little group surrounding him is hanging on every word. The Cámara look-alike glances our way to see if we notice.

But our fascination is the booth, with its smells of fermentation—sultry ripeness with undertones of mold and herbs. There is the odor of leather, too, and some kind of smoky duskiness mixed with an odor of mountain grass.

Looking about, I see *Cadí* butter, revered by chefs throughout Europe. Its richness and creamy taste are without peer. The Cadí cooperative is located in northern Catalunya where they also make cheese.

The Cadí cooperative, established in the Catalan Pyrenees in 1915, produces butter, *Serrat Tupí* and *Mató*, the oldest documented Catalan cheeses, going back to the tenth century—originally made by shepherds and farmers for their own consumption.

Cheese, butter, milk, and yogurt, especially from goats, benefit health when the products are from animals that are free from growth hormones and feed on grass. We will talk about the nutritional benefits

Healthy Gut Bacteria May Thwart DNA Programmed for Disease
Food scientists have found that gut microbes are a direct link to our genetics, meaning that foods rich in bacteria, such as milk from goats, might thwart DNA programmed for disease. To find out more, see the YouTube presentation by Professor Simon Harding.

of these foods in a moment.

But first, I must tell you about Eulàlia Torras, a privileged lady who lived in an upscale Barcelona neighborhood filled with architectural masterpieces and designer stores. Tired of the pampered life, Eulàlia moved to the Pyrenees in 1976 to milk goats and make cheese.

And, yes, she traded couture for milking buckets.

Eulàlia, a hardworking and entrepreneurial woman, somehow turned a small herd of goats into Cal Codina, a highly respected cheese-maker that ultimately developed Catalunya's prized *Serrat Gros*.

According to a 2011 study conducted at the Universidad de Granada, milk from goats has 13 percent more calcium than cow's milk and improves bone formation, helping prevent osteoporosis.

Milk from goats also protects DNA and supports the development of gut probiotic flora, strengthening our immunity. And finally, goat's milk helps prevent heart disease by lowering harmful LDL cholesterol.

Cheese has been eaten in Spain for a long time. Aragón, Navarre, Cantabria, Asturias, and Galicia produce an impressive array of cheeses made from goats, sheep, and cows as well as mixed-milk cheeses such as *Valdeón* and *Gamonedo*. In most cases, when the seasons permit, animals roam freely and feed on grass. There is archaeological evidence that La Mancha's Manchego cheese was made as far back as the Bronze Age, from a breed of sheep known as Manchega.

Saturated fat in cheese, particularly from animals that are grass as opposed to grain fed, is higher in nutrients and better able to fight inflammation because of a better balance of omega-6 to omega-3 fats. Cheese from grass-fed animals is an excellent source of another protective fat, conjugated linoleic acid or CLA, which enhances immunity and boosts metabolic function, meaning this fat also helps us lose weight.

More in a moment.

When milk for cheese is produced from animals during summer, it is higher in antioxidants and fatty acids. Grass provides nutritious substances as opposed to hay, which the animals eat during winter.

If you are worried that cheese will make you fat, relax.

Even Walter Willet from the Harvard School of Public Health agrees. In an interview with Newscience.com, Dr. Willet said that consuming one to two servings of full-fat dairy a day means we are less—not more—likely to pile on the pounds.

Unfortunately, pasteurization laws in the United States prevent the import of many types of Spanish cheese. This is because U.S. law requires that cheese from cows, sheep, and goats must be aged a minimum of sixty days to avoid pasteurization before entering the country. But despite this, there are many kinds of Spanish cheese that we can buy in the USA.

No food is more connected to the earth than artisanal cheese.

Let's get to it.

Here is *Mató*, also called *Recuit*. Mató is similar to cottage cheese in texture and served fresh with honey for dessert, as it has been since the tenth century when it was noted in the texts of monks and nuns, who loved to eat.

Don't miss Eulàlia's award-winning raw goat's milk *Serrat Gros*.

Do you see that this Galician *Tetilla* is shaped like a small breast? Tetilla is a buttery cheese that one finds back home. The flavor is similar to Monterey Jack, but with more character.

Notice this *Gaztazarra, queso viejo*, (*queso viejo*an aged Basque sheep's milk cheese that has been fermented. And there: *Garrotxa*, an aged Catalan goat's milk cheese that has a sweet nutty taste, also available in the states.

Vall d'Aran, another cheese produced in Catalunya, is a creamy, smoky cow's milk cheese. Look, here is *Taramundi*, a

According to a 2013 article in the *British Medical Journal*, "Recent studies have not supported significant association between saturated fat intake and risk of cardiovascular disease. Instead saturated fat has been found to be protective."

On the next to last weekend in October, if you find yourself in Seu d'Urgell in the Pyrenees, you will see more than 100 different kinds of cheese to sample, made just in the vicinity of this little village.

Dulce de Membrillo Quince, common to the Mediterranean, is a fruit that is extremely high in fiber and contains cancer-bashing antioxidant tannins. Dulce de Membrillo made from slow-cooked quince and a touch of cane sugar is an ideal way to benefit from this healthy food. A sliver on a slice of Manchego, in salads, or layered with greens on a sandwich with chicken, cheese or a little jamón, is so tasty that including membrillo in small amounts helps us maintain a healthy pattern of eating by adding interest to our meals. Spain's Mediterranean diet existed for centuries and this healthy pleasure was always enjoyed in small amounts here.

blend of cow and goat's milk cheese that can be melted, and also available from Spanish importers.

Many of Spain's finest cheeses are made in Asturias. Her blue *Cabrales* is ripened in caves. A mixture of cow, goat, and sheep's milk, Cabrales is smoother and less sharp than French Roquefort, and I think you will like it more.

Look—*Roncal* from Navarre, a sheep's milk cheese that can also be found in America. The taste is sharp, piquant, and pleasing. Let's take a closer look at this *Idiazábal*, or Basque shepherd's cheese, for it too is available back home. Idiazábal is aged sixty days and has the full taste of ripened sheep's milk with a distinct yet gentle smokiness.

Now the Cámara lookalike strolls over, offering us a sample of the Idiazábal he saw us discussing.

He looms so close I smell his aftershave. Something woodsy—vetiver? The taste has a jolt of buttery smokiness.

"Yes, it is excellent," I tell him, stepping back a hair.

Clearly he wants to talk, but we take our leave, eager to see more of the market.

Besides, I'm thirsty. So we backtrack to find the booth offering fresh juice we saw yesterday.

On the way I spot *membrillo*, a staple of the Spanish Mediterranean pantry. Membrillo is a tart, slightly sweet, fragrant fruit paste, usually made from quince, a fruit so old that it predates the apple. The tradition of fruit paste dates back centuries. Membrillo is also made from pears and plums. Upon opening the container, the jellied fruit gleams like dulled stained glass of a medieval church. The delicate perfume of membrillo invokes a grove of heritage fruit trees after a summer rain.

When membrillo is matched with Spanish cheese and olives, you have big as the world Spanish Mediterranean flavors to share with friends. Membrillo is delicious in salads, thinly sliced on sandwiches of cheese, ham or meat, and it can be diced in small pieces to glaze roasted poultry or pork. And sometimes I mix membrillo with French mustard, to glaze roasting meat.

Right now, I'm craving watermelon juice, so I hope the fruit stand we are approaching doesn't disappoint.

Oranges and clementines are an important part of Spanish cooking and eating. When in season, a vanguard chef might feature clementines in every course of the meal, from appetizer to desert.

We see many types of fruit so numerous it will be a challenge to discuss them all. What's more, the stall is packed, so to the end of the line we go—the custom here at *la* Boqueria.

I see watermelon but no juice. So I choose papaya instead. Knowing that it is rich in vitamin C is comforting. I taste. There is mango mixed in the juice, an added benefit. According to research at Texas A&M University, extract of mango kills breast cancer cells without harming healthy ones.

The stall offers plenty of freshly squeezed grapefruit juice. As with all citrus fruits, grapefruit contains compounds called monoterpenes, which help eliminate cancers before they form. Also present are beta-carotene and folic acid, and in pink grapefruit, lycopene.

The two young women standing beside us are enjoying a drink so fragrant it startles. Of course. Valencia orange juice. The smell is potent. It's as if we are in a grove of trees.

One of my favorite ways to eat oranges is segmented in salads with lettuce and olives, and tangy vinagreta. Another Spanish salad of orange segments, tomatoes, and manzanilla olives, topped with a touch of honey and extra-virgin olive oil is also filled with distinctive taste.

Oranges are rich in pectin, which blocks the absorption of cholesterol as well as a protein called galectin-3, a substance that scars the heart and is linked to congestive heart failure, a condition almost impossible to treat with drugs.

The Moors introduced oranges to Spain hundreds of years ago and today, as with olive oil, Spain leads in world production. Organic oranges play a greater role every year.

Orange Salad with Spanish Cheese, Olives, and Sweet Onion

Combine Valencia orange sections with gem lettuce, thin slices of fresh, sweet onion, olives, and Manchego, Idiazábal, or *Petit Basque* cheese, all seasoned with olive oil and white vinegar.

———◆———

It's not only Valencian oranges that are prized. Clementines are too, and the best are believed to be from the Catalan *Terres de l'Ebre* region.

On the counter in little cups, glistening blood-red pomegranate seeds beckon. They are used in Spanish Mediterranean cooking in unique ways. Try pom seeds with roasted cauliflower and tossed into cooked rice or quinoa, with toasted almond slivers. A rainbow fresh surprise.

Moving through the stall, suddenly strawberries emit fragrant perfume. The aroma and plump lushness is a reminder we should eat all kinds of berries often. The American Institute for Cancer Research reports that strawberries, raspberries, blueberries, and cranberries can help fight cancer due to the antioxidant pterostilbene.

Berries also offer protection from cognitive decline and help prevent glaucoma, with black currants preventing the spread of glaucoma better than any other drug on the market as claimed by a study from Japan.

Try black currant coulis with grilled venison.

Make Poms Your Game Changer A 2010 study in the *International Journal of Oncology* reported that a compound in pomegranate supported apoptosis, or programmed cancer cell death. Another study reported in *Breast Cancer Research and Treatment* found that pomegranate seed oil showed a 90 percent inhibition of MCF-7 breast cancer cells. According to Dr. Michael Aviram from Technion Institute in Haifa, Israel, just eight ounces of pomegranate juice a day can help dissolve plaque buildup (caused by oxidized LDL cholesterol) from arterial walls and, in some cases, actually reverse it.

Black Currant Coulis to Sauce with Grilled Meat

In a medium saucepan, sauté a few minced shallots in EVOO. Salt lightly and add a grind or two of white pepper. When caramelized, add ½ cup of chicken stock and ½ cup red wine. Bring to a boil, simmer for 5 minutes, then add several pinches of dried thyme and a bay leaf. Cook for 5 minutes more. Next, add 3 cups of rinsed, destemmed black currants, 2 tablespoons honey, and ½ cup black currant vinegar. Crush in the berries with a wooden paddle. Salt lightly and cook on medium for 10 minutes. At the last moment, remove the bay leaf and add 1 teaspoon of butter and a grind more of pepper. The sauce can be strained or served rustic style.

Black Currants: Heavy Nutrition Hitters Black currants, which resemble tiny grapes, are antioxidant powerhouses extremely high in vitamin C, as well as a source of B vitamins, calcium and zinc. They also contain anticancer anthocyanin. A 2015 study shows that extract of black currant can help protect against breast and endometrial cancers by binding to the receptor site of estrogens. In other studies, they have been found to be good for vision and to help reduce discomfort from arthritis by their inherent anti-inflammatory properties. Herbalists have used black currants since medieval times, especially to heal the liver.

Blackberries, or *moras*, are a food that everyone should eat often. They are rich in antioxidants, protecting the heart. Also abundant in ellagic acid, a compound that is antiestrogenic, moras help ward off estrogen sensitive cancers.

The many types of grapes we now encounter takes up more floor space than any display we have seen in two days. They all reflect a distinctive Mediterranean luster.

Dios mío. The Spanish eat a lot of grapes!

I want you to know about three in particular. Those dark-skinned ones contain resveratrol, an antioxidant (also present in red wine and dark chocolate) that inhibits enzymes that initiate cancer cell growth, increases immune response, and protects the heart. They are a good source of potassium and vitamins K, C, and B1. The pale whites are Moscatel, and don't miss the *Uvas pasas* from Málaga, for they are dried to make raisins so first-class, they are famous throughout the culinary world.

At our feet, we admire bushel baskets spilling with apples, pears, and peaches. Apples are a source of calcium d-glucarate, the compound that researchers have found in animal studies to help prevent mammary cancer. This is because CDG is a detoxifier of harmful xenoestrogens.

Spanish people have many varieties to choose from, but according to a recent article in *Foods and Wines of Spain*, those from the North are superior, especially Basque *reinetas*. Another venerated Basque apple is the *errezila*.

This discussion of apples reminds me of a story.

The Basque restaurant Rekondo, in Donostia/San Sebastián, is known for its famous wine cellar, and the retired owner, Txomin Rekondo, who still visits the restaurant every day is a bullfight aficionado. Photographs of famous matadors in life-threatening action adorn the walls of his beloved restaurant, now run by his daughter Edurne. One brutally handsome matador sports a shocking scar that slashes the entire length of his proud face.

Rekondo's young chef makes an apple tart from reinetas, so thin and flaky it could be a giant airy cookie. In true Basque fashion, the tart is starkly simple, with dreamt-of taste. I told Edurne "Bullfighters must love the food at your restaurant." With a tilt of her head, Edurne's dry reply: "Bullfighters love their women more than their food."

Edurne's tart reminds me that apples are prepared in many delectable ways in the North, including as a beverage in Asturias and the Basque country. Catalans love to roast apples with goose, duck, or pork; and sometimes substituting pears, which are high in anticancer flavonols.

The ones here are *Puigcerdà*, grown just north of Barcelona.

Apples Stuffed with Ground Pork

Popular in Catalunya, cored apples are stuffed with ground pork, seasoned breadcrumbs, chopped apple, pine nuts, sautéed onions, garlic, and thyme, and all combined with beaten eggs. The mixture, after seasoning with salt and pepper, is stuffed into scooped-out apples and placed on a baking dish coated with EVOO. White wine is spooned around the apples. They are then covered with foil and baked in a 350°F oven for about an hour, depending on how large the apples are. The foil is removed for the final 10 minutes of cooking. The roasting pan can be deglazed with chicken stock to combine with the bits at the bottom to make a sauce.

Roasted Sausage with Pears

Any type of artisan sausage can be used. Place sausages in a baking dish coated with EVOO and cut pears into medium-sized chunks. Arrange pears on top of sausages, and tuck in cloves of peeled garlic. Lightly spoon a splash of chicken stock into the baking dish, cover in foil and roast in a 325°F oven for an hour. Remove the foil and continue cooking for 15 more minutes. Pear chunks should caramelize to a delicate golden.

———•———

What's interesting about the peaches here are the ones we don't see. Blush-toned *rouge de roussillons* are so delicate they must be eaten within hours of picking.

Cocina Rápida

Peaches Poached in Rosado Wine Topped with Frozen Yogurt

Wash and slice ripe summer peaches and put in a saucepan. Cover with a little rosado wine, add a very small stick of cinnamon, and bring to a gentle boil. Cook for 5 minutes and serve with plain frozen yogurt.

Figs, an Excellent Food for Health

Figs are rich in potassium, which guards against high blood pressure, and they contain a good amount of calcium. The insoluble fiber and antioxidant phenols in figs help guard against breast and colon cancers. Figs contain fifty times more phenols than any other fruit.

Figs. So many varieties before us—lime green, purple, and almost black, just to name a few, confirming the strong presence figs have in Spain's Mediterranean diet.

Dried, roasted, or fresh, the Spanish eat figs often. Cheese and olives, and savory dishes such as roasted pork are complemented by figs. Ripe figs are peeled and sliced, to serve with serrano ham for tapas. Then there is the recipe that I told you about earlier, oliago gazpacho, which is also served with ripe figs.

Cocina Rápida

Slow-Roasted Figs

Deep purple figs, oven roasted for dessert. Rinse and slice figs, dust lightly with sugar, spoon a little anisette liquor on the top, and roast uncovered in a 275°F oven for about 40 minutes.

Now I spot kiwis, pineapples and bananas.

Kiwifruit actually contains even more vitamin C than oranges, and is known to protect DNA against oxygen-related damage.

Pineapples, another vitamin C-rich fruit, contains bromelain, an enzymatic compound that supports digestion.

These bananas remind me of a distinctive Catalan salad. *Ensalada Islas Canarias* is composed of sliced bananas with coconut flakes, orange segments, and slices of red pepper with olive oil and sherry vinegar. Simple, bold and natural.

More culinary dreams. This extensive, gorgeous display of dried fruit near the register dazzles. It reminds that dried black currants, raisins, figs, as well as cherries, apricots, prunes, and pears all play an important role in Spain's gastronomy. As you see, dried figs are well represented in this display. Fresh or dried, figs contains nutrients that benefit lung and heart function, as well as bone strength and immunity.

Bananas Lower Blood Pressure and Protect the Heart Bananas are rich in vitamin B6 and potassium, which benefit the cardiovascular system. Just one contains over 400mg of potassium. Many studies also show that potassium-rich foods help lower blood pressure.

Let's talk raisins and currants.

In terms of cognitive health, recent studies have shown raisins and currants contain antioxidant properties and aid the memory, a finding that may help delay the onset and severity of Alzheimer's disease.

As for prunes, Catalunya is one of the biggest producers in Spain, and chefs here revere them. Prunes are cooked in dishes that include duck, chicken, capon, and pork.

Consider the following recipe inspired by Ferran Adrià.

Easy Rotisserie Roasted Chicken with Dried Fruit Sauce

Cut a cooked rotisserie chicken into 8 pieces, set drippings aside. Heat a sauté pan with 1-2 tablespoons of EVOO. When oil is heated, add 1 large minced leek and several minced shallots. Sauté until light golden. Next add ½ cup of the following dried fruits: cut-up pitted prunes and apricots, and black currants. Cook fruit on moderate heat until slightly brown and then add ½ cup white wine, a small stick of cinnamon, and freshly ground nutmeg. Add the drippings and bring to a low boil. Cook for a few minutes then set aside. Toast 2 tablespoons of pine nuts until golden. Arrange the chicken on a platter and spoon on the fruit sauce. Garnish with toasted nuts and serve.

Walking slowly past a booth displaying chocolate, I am reminded that Barcelona makes my favorite chocolate in Europe. Chefs who cook in the new style create standout desserts and some ancestral dishes incorporating chocolate, which contributes a unique but understated dimension to poultry or game. Penelope Casas, in her classic *Food and Wines of Spain*, said, "The flavor of a sauce with chocolate in it will be subtle and difficult to place."

Chicken in Chocolate Sauce

Inspired by Penelope Casas's Partridge in Chocolate Sauce, in her book, *¡Delicioso!*, my recipe substitutes chicken. Begin by sautéing a cleaned, dried, cut-up chicken with a generous handful of chopped onions, a minced shallot, and three cloves of minced garlic in a glug of olive oil. Season with salt and pepper. Be sure the bird is browned and onions wilted. Then add 1 tablespoon of flour, ½ cup dry white wine, ½ cup of chicken stock, 2 tablespoons of vinegar, 2 bay leaves, and 2 cloves. Cover and simmer for 45 minutes. Remove chicken from pan and set aside. Add a teaspoon of grated bitter chocolate to the sauce. Dissolve the chocolate into the sauce by stirring with a whisk. Return the chicken to the casserole and cover. Continue cooking for 10 minutes more.

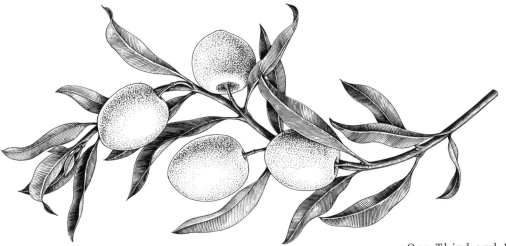

Now a spice booth begs attention.

The environment is like stepping into an 1890s painting by the Catalan Santiago Rusiñol, executed in his elegant, aloof style. The booth seems an old shop of curiosities begging exploration. Diffused light and shade dance over everything.

The long worn iron table, topped with a slab of beat-up old marble at the center of the booth, holds mysterious-looking items. We admire oversized vintage apothecary jars filled with tea, and what appears to be dried flowers. There are smaller glass jars, too.

Traversing the table, I smell something tangy.

Of course—see the jars with honey? Others are filled with marmalade. All have labels that beg examination.

Tins of pimentón also beckon. With vintage labels, they seem old-world treasures.

The booth is arranged near an outside wall of the market. Light from the unwashed window softly illuminates all the table holds.

Farther along the table, the fragrance changes to that of smoky paprika, tea leaves, and lavender honey.

Glancing beneath the table, we see bins made from wooden drums. Inside, boxes of teas, tamarind and tiny glass jars filled with saffron. Spoils from a forbidden land.

The vendors are Japanese. The man, who is handing money to a younger man, perhaps his son, does not notice us, but a

> **Health Benefits of Saffron** Studies have determined that saffron can slow and even reverse cancer growth, help prevent cardiovascular disease, improve vision and mood, and may help prevent kidney damage for those with diabetes.

> TIP: **Cooking with Saffron Threads and Powder** Before adding to recipes, cooks sometimes warm saffron threads gently for a few minutes in a preheated oven. Warmed or not, crumble threads lightly and infuse in warm chicken or vegetable broth, or warm water for a few minutes. Then add to your recipe. Or crumble a few threads in your fingers and add toward the end of cooking, which is what I often do when steaming vegetables and preparing whole grains such as brown rice. Powdered saffron can be put directly into recipes.

woman—maybe his wife—looks our way. Though her body is slender she seems strong.

Watching her unpack a carton of tea, we say *¡Hola!* She brushes her hair from her face and answers, but her voice is so soft I barely hear.

Her eyes reveal nothing.

Once again, we are left on our own.

Though all the items on the table summon, the reddish saffron threads grab me first.

Saffron, endemic to Spanish Mediterranean cooking, harmonizes recipes with its aristocratic taste and is a benefit to health in numerous ways. Saffron helps prevent cancer, improves mood, and protects vision. Consumption of saffron also supports those who suffer from diabetes, since it protects the kidneys.

And this saffron has a strong red color, meaning it is rich in carotenoids.

Saffron is used to flavor *suquet*, an iconic Catalan stew prepared along the Costa Brava made with all sorts of seafood, including sea urchin. Suquet was Truman Capote's favorite during the years he wrote *In Cold Blood* in Palamós, a northern Mediterranean fishing town renowned for excellent seafood.

The rhizomes (roots) in the baskets below are turmeric, which is also available in powder form, so there is every reason to cook often with this anticancer superstar. In addition, turmeric reduces inflammation. On the culinary front, this spice is basic to curry powder, and enlivens chicken or fish, and transforms sautéed vegetables with character. Fresh turmeric rhizome can be peeled easily with the tip of a spoon.

> Turmeric inhibits the production of the inflammatory-related enzyme COX-2, of which levels are high in certain inflammatory cancers. It is believed to impede cancer-causing substances called nitrosamines.

Research shows black pepper enhances the benefits of turmeric. Black pepper, which contains its own inherent anticancer compound piperine, has been shown in many studies to prevent cancer cells in vitro.

Cumin, a standout spice in the Spanish pantry, has been shown in research to support the liver's production of detoxification enzymes, crucial in eliminating harmful estrogenic hormones. Studies show that cumin can protect the stomach and liver from developing tumors. Studies have been so promising surrounding cumin that researchers think this spice may be even more protective than we know it to be today.

Cumin appears in many Spanish recipes, from fried cod with honey to gazpacho to *mojo picón*, a sauce that originated in the Canary Islands, made from EVOO, vinegar, garlic, chili pepper, and paprika. It is spooned over little red potatoes, vegetables, chicken, or fish, and makes an excellent dipping sauce for little skewers of grilled meats, as when serving tapas.

Mojo Picón Sauce

Makes about one 1¼ cups

INGREDIENTS: 2 teaspoons of ground cumin, 6 cloves of garlic, 2 pinches of dried oregano, 1½ teaspoons sweet pimentón, ⅓ teaspoon salt, 2 dried ancho peppers reconstituted in hot water, 1 small dried chili pepper (remove seeds), ¾ cup EVOO, ½ cup sherry vinegar, and ¼ cup water. Using a mortar and pestle, crush garlic with salt, cumin, dried chili pepper, pimentón, and oregano. Slowly mix in half the EVOO. Mince the reconstituted ancho chili and work into the mixture along with the vinegar and water, and the remaining EVOO. Taste and adjust salt. You may want to add a pinch or two of hot red pepper flakes.

———•———

Don't miss the black cumin. It is known to have antiviral properties. *Nigella sativa* is the Latin name. Seeds from black cumin contain the compound thymoquinone, which has been found in studies to have an inhibitory effect on cancer cells.

Admittedly, black cumin seeds are a challenging taste to develop. Perhaps best ground lightly over curried potatoes.

But look—here is something you will like more. *Piment d'Espelette.*

The sweet gentle-hot taste of this French Basque spice cannot be resisted. Though not usually associated with the cooking of Spain, Piment d'Espelette crosses the border into the Basque and Catalan regions of the North.

Several pinches of Piment d'Espelette flavors many dishes with character. Oxtail stew is no exception.

TIP: Black Cumin Seed: If you wish, grind black cumin seeds over food as you grind pepper, or mix crushed seeds into a glass of water, or combine into a health shake.

Oxtail Stew with Piment d'Espelette

Heat a glug of EVOO in a large, heavy pan. Add 4 pounds of oxtails, dredged lightly in flour seasoned with salt and pepper, and begin browning. Add 6 cloves of garlic and 2 large chopped shallots. Turn oxtails as they cook—brown on all sides. Add 1 large chopped onion, 1 large chopped carrot, and 6 more whole shallots. After onions start caramelizing, which takes about 10 minutes, add more EVOO, 4 medium chopped tomatoes, another clove of garlic, 4 sprigs of fresh thyme, 2 bay leaves, and 2 cloves. Cook for about 5 minutes and then pour in 2 cups of Spanish red wine and 1½ cups of water. Cover, and simmer for approximately 2 hours. Remove the lid to finish cooking; perhaps 40 minutes more will be required. The final 5-10 minutes, add 1 teaspoon of Piment d'Espelette. You will know the oxtails have finished cooking when the meat begins to pull away from the bones.

Now here is something iconic. *Pimentón de la Vera.*

My nose prickles in anticipation.

Pimentón is made from ground red capsicum, a kind of pepper that possesses fat-soluble, cancer-protective antioxidants. Try a dusting of this smoky spice on salmon salad, grilled cod or shrimp, and sautéed potatoes and cabbage. Pimentón also works with beans.

Pimentón is delicious by itself to flavor grilled squid, for instance, and other times in combination with spices to add culinary dimension. I particularly enjoy pimentón with thyme, garlic, and olive oil.

Now I see cinnamon, nutmeg, cloves and juniper berries.

Cinnamon, another defining Spanish spice, is used in many desserts. But it is not just about dessert here. Catalans have known since medieval times that a touch of cinnamon can flavor savory dishes, too, as noted in *Llibre de Sent Soví.*

Recent studies show that cinnamon can lower blood sugar significantly, something that should be of interest to those concerned about managing diabetes. It is also full of antioxidants, so consumption of this spice benefits us all.

Nutmeg is known to boost collagen production for strong skin. Freshly grated, it has a bright, nutty taste that you will come to crave. I use freshly grated nutmeg often, especially over root vegetables or pumpkin roasted with a drizzle of honey. Cinnamon flavors *crema catalana* and other defining Iberian desserts, such as Asturian rice pudding.

It's interesting, as a devotee of culinary history, that in addition to cinnamon, Catalan chefs have traditionally used nutmeg in unexpected ways, as when flavoring certain sausages. This is mentioned in *Llibre de Sent Soví.* Nutmeg and cinnamon, when used in savory recipes, transport us back to medieval Catalunya.

Pimentón, Better than Paprika In 2007, the journal *Scientia Horticulturae* reported that Pimentón significantly increased activation of the antioxidant enzyme, glutathione, and that two to three teaspoons a week of pimentón de la Vera detoxifies the body and doubles antioxidant defenses.

Now cloves.

Studies show clove extract can inhibit the effects of skin, stomach, bone, and blood cancers. A 2012 study reported in the journal *Molecules* found that eugenol, a component in cloves, has antioxidant and anticancer potential and binds to heavy metals, such as mercury and lead, removing them from the body.

Juniper berries are often used to flavor wild game.

Venison Steaks with Juniper Spice Rub in Pomegranate Sauce

Pound 1 teaspoon of juniper berries in a mortar, with a pinch of coarse salt, 1 pinch dried hot pepper flakes, 2 tablespoons EVOO, and 2 cloves of garlic. Rub mixture over venison steaks 2 hours before cooking. Meanwhile, in a small pot, add a little EVOO, heat, and add ½ cup minced onions, 1 clove minced garlic, and season with salt. Sauté until onions just turn golden. Turn the heat up and add ¾ cup of red wine. Bring to a boil and quickly turn down. Reduce for 5 minutes on simmer. Add pomegranate seeds and juice from 1 large pomegranate, along with a ½ sprig of fresh rosemary. Simmer for 5 minutes. Melt 1 tablespoon of butter into the mixture, season with salt and pepper. Taste and adjust salt.

Juniper Berries, Tiny Treasures with Giant Benefits Juniper berries offer antibacterial properties and are rich in antioxidants as well as the life-extending substance, 4-terpene, which is thought to lower levels of uric acid and help keep *herpes simplex* virus at bay.

Heat a large pan with EVOO. Slice one or two large shallots into vertical pieces and place in pan. Sauté for a couple of minutes to soften, then just before the shallots brown, add the spiced venison and sear. Cook 3 minutes on each side for medium rare, 4 minutes for medium well; however, cooking time depends on how thick the steaks are. When meat is done, set aside to rest. Serve with sauce.

Honey. The colors shimmer through glass jars. Molten unguents. As we lean in, scents of lavender, orange blossom, chestnut and rosemary whirl.

We examine jars that contain heather, chestnut, rosemary, lavender and propolis-rich amber honey from the mountain forests near Valencia, where the earliest record of beekeeping in the world was found some 8,000 years ago. There is also orange blossom honey that contains propolis, and bee pollen and royal jelly. Substances that have been shown to benefit human health in many ways.

A light application of honey over eggplant sticks that were fried in EVOO is extremely popular in Catalunya and Andalusia, as tapas. Use coarse wheat flour, shake off the excess, and as always, fry in good EVOO. After the eggplant turns golden, season with salt and a little honey.

Pure natural honey offers antitumor, antibacterial, and antimicrobial properties. It contains vitamins, enzymes, and approximately eighteen essential and nonessential amino acids, which form the building blocks of protein such as glutamine, cysteine, and tryptophan.

Don't miss the vinegar, for the cooking of Spain would not be the same without it.

Nutrition science has made it obvious that there are benefits to consuming vinegar, something that traditional healers have always known. For one thing, traditionally it has been understood that consuming vinegar helps break down bile in the liver.

Returning to the culinary, vinegar is combined with EVOO to dress salads, make gazpacho, and to flavor cold fish and seafood salads, all of which the Spanish eat often. And of course, vinegar is used to deglaze pans to make sauces.

Red and white vinegar, and sweet and sour yellow vinegar from muscatel grapes is before us. Look, here are Jerez sherry and Cava vinegars. Through the glass, colors are muted and old-world.

Here is a historic recipe that I bet you will like.

Muscovy Duck Breast or Chicken with Sweet-and-Sour Fig Sauce

For the sauce, sauté ⅓ cup of chopped shallots seasoned with salt in EVOO until caramelized. Separately, reconstitute 3 chopped dried figs in a bowl with some very hot water. Add to the shallots along with 1 cup chicken broth, 2 tablespoons of honey, 2 tablespoons of balsamic vinegar, several pinches of ground allspice, 1 clove, several pinches of cayenne pepper, and salt. Bring to a boil, reduce heat, and simmer for 20 minutes. Set aside.

Score the skin of the duck breast lightly with a knife, taking care not to cut through to the meat. Season delicately with salt and allow to sit for 10 minutes. Then season with allspice and sauté in a heavy pan coated with olive oil or duck fat. Cover for five minutes. Many chefs cook Muscovy duck breast to medium rare or it won't be juicy, so this will take approximately 12 minutes. When juices from the duck appear on the surface, it shows that the duck is medium rare. Spoon over sauce and serve.

———•———

Just now, looking through the unwashed window, it is apparent that the afternoon is drawing to a close. I tell the vendors *Adéu*, in my best Catalan accent.

Taking our leave, as we stroll through the giant building toward the entrance, we encounter a booth with an impressive display of Spanish wine.

The prices look good. One doesn't have to spend a lot on Spanish wine for selections that are memorable. Indeed, Spanish wines are highly regarded, and have been since early Roman times when even the conquering Romans brought wine with them from Spain in their amphoras. Spanish wines are so good and generally represent such great value, even the French buy wine from Spain today.

Wine drinking is not about snobbism or false elegance in Spain, and the Spanish know many wines are meant to be drunk young. These inexpensive varietals are among my favorites.

Standards are high for production of wine in Spain. On the subject of health, some believe that moderate consumption of red wine as part of the Mediterranean diet has been shown to be healthy.

Bioflavonoids in red grapes help prevent cancer, and resveratrol, which inhibits enzymes that stimulate cancer cell growth, is protective too. The polyphenols in red wine protect the heart by keeping blood vessels flexible, and they help prevent cancer as well. This antioxidant also supports brain function and reduces the risk of blood clots. A 2015 study found that resveratrol in wine could help prevent osteoporosis.

As we approach the entrance to go our separate ways, I am recalling what Ernest Hemingway said about wine.

When living in Paris as a young writer, Hemingway saved his money so he could vacation in Spain. He attended *Sanfermines* in Pamplona, to take part in the running of the bulls, and then went into the mountains and great forests of Navarra, to the river Irati, to fish. Ernesto, as the locals called him, loved his secret fishing spot but never revealed it. Hemingway loved the local food and wine. His favorite wine, *las* Campanas *rosado*, hails from Tiebas, south of Pamplona in Navarra, named after the pair of bells that grace the tower of the town's church.

Among other things, Hemingway said, "Drinking wine was not about snobbism, nor a sign of sophistication, nor a cult; it was as natural as eating."

As with her wines, the cooking of Spain offers an unpretentious way of eating that is tied to the earth. With this lack of affectation, there is genuineness to her recipes, which belong to all people, rich or poor, who know that good food is something to be shared. Many recipes were born from the farm, the banks of a high mountain river, or on a fishing vessel, all of which I am certain appealed to Hemingway. This rustic authenticity, expressed with basic ingredients so good they can stand for themselves and unfussy seasonings designed to let the true taste of food shine, offers the promise of life.

There is ingenuity to Spanish cooking, too, expressing culinary knowledge. Flavor can be coaxed from ingredients by cooks who understand the value of something as simple as a mortar and pestle.

And there is Spain's ineffable history, offering inspiration from all sorts of recipes that span the ages. What better way to realize this truth than to spend time as we have, here in *la* Boqueria, in this icon of the Spanish Mediterranean diet.

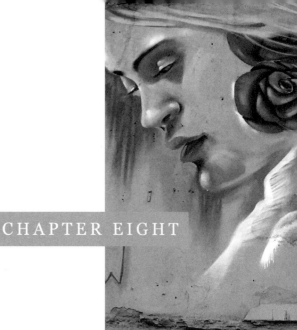

CHAPTER EIGHT

Interviews with Celebrated Chefs Carme Ruscalleda and Elena Arzak ... and Their Recipes

"The boom that gripped Spanish cultural life after Franco, producing figures like filmmaker Pedro Almodóvar, has taken hold in Spanish kitchens."

– Anya von Bremzen, author of *The New Spanish Table*

Make no mistake, women have played a crucial role in the gastronomy of Spain, with the most well-known being Michelin-starred chefs Carme Ruscalleda and Elena Arzak.

I am honored by the participation of Chefs Ruscalleda and Arzak, both of whom have generously given of their time in order for us to discover some of their views on cooking and health.

———•———

Interview with Chef Carme Ruscalleda

Carme Ruscalleda has the distinction of being the only female chef in the world awarded seven Michelin stars—spread across her two restaurants in Catalunya and, yes, a third in Japan, which has two stars. Ruscalleda's gastronomic journey, a passionate embracing of Spanish Mediterranean cooking, began with her husband, when she took over her parents' small food store, developing it to offer a wide range of specialty items such as prepared vegetables and foie gras. Later, Ruscalleda could not resist the lure of her own restaurant when she acquired an old hostel, Hotel Sant Pau, that was in front of the family farmhouse. This was in 1988 in the Maresme region, in her hometown Sant Pol de Mar, just north of Barcelona. (After 30 years, Sant Pau closed in 2018.) Ruscalleda brought her Catalan sensibilities to Japan in 2004 when she opened her restaurant Sant Pau in Tokyo, initiating what has become a successful cross-cultural gastronomic exchange. Later Chef Ruscalleda added the acclaimed restaurant Moments in Barcelona's Hotel Mandarin Oriental to her crown of stars. There, with her son Raul at the helm, Ruscalleda offers an antiaging menu reflecting her lifelong commitment to health. "Ruscalleda's attempt to point her diners to a healthier lifestyle is an effort toward initiating conversation about living well by eating well," says Geeta Bansal, in a profile of the chef published in the *Examiner* (2015).

With dedication to nutrient-dense chemical-free cooking and the author of over a dozen books geared toward the home chef, Carme Ruscalleda is someone Americans need to know.

RK. It is a thrill to interview you, a remarkably distinguished chef who has maintained the rebelliousness of a self-taught person. Tell us about your family home and how you became involved in the restaurant business.

CR. First may I point out that I was born in my parents' farmhouse in the middle of Sant Pol de Mar. I grew up there—in a fishing and farming village. Our farmhouse looked out towards the sea, and there I learned to cook. It was a beautiful, natural rural environment. We raised chickens and had a shop in which we sold milk, wine, pulses, and vegetables. The farm taught me the value of ceaseless toil but also the beauty of the seasons. In 1975, I married Toni Balam, and a couple of years later we launched our own take-away business in my parents' store.

RK. So from this rural Mediterranean life, your philosophy as a chef was born: the melding of nature, creativity, and technique. I know you have an interest in the arts, which I wish to discuss in a moment, but for now, please tell us about your first restaurant.

CR. Well, very near our family farm and business, a property became available that was perfect for a restaurant. I could not resist. This was in 1988. The property had views of the Mediterranean and a garden! Our practices in the kitchen at Sant Pau conveyed the values of the vegetarian world: very simple, very pure techniques and excellent products.

Before we proceed, I wish to offer insight into how pure is the marine culture of El Maresme. For example, when noodles or potatoes are added to a fish or shellfish dish, the broth must be closely related to the seafood in the dish. So if we prepare broth for suquet, Catalan seafood stew—customarily made from monkfish and shellfish—the broth must be cooked with monkfish so there is a conjunction of pure flavor. We want the essence of the flavor to be unchanged so that it does not confuse the brain.

RK. Thank you for this culinary insight. Over time your first restaurant became distinguished. How did you catch the attention of diners so soon?

CR. Dining guides began to include the Sant Pau restaurant in their lists of local endorsements, and three years later, in 1991, we received a Michelin star.

RK. That was only the beginning! Sant Pau received her second star in 1996 and a third in 2005, making your restaurant one of the most important in Spain, equal to Ferran Adrià's El Bulli. There have been many other awards after this distinction as well as almost a dozen books that you have authored, not to mention your restaurant in Japan. You remain busy and yet you maintain abundant energy. Your secret?

CR. I confess that I have a very committed professional life, so I am focused on maintaining health. My key is adequate sleep. I try to sleep about seven hours a night. Exercise is important, too. So at least two days a week I practice invigorating gymnastic exercise.

RK. Give us an idea of your daily life. What is your schedule like?

CR. I eat a simple breakfast by 7:30 in the morning, say a piece of fruit with yogurt and cookies that I make from whole grain flour, almonds, and sesame seeds sweetened with a bit of sugar. I am disciplined, so I eat no more than three. With this, I take a daily vitamin complex and a calcium supplement. Oh, I always have coffee with soymilk. It's my take on latte. Then, around 11 am I enjoy a piece of chocolate—70 percent cocoa. By midday I have a lunch consisting of lots of varied, fresh vegetables with a bit of meat or fish. I believe in naps, too. I sleep for about twenty minutes, and when I awake I drink Hojicha tea and have a piece of fruit. My dinner at 8 o'clock usually is vegetarian. Holidays, Sundays, and Mondays I dine with family. For nourishing my artistic spirit, I read and I draw.

RK. Yes. I saw an online video of you creating a drawing for a specific dish. You used color ink pens, and your style is simple, elegant, and shows a joy of color. You embrace color in your gastronomic creations, too. Returning to the subject of self-nourishment, in your book *Cuinar per ser feliç*, which translates as "Cooking: A Source of Joy," you claim that the "kitchen is a source of tenderness." Tell us more.

CR. I am convinced that besides benefiting the body, cooking good food nourishes our emotions in the way that music does. Just as a melody can move us to intimate memories, so can the essence of taste. A pleasant meal can give us sentimental pleasure as well as create an excellent state of mind. A nice meal also nurtures creative energy, which can lead to expressing our talents, whatever they might be.

RK. Speaking of talent, not only are your culinary presentations similar to contemporary paintings, but many dishes that you have created are three-dimensional works of art. Your chocolate dessert "The Dragon" is original, humorous and incredibly beautiful. Do your presentations reveal your personality?

CR. A creative work is a reflection of the person who has created it. Our philosophy at Sant Pau, in Spain and Tokyo, as well as at Moments represents our desire to advance emotions through food but also to offer experiences of "fun" or "joy." In addition, we wish to offer health and happiness.

RK. Your culture is central to your gastronomy. Please offer insight into the Catalan expression "el seny i la rauxa." From what I understand, rauxa means passion, a lot of heart, and *seny* means judgment and prudence. How do you nourish your own seny and rauxa?

CR. My seny is expressed by my daily commitment to my clients and staff. My rauxa, or playful moments, are times spent with family and friends, as well as taking walks, going on trips, and attending the cinema or theatre.

RK. Returning to the subject of your work, your success confirms that you are an incredible motivator of people. How do you encourage those around you to work as a team, yet share the best within?

CR. For me, this is a natural process. I work side by side with my staff. We share research, inspiration, schedules, service—we share everything. One could say that we are together through thick and thin.

RK. What advice would you give women who want to become chefs?

CR. First and foremost, a woman must believe in herself. We are not second-class human beings. We must feel our inherent inner strength and act with conviction and passion. And, of course, a natural gastronomic and creative ability is key. But we must be prepared to join a profession that requires challenges to one's schedule. We can achieve our goals by working without laziness and by entrepreneurship.

RK. We share an affinity for Japanese products such as miso and umeboshi plums. These, among other Japanese foods, are considered to be supportive to health, as believed by those who follow macrobiotics, which, as you know, is a Japanese healing philosophy. Through your restaurant in Sant Pau, Tokyo, you must have incorporated Japanese products into your kitchen. Can you speak to this?

CR. Yes. I am inspired by natural products—in addition to being healthy, they provide contrast and flavor to recipes, so miso and umeboshi have worked their way into many of my dishes. Both miso and umeboshi are highly appreciated products for us.

RK. Speak about your admiration for the products of your land.

CR. I am excited to speak about the nutritional and culinary advantages of our healthy products. I believe that we are children of the earth, so we must honor ourselves and the earth by embracing organic. And, of course, organic products are very healthy, so when we eat them we feel healthy. For this reason, in my restaurants, I offer a seasonal cuisine that shows my commitment to nature. Also, because we are "heirs of a culinary culture" with a large presence of pork—one of the most attractive products of our culture—is Iberian ham, which offers unique benefits to human health.

RK. Yes, Iberian ham is nutritious and it tastes incredible. I can't wait to hear about your recipe for croquettes made from Iberian ham, but since sofrito is a Catalan invention, I am eager to ask—Carme Ruscalleda, Catalan chef par excellence, how do you use sofrito in your home?

CR. Sí, sofrito is the basis of very, very tasty dishes! At home I make many types of sofrito. Since they are easy to prepare and to freeze, they could not be more convenient to have on hand. In fact, I make sofritos in advance. I will tell you how. Just sauté each ingredient individually, and when you're ready to cook, you can defrost and combine as you like.

Once I am done, I keep individual bags of these sautéed vegetables and then use them for different combinations. For example, one day I might grab onion and tomato. Another leek and red pepper, or leek, tomato, and green pepper, and so on.

RK. Could you speak to the passion you have for fresh vegetables, as with salads? How does your culinary aesthetic embrace the importance salads have on the spirit of your cooking?

CR. Produce is integral to the art of cooking. For example, from the beginning, our salads grow more and more elaborate, more attractive, more entertaining, and more daring.

RK. Thank you, Chef Ruscalleda, and our gratitude for sharing your recipes for jamón ibérico croquettes and sofrito.

Carme Ruscalleda's Sofrito Prepare the following individual ingredients in extra-virgin olive oil, lightly salt, and separate into small freezer bags:

Onions—Finely chopped sautéed until lightly golden

Ripe Tomato—Grate tomato and sauté slowly

Green Italian Pepper—Skin the pepper, chop into small pieces, and sauté slowly for a long time

Leeks—Mince finely and sauté on medium heat until light golden.

In 2022, Ruscalleda joined the gastromomic innovation team at CUICK, an organization having the objective of providing support to professional and home cooks alike through the offering of sofrito bases and cooking stock made with the highest quality fresh and local ingredients.

Carme Ruscalleda's
Irresistible Ibérico Ham Croquettes

(Makes about 40 croquettes)

2 cups Ibérico ham, chopped fine
¾ cup finely chopped leek, white part only
1 quart milk
1 cup white flour
½ cup cornstarch Maizena
    (a gluten-free natural product that adds lightness to croquettes)
Couple pinches of salt

FOR THE BATTER:
Wheat flour, 4 beaten eggs, panko Japanese breadcrumbs
extra-virgin olive oil

METHOD: In a sauté pan, add a little olive oil and chopped leeks. Delicately season with salt and pepper. Leeks must be well cooked. Meanwhile, in a large bowl using a wire whisk, mix milk, flour, several pinches of salt, and cornstarch. Add to this mixture the chopped Ibérico ham and the sautéed leek. Using two tablespoons to form, mold croquettes. Roll them in flour, beaten egg, and finally panko. Can reserve in the fridge. To fry the croquettes in extra-virgin olive oil, using a thermometer, heat the oil to 350°F. The oil should not smoke. The croquettes should be golden, crispy, and hot.

TIP: If you don't have a thermometer, stick the tip of a wooden spoon into the heated oil. Once bubbles form and float to the surface you are ready to fry.

Interview with Chef Elena Arzak

Elena Arzak studied with her father Juan Mari Arzak, and Ferran Adrià, who calls her "one of the most important chefs in history." Selected as the top woman chef in the world by *Restaurant* magazine in 2012, Chef Arzak also won the Augie Award from the Culinary Institute of America in 2015.

Elena travels often, but this three-star Michelin chef can frequently be found in her family's San Sebastián restaurant, which opened at the end of the nineteenth century as a roadside tavern. She now shares the helm with her father and loves to develop avant-garde ideas while maintaining staunch devotion to the Basque code of flavors. Elena Arzak is one of six women in the world with at least three Michelin stars.

> "What we eat, how we eat defines our culture. We are Basque and we cook unconsciously with this identity."
>
> – Elena Arzak

RK. Thank you for taking part in this book about health. It is an honor to interview you. Basque cooking is something that every follower of gastronomy wants to know more about. Tell us, Chef Arzak, what makes Basque cuisine so special?

EA. Call me Elena. Let me first say that Spain and Portugal are a collection of diverse regions—a mosaic, if you will, of excellent food cultures, all unique, yet we influence each other. Each region offers its own specialties. For example, Galicians are known for seafood and Navarre for vegetables. Food has always been very important in Spain. Mothers teach their children how to cook, and on the weekends everyone gets together to cook and to eat. But also, simple foods are ingrained into our culture. It is common for women to know how to prepare dried lentils and chickpeas, and also broad beans (*favas*). Since there is a lot of land, there are many gardens, and we eat all types of greens. The Basque region where I am from, San Sebastián, is privileged in that we have the best foods from the land and the sea, and land products are grown with care. Small producers sell their fruits, vegetables, and artisan cheese, and are supported. Freshness is assured. But also, we Basques keep cooking interesting. For example, we love recipes from every part of Spain!

RK. What about your favorites? I know you love vegetables. Tell us more.

EA. Sí, I love vegetables. I don't know what my life would be like without them! Not only do I eat lots of salads but when in season, I also adore asparagus and peas. In the winter I eat plenty of cabbage. But even if you eat a vegetable as healthy as cauliflower all of the time, it's not enough. I believe that we need a wide variety of vegetables to be healthy. Vegetables have lots of nutrients, minerals, and anticancer compounds, but we need the widest spectrum we can get. Variety is key. I am the type of person who eats a little bit of everything, including jamón Ibérico.

RK. I love jamón Ibérico. This brings me to my next question. In general, what type of diet do you follow?

EA. We are all different, so there is no one ideal diet. I believe that our needs change as we age, too. Someone who is very young and physically active will need to eat many calories. Some people have allergies. I am forty-seven. When I was very young I ate a lot of meat. Now I am older so instead of meat, I eat more fish. In general, I will say that I think women need to eat more fish. This is for the omega-3. Besides, it is normal for Basques to eat a lot of fish.

RK. I want to hear more about fish in a moment, but I must ask you now, what makes the Basque people so excited about cooking?

EA. (*Laughing*) No one can explain why, but we love to eat!! And so we cook. Basques begin cooking when we are very young. We teach our children to cook, and for me this is important. But also it is our way of life to be attached to the seasons here, so we love local products, which of course reflect the changing seasons. It is exciting and defines our way of life.

RK. Do you have any special tips for cooking fish? I know that you have been experimenting with quick methods, and I know that Basques don't eat burned or charred foods, so what do you suggest for cooking fish?

EA. No. Basques don't like burned foods! We follow specific cooking techniques and sauté with finesse. For example, here is a simple, delicious recipe for cooking fish, but I don't recommend that the olive oil be extremely hot else it loses its flavor, aromas, and benefits to health. Okay, Bueno—fish filets with the skin on are easy to cook, but because the skin is left on, the taste is made even more delicious. But of course the scales must be removed. Step one—infuse the extra-virgin olive oil with chunks of garlic. It is easy. Just leave as much garlic as you like in a little bowl with extra-virgin olive oil on your counter overnight. If it is summer and your kitchen is hot, put the oil and garlic in the refrigerator. When you are ready to cook, heat a small amount of the garlic-infused oil, but remember, do not allow the oil to get extremely hot. Place the fish filet, skin side down, and cook in the hot oil for 1–2 minutes. Flip over and finish cooking for several minutes more, depending upon how thick the filet is. Also, Basques love "fish breaded and coated in egg." Again, very simple. Just dredge the fish in a little flour and coat lightly with a whisked egg. Then fry the fish quickly in oil again— that is not too hot. Afterward, use paper towels to drain the oil from the fish.

TIP: On searing fish, Jenny Chandler, author of *The Food of Northern Spain: Recipes from the Gastronomic Heartland of Spain*, tells those of us who like our fish rare to allow fish to "come up to room temperature otherwise the center will be cold." And coatings on nonstick pans can be toxic. Enameled cast iron or ceramic are better choices.

RK. What about those tender Basque potatoes? They are so delicious, and I have never had anything like them. I would love to know how to make them.

EA. In Spain, everyone adores potatoes, which is good since potatoes are a healthy food, no? The Basque approach you speak of is what we call confit of potatoes. To begin, slice the potatoes very, very thin and place them in a shallow casserole, salted, with a small amount of extra-virgin olive oil to cover. Take care not to use too much salt. I like chives and fresh onions cooked with the potatoes, so you might want to add them, too. Cover and roast in a 200°C (350°F) oven for 30 minutes. Of course, if you slice them thicker you will need to roast them for more than 30 minutes. Be sure not to let the oil get to high temperature. After the potatoes are cooked, it is very important to strain away the oil. At this point if one likes, one can garnish the potatoes with minced garlic.

Elena Arzak's Gem Lettuce

Grilled Gem Lettuce: Wash and dry lettuce. Salt lightly. Using a flat grill-like pan, coat with extra-virgin olive oil and place lettuce clusters in pan. Cook on medium-high for several minutes. Turn lettuce over, and cook for several minutes more. Serve with fish.

RK. Let's talk about when you first became interested in cooking.

EA. My sister Marta and I used to go to the restaurant to watch our grandmother, father, and mother cook. Ever since I can remember I recognized if something tasted good just by the smell. My grandmother was an excellent chef. I especially liked the way she taught me to love cooking vegetables. She would prepare each one separately and, at the final moment, mix them together. I asked her, "Why don't you cook the vegetables together?" My grandmother told me it "wasn't the same"and "for really great cooking you must be patient." Vegetables were very important to my grandmother. She used to eat plates of cardoons in the winter. Cardoons are known to be a very healthy food, and Basques love the flavor. They have high water content and make you feel very good when you eat them. Also, artichokes are another very healthy food that we love. The flavor of artichokes is intense, but we Basques also believe that one gains physical power from eating artichokes.

RK. How interesting. Let's talk about olive oil, another food that we gain physical energy from. It sounds to me that you are careful to drain away heated oil from your food, but do you have any special habits for consuming unheated extra-virgin olive oil in your diet?

EA. We Basques like Vinagretas, and for breakfast I enjoy a spoonful of extra-virgin olive oil on my bread every morning. I like whole grain bread slightly toasted with a drizzle of olive oil.

RK. Like Carme Ruscalleda, you are active and vibrant so I guess that you have always eaten well. Is this true?

EA. People tell me, "Elena you are so full of energy." Yes, for the most part I am very healthy. I attribute this to the fact that I have always eaten well. I believe this with my brain and with my heart. But also, remember food is about pleasure! Sometimes we need a piece of chocolate, sí? We must not forget that delicious food is good for the soul.

RK. Sí, Elena. Delicious food is good for the soul.

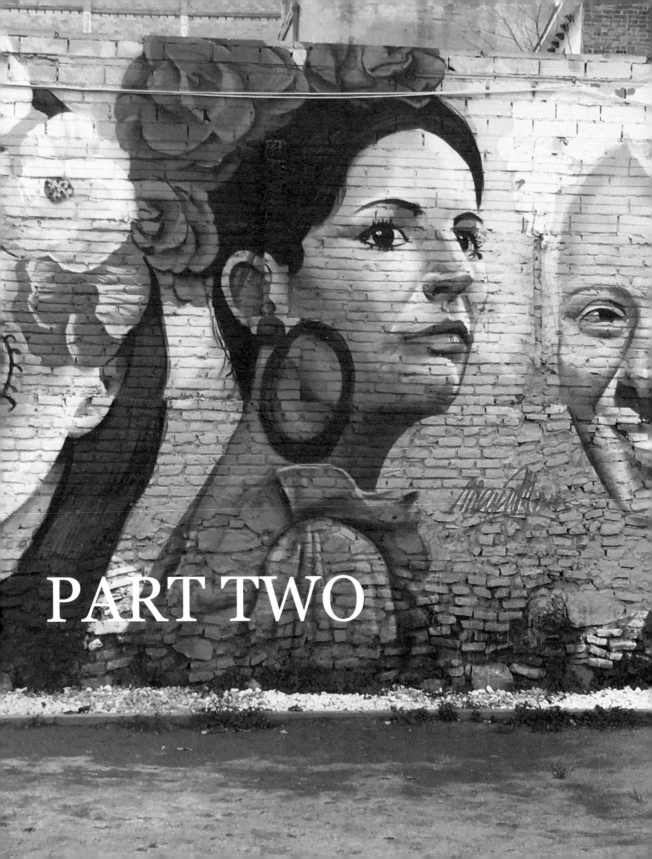

PART TWO

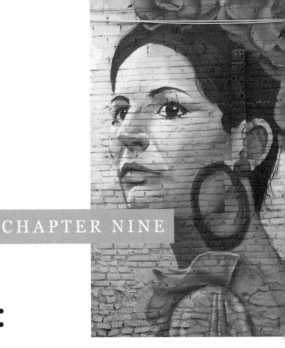

CHAPTER NINE

The Spanish Pantry:
A Delicious
Path to Health

"Spanish cooking has remained vigorous and individual, a good basis for its current renaissance."
– Charles Perry, "Ghosts of the Past, The Roots of Spanish Cooking,"
The LA Times, July 16, 1992.

R ecommendations from the medical community regarding health are often retracted. Consider, for instance, the 2022 report that taking an aspirin a day to lower risk for cardiovascular events is no longer necessary and may even be harmful. Or another 2022 report that we don't need to follow a low-fat diet for heart health after years of recommending the opposite. After countless studies, the same cannot be said of olive oil, whose thoroughly documented benefits open the door to the life-extending Mediterranean diet.

To develop a Spanish Mediterranean pantry, keep in mind that ingredients must be first rate, whether bread, chocolate, produce, or olive oil.

For Spanish tuna, olive oil, and cheese, please refer to Spanish food importers in the Resource Guide. Certain products such as cheese undergo stringent production protocols to assure excellence. Look for the government "PDO" seal, which signifies the product has been certified to come from a Protected Designation of Origin, meaning these protocols are in place.

Regarding flavor, generally speaking, Spanish cooking does not rely on spicy taste. Flavors are bold, citrusy, savory, nutty, earthy, piquant, or herbal. Even pungent. Consider dried ñora peppers. After reconstituting, there is an earthy, delicate sweetness to the flesh, that is also slightly pungent. Mediterranean *Salmoretta* Sauce, flavored with ñoras, is the basis for all sorts of appetizing rice and seafood dishes, and a topping for baked fish:

Mediterranean *Salmoretta* Sauce

Reconstitute 2 dried ñora peppers by adding boiled water to cover for about 30 minutes. Scrape out the pulp. Roast two halved large tomatoes. Remove the seeds and scrape out the pulp. Combine the pulp with a small handful of chopped parsley, a little minced garlic, the reconstituted pepper pulp, a splash of olive oil, and vinegar. Salt lightly. Combine in a food processor or by hand with a mortar and pestle. Taste. Adjust salt.

———— • ————

Food historian, scholar and food writer, Charles Perry, who translated the 14th century classic *The Anonymous Al-Andalus Cookbook* first from Arabic into Spanish and then into English, reminds us Spanish recipes are expressive and that they give form to "an existential sort of cuisine with a tough, dogged, living-on-the-edge character." *Pa amb xocolata*, the Catalan snack, is such a recipe. Melted chocolate on a slice of good bread finished with a sprinkling of coarse Spanish sea salt, *Pa amb xocolata* was developed during the Spanish civil war when ingredients were hard to come by. This recipe is kept alive today by Catalan chefs who create variations based on the original.

Remember that the Spanish Mediterranean diet is plant-based, which means fresh seasonal produce is fundamental. A basic pantry should be built on the items listed below. Some of you may be surprised to see bread. In recent decades, there has been hesitation about consuming bread, which in my eyes is a shame. Bread will always be basic to the Mediterranean diet, which remains the gold standard for health.

Donnie R. Yance pointed out in a recent blog, "The Many Health Benefits of Bread" that "the trouble with wheat is that most people consume it in unhealthy forms. This isn't the fault of the grain or the bread, but what we have done to it."

And so I say, look for whole-grain, crusty bread from bakeries that turn out fresh product and mill their own grain. Such bakeries can be found in every city and village in Spain. Because Spain is one of the leading countries worldwide in organic farming, whole grains will be grown with care.

Those who are bakers may want to explore and mill whole grains to maximize freshness and boost the nutritional value of bread, which has the potential to be vast.

The Pantry

- **Extra-Virgin Olive Oil**

  Spain has many great olive oils, so collect a few. Don't overlook oil made from Arbequina and Picual olives, which contain the highest amount of antioxidants. Also try olive oils from the Tarragona and Jaen regions.

- **Seasonal Produce, Fruit and Berries, Including:**

  Tomatoes
  Potatoes (all types, including miniature and purple)
  Sweet potatoes
  Green, red, orange and yellow bell peppers
  Flat-leaf parsley
  Chard
  Cabbage
  Leeks
  Dandelion greens (and wild greens, including dandelion)
  Onions (Mild or sweet for salads, and regular for cooking)
  Fennel (Often eaten as well by the long-living people of Sardinia)
  Eggplant
  Asparagus
  Mushrooms
  Hard squash
  Pumpkin
  Root vegetables, including rutabagas, parsnips, turnips
  Courgettes
  Lemons, oranges
  Strawberries, raspberries, blueberries, etc.

- **Vinegar**

  As with olive oils, Spain has several great vinegars. Make sure to include young sherry vinegar, *vinagre de Jérez* and red wine vinegars.

- **Salt**

- **Olives**

  There are many varieties of olives in Spain including Arbequina, Picual, Manzanilla, Gordal, and Empeltre, just to name a few.

- **Garlic and Shallots**

- **Cheese (Sheep, Goat and Cow's Milk)**

  Manchego (both young and aged), Cabrales, Valdeón, Roncal, Idiazábal, and Mahon for melting are among favorites. Aged Manchego can be used in recipes instead of parmesan. See Cheese Chart in Appendix A.

- **Yogurt (Goat, Sheep and Cow's Milk)**

- **Whole-Grain Crusty Bread**

In addition, explore the many types of artisan bread from Spanish food importers.

- **Saffron**

- **Nuts**

  Almonds, Marcona almonds, pine nuts, walnuts, hazelnuts, pistachios, and chestnuts

- **Beans (Dried, Jarred or Canned)**

  Lentils, chickpeas, white, navy and kidney beans

- **Dried Ñora and Choricero Peppers**

- **Spreads**

  Mayonnaise
  Allioli

- **Capers**

- **Eggs**

- **Bay Leaves**

- **Thyme**

- **Rosemary**

- **Chives**

- **Dried Lemon and Orange Peels**

- **Rice, Grains and Pasta**
  Fine noodles for fideuá, along with regular pasta
  Rice, including *bomba* for paellas
  Buckwheat
  Couscous
  Kamut
  Farro
  Quinoa

- **Canned, Jarred, Packaged and Frozen Goods**
  Canned tomatoes, tomato paste and sauce
  Canned or jarred tuna, sardines and anchovies (in EVOO)
  Tinned fish and shellfish, for tapas and more

- **Fresh Fish and Seafood**

- **Meat**
  Naturally raised is best. Chicken, turkey, pork, beef, lamb, jamón, and rabbit

- **Honey**

- **Molasses, including Pomegranate**

- **Rosewater**

- **Spices**

  Cumin
  Coriander
  Ground pepper
  Nutmeg
  Pimentón de la Vera, DO (sweet, bittersweet, and hot)
  Basque pimiento de Espelette
  Juniper berries
  Anise seeds
  Turmeric
  Cinnamon and nutmeg are often used in desserts, however, aniseed and anise liqueur are most commonly used in traditional baking recipes.

- **Dried Fruits**

  Figs, currants, raisins, prunes, apricots, and so on.

- **Cellar**

  Wine (white and red)
  Brandy
  Anise Liqueur
  Sherry
  Vermouth

- **A Taste of Sweetness**

  Candy, cookies, marmalades, chocolate and other treats are eaten in small amounts in Spain. Ingredient lists are refreshingly short. No coloring or preserving agents. Marmalade speaks for itself. Just try Valencia orange marmalade and you will understand. The taste hits true.

All natural creamy turrón
Crisp Marcona almond and honey turrón
Candied nuts, covered in yogurt or chocolate
Various Spanish chocolates, including dark
Dried fruits dipped in chocolate
Spanish pastries
Holiday cookies
Fig cakes
Dark chocolate covered orange peel
Crispy cinnamon tortas (made wth EVOO)
Marcona almond butter, if you can find it!

Optional Pantry Items

Jarred Guindilla peppers
Jarred Romesco sauce
Packaged seafood broth
Packaged bone broth, to add to soups
Jarred *piquillo* peppers
Jarred sofrito for quick casseroles or paella
Jarred garlic spread, known as allioli
Cantabrian white anchovies in olive oil
Sardinillas (small sardines)
Squid ink (Nortindal brand is my favorite)
Cockles, mussels, baby squid, razor clams, and more
Galician bread ready to bake, can be shipped to your door.
Pommery Moutard de Meaux
Frozen croquettes from Spain

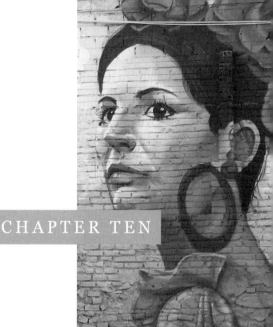

CHAPTER TEN

¡Vamos! ¡A Cocinar!
Let's Cook!
Spanish Recipes Adapted
to the American Kitchen

"To know how to eat is to know how to live."
– Ancient Basque proverb, anonymous

"My kitchen year started in a time of trouble, but it taught me a great deal. When I went back to cooking, I rediscovered simple pleasures, and as I began to appreciate the world around me, I learned that the secret to life is finding joy in ordinary things."
– Ruth Reichl, *My Kitchen Year, 136 Recipes That Saved My Life*

On any given day in my kitchen, you will see me cooking with traditional Spanish ingredients—such things as pimentón, bay, thyme, and extra-virgin olive oil, which by the way can commonly be found in grocery stores. But you may also find me using *Pommery Moutard de Meux* and tamari sauce. These so-called global ingredients, and others, occasionally make their way into my cooking, and some of the recipes in this chapter are no exception.

Obviously, I am not placing myself in the category of Ferran Adrià, but like this mastermind who shares his own global pantry in *The Family Meal: Home Cooking with Ferran Adrià*, using a few non-Spanish ingredients on occasion keeps cooking fresh.

On the subject of health, my recipes and menus embrace the guidelines of Dr. Ramón Estruch, lead researcher of the Spanish PREDIMED study:

- Four tablespoons each day of extra-virgin olive oil.
- Three servings a week of nuts (walnuts, pecans, peanuts, etc.)
- At least three servings of fresh vegetables each day.
- At least three servings of fish and seafood every week, especially fatty-rich fish such as salmon, tuna, sardines, and anchovies.
- Three servings of beans/legumes every week.
- Limit red meat.

Staying with health, a 2022 report evaluating recent studies found that ultraprocessed foods, because of their assorted problematic ingredients including artificial flavors, colorings, emulsifiers, and thickeners, are linked to inflammation in the body, which ignites health problems. There is increasing awareness about the dangers of inflammation, tying it to cognitive decline and cancer. The report also pointed out that consumption of ultra-processed foods means we are eating foods that lack nutrients for which there is no compensation. You can't make up these deficiencies by including whole foods in your flawed pattern of eating. Just one more reason to cook from scratch.

If that weren't enough, the typical American adult gets one of every five calories from a restaurant, and probably too much salt. According to a recent study by researchers at the Friedman School of Nutrition Science and Policy at Tufts University, eating out is a program for meals of poor nutritional quality.

Do I think poor nutrition sets the stage for increased use of prescription drugs? Sure I do. Moreover, prescription medication is a leading cause of death in the United States.

Bettering our diet is crucial.

The Heritage of Spain's Mediterranean Diet: Jewish and Arabic Influences

For hundreds of years, Christians, Muslims, and Jews lived together in peace on the Iberian Peninsula. This melding of cultures contributed to the infinitely rich legacy known today as the Spanish Mediterranean diet.

As the scholar Luis Benavides-Barajas pointed out, "There can be no doubt that long before even the Visigoths ruled Spain, it was the Jews who influenced Spanish cooking." However, the Muslim presence had a profound impact on gastronomic Iberia, too, even in parts of the peninsula where its presence was brief.

For more on this saga, I recommend *The Story of Spain: The Dramatic History of Europe's Most Fascinating Country*, by Mark R. Williams. His book describes the invasions, expulsions, and conversions that took place under the Catholic monarchs Ferdinand and Isabella during the late 1400s.

Among the numerous culinary contributions that the Jewish people, also called Sephardim, made to Spain, are a variety of stuffed vegetable and fish recipes. In addition, the Spanish national dish, *olla podrida*, a casserole of vegetables, aromatics, chickpeas, lamb, chicken, and beef meatballs, along with beef marrow bone or lamb shank, is believed to originate from the Sephardic *adafina*. It's meant to be slow-cooked on Friday and eaten on the Sabbath. Lighter fare falls under their influence, too, such as salads, lentils, and chickpea dishes. Breaded and fried zucchini and eggplant recipes are also credited to Sephardic legacy, as are fried onions, garlic, lemon, cumin, and sweet and sour tastes in the same dish.

And always, olive oil was used for frying and cooking foods, whether it be Sephardic or Arabic.

Arabic influence includes clay pot cooking, skewered roasted meats, meats cooked with fruit such as pears and apples, vegetables stuffed with rice and chopped meat, sauces thickened with ground almonds and hazelnuts, and garnishes of pine nuts and raisins. Saffron is central to Arabic impact on Spanish gastronomy. The Arab people also brought rice, artichokes, spinach, carrots, bitter oranges, and sugar to Spain.

¡Olé! A Few Useful Tips

You may have observed that many recipes I've offered up to this point do not use exact measurements, an approach I urge you to develop. This encourages creativity, which makes cooking more meaningful.

Before I share recipes, let me begin by urging you to reject commercial table salt, and avoid oversalting. The Spanish don't have salt shakers on the table. Proper amounts of salt are used to season food during preparation, but also the Spanish don't like salty foods. Moreover, salt in Spain is natural sea salt, which unlike commercial salt in the United States, contains minerals, is relatively lower in sodium, and is chemical-free. And finally, the right type and amount of salt are healthy for us. Even necessary.

Our high-salt diet is a reason that the United States is ranked with nations that have the worst diets. Think of all the salty snacks Americans regularly eat such as chips and pretzels. In September 2022, as reported in *Nature Food*, researchers at Tufts University gathered data from 185 countries listed in the Global Dietary Database and found that "the diet of Americans is just as unhealthy now as it was 30 years ago."

Moreover, there is reason to believe that the poor quality salt used in the United States to preserve meats contributes to the reasons that, for instance, commercial sausage and other meat from pigs, are linked to cancer here. So, be sure to cook with the best salt you can find.

Here are a few more useful tips:

WATER: You may have noticed that some Spanish chefs recommend mineral water in recipes, meaning that water is considered an ingredient. Mineral water avoids chemicals that alter the taste of food, and toxins that threaten our health. As a practical alternative to bottled water which is expensive, I use a solid carbon block water filter at the kitchen tap and change the filter regularly.

EXTRA-VIRGIN OLIVE OIL (EVOO): Cook and dress salads with it and add lightly over vegetables, fish dishes, soup, stews and beans. Recently I was delighted to see a big box store carrying Spanish EVOO at a great value. Also, look for special offerings from Spanish importers listed in the Resource Guide. As previously mentioned, try combining 2 parts EVOO with 1 part dry Spanish sherry or vermouth. This mixture adds a sophisticated note to roasted fish and seafood recipes.

GARLIC: As discussed earlier in *The Iberian Table*, crushing garlic and allowing it to oxidize for at least 10–15 minutes before use strengthens the anticancer compounds, as reported by the American Cancer Institute, November 7, 2013.

VINEGAR: The average person in Spain consumes between 1.4–2 liters of vinegar a year, a good thing because vinegar is a boon to health. Traditional healers have always believed this, so it is encouraging that a study by the American Institute for Cancer Research (February 2015) has shown that vinegar consumption lowers blood sugar, especially when

Olive Oil: Flavors and Uses

In general, **delicate-tasting oils** are smooth, buttery, mellow and rich with a subtle, grassy note. These oils are for salad greens, fish, baking, eggs, and to make mayonnaise.

Medium-tasting oils are pleasantly pungent, bitter, and fruity. These are appropriate for gazpacho, grilled chicken, salads, lamb, vegetables, fish dishes and slow-roasted meats.

Robust-tasting oils are intense, spicy, and strongly grassy. Use for dishes that require bold flavors such as seafood paella and garlic mashed potatoes.

people consumed a high-carbohydrate meal. Chefs in Spain like sherry, chardonnay, apple cider, red wine, cava, and champagne vinegar. Aged Spanish sherry vinegar is a welcome alternative to sweet balsamic.

CAPERS: Spain is the largest producer of capers, a food richest in anticancer quercetin and selenium. Add capers to salads, seafood dishes, tapas, and more. If salty, rinse lightly before using and pat dry. Ballobar capers from the Huesca region of Aragón are considered the best.

FISH BROTH: Used frequently in Spain, the health benefits are many, especially when made with not just the bones, but also the head of the fish. Head or not, several recipes in this chapter call for fish broth, and Appendix C has a recipe for *Caldo de pescado*. Spanish fish broth can be found in some health food and grocery stores.

COFFEE: Two studies in 2017 reported that drinking coffee could lead to a longer, healthier life. The Spanish drink coffee often and don't like fancy syrups. Many of these flavored syrups are high in additives and sugar. *Café con leche*, or coffee with hot milk is favored. The Spanish make coffee the healthiest way: high pressure, high heat, and no filter. Medium-roasted beans are richest in anticancer polyphenols.

CAZUELA COOKING: Clay pot cooking is said to improve the flavor of food, which from my experience is true. Cazuelas, the most natural cookware available, are lead free. Recently I made turkey meatballs with wild mushroom sauce in a cazuela, starting on the stovetop and finishing in the oven. The cazuela helped hold the meatballs together but did not dry them, and the transition from stove top to oven was made with ease. Paula Wolfert pointed out in her classic *Mediterranean Clay Pot Cooking: Traditional and Modern Recipes to Savor and Share*, "I specify Spanish cazuelas. That's because they're well made, stronger than most others and totally lead free."

Cazuelas can be used on a gas stovetop (if necessary, with a flame diffuser) or in the oven for when roasting. To protect the clay vessel, do not subject it to extreme changes in temperature. Frequent use also helps to prolong the cazuela's life. Janet Mendel, the author of some of my favorite books on Spanish cookery, advises: "Soak your new pot in water for 24 hours. Dry well, then coat the inside with olive oil and place in a medium-low oven for 40 minutes." If you live in a dry climate, on occasion, you may want to re-soak your cazuela.

NUTS: My pantry is always stocked with a variety of nuts. Nuts are not costly, and they add an earthy depth to recipes. If you want to embrace tradition, purchase a mortar and pestle, and don't miss the fun. Roasting, then grinding nuts right before use in a recipe, ensures fresh, deep taste.

SAUSAGE: Quality sausage is made from good cuts of pork, with fat, which keeps it from drying out, and high-grade salt. My favorite is hormone and antibiotic free. On occasion, I use a little sausage to flavor a pot of bean or legume soup. Good quality sausage can be purchased from Spanish food importers. All-natural chorizo with no preservatives can also be added to potatoes with peppers but because *chorizo* is salty, I use it as a flavoring and I cook with much less salt in the recipe. Balance is key. Many times chorizo is offered as a tasting, as when cooked in apple cider. This makes a

Picada is made from nuts and can be mixed into all types of stews, adding nuances of flavor. Experiment. And remember, don't worry about exact measurements. Much tastier than a roux, picada is a thickener and flavor enhancer. Colman Andrews has said that picada should not stand out but when it is missing, you can tell. Although I offer a couple more picada recipes later, let's start with this one.

Picada Method: Preheat oven to 350°F. Place one slice of crustless country-style bread, and a handful of skinless hazelnuts, almonds, or both, on a baking sheet and toast until each is lightly golden, about 6 to 8 minutes. Once toasted, sliver the nuts and cut the bread into cubes. On the stovetop, toast 2 pinches of saffron threads in a small pan over medium heat. Transfer to a mortar and pestle, grind the saffron with a pinch of salt, and work in 2-3 cloves of minced garlic, chopped parsley and the toasted nuts and bread, adding a splash of EVOO as you go. Taste to adjust salt, and add the picada to your finished stew to thicken, as a final step.

tapas known throughout Spain. *Morcilla* sausage (delicious in fabades) has a soft texture and subtle flavors of nutmeg and cinnamon. Juicy, mild Catalan *Butifarra* is seasoned with black pepper and garlic. Popular in Aragón, *Butifarras* are delicious grilled and served with white beans. *Fuet*, another Catalan sausage, is a thin, air-dried sausage that is sliced and added to soups and stews. Fuet can be served right at the tapas table, on a cutting board with a knife. Asturian morcilla black (blood) sausage, usually made with onions, can be grilled and sliced as an appetizer. If you can locate artisan sausage from a local farmer's market, and can afford it, this type of sausage is an excellent choice, but make sure it is free from hormones and antibiotics.

MORE ON CHORIZO: Monika Linton points out in *Brindisa: The True Food of Spain* that in Spain "people tend to be more judicious in their use of chorizo, the argument being that not only is it quite rich and fatty, but if they are combining the sausage with other subtle ingredients, they don't want these to be blasted by powerful flavor."

MEMBRILLO PASTE: This natural, subtly sweet/tart fruit paste is a refreshing complement to roasted poultry, and to Spanish cheese for tapas. It is also excellent with salads, especially ones that contain toasted pine nuts. Included in this chapter is a recipe with membrillo and pine nuts hails from Barcelona. Recently, I have been layering thin slices of manchego with thin slices of membrillo on a plate, then stacking salad greens and tomato on top, to be finished with a little tangy vinagreta.

PIMENTÓN: A dusting adds magic to stews, bean dishes, tomato soups, roasted salmon, sautéed potatoes with onions, and more. I like pimentón to show its smoky character, as when flavoring wild salmon salad. I also use the spice with cumin, to provide sultry background. There are three types of pimentón: *dulce* (sweet), *agridulce* (bittersweet and a little hot), and *picante* (hot).

RICE: Never wash rice for paella or you will have a mushy dish. Bomba medium-grain holds up well in paella and, as advised earlier, is excellent for soupier recipes. Long-grain is ideal for pilafs.

BEANS: *Asustar* them, which in Navarra means to shock the pot with cold water and never allow beans to boil. Interestingly, this happens to be the macrobiotic method for cooking beans as well. This method helps the acids and pectins in the beans to become smooth, producing a pleasing sauce. *Choricero* peppers (dried and reconstituted) add a sweet depth to beans. More on choriceros in a moment.

SALT COD: To prepare, rinse dried salt cod and cover with water. Refrigerate for 24 to 48 hours, changing the water two to four times. To test for saltiness, break off a small piece and taste it. The whiter the salt cod, the better the quality. Thicker pieces are preferred.

ANCHOVIES: Outside Spain, fresh anchovies are difficult to find. Look for tinned anchovies imported from Spain packed in olive oil. Oil-packed anchovies can be used from the tin without rinsing, but when you buy them packed in salt, rinse quickly in a little spring water and pat dry. *Boquerones* are anchovies packed in light vinegar. They are exceedingly tasty, too.

CUTTLEFISH AND SQUID INK: A tasty and sophisticated addition to rice, this substance also makes a tasty sauce for seafood dishes. A few teaspoons add a savory complexity. I usually buy it in 3 oz jars from Spanish importers. Sometimes fishmongers offer it in small packets; however, I have found it inferior. For a recipe for two, use ¼ ounce, and for six, use ¾ of an ounce.

SAFFRON: Often I crush saffron threads with my fingers and add directly to recipes in the final moments of cooking, such as vegetables sautéed with garlic in EVOO or whole grains such as buckwheat, brown rice or quinoa, which actually is a seed. If you wish, infuse saffron threads in warm water for 5-20 minutes, then add the saffron and soaking liquid to the recipe. (By the way, saffron powder, which adds uniform color, can be added directly as you cook with no soaking.) For toasting, place saffron threads wrapped in parchment-lined foil in a hot oven or in a small skillet over medium heat, either way for less than two minutes. Then, crumble directly into recipes with your fingers, or use a mortar and a pestle to grind the toasted saffron threads before adding to recipes.

Liver Detox Tea. Place trimmed artichoke leaves and stems in a pot. Cover with water, bring to boil, reduce to simmer. Cook for 20 minutes. Remove from heat and steep for ten minutes more. Drink at room temperature.

ARTICHOKES: Artichokes can be braised with a sauce, sautéed, stewed, baked, stuffed or roasted. To prepare, trim off the tough outer leaves. Then remove the stem that you have trimmed leaves from and discard. Slice off the top ⅔ of the artichoke and cut into pieces—chefs sometimes cut them into four or six pieces. Or, precook artichokes, which is ideal for when you stuff them. First, as described, discard tough outer leaves and cut off the stem, leaving about a half inch at the bottom. Trim off prickly tips with sharp shears. Working quickly, place trimmed artichokes in a bowl with water and a bit of lemon juice so they don't darken. Bring pot of water to a boil with a little lemon juice, olive oil, and salt. Add artichokes, reduce heat, cover, and simmer gently for around seven minutes. Remove with tongs, drain, cool, and cut lengthwise. Dig out the prickly yellow leaves and fuzzy chokes with a paring knife. Stuff with a mixture of breadcrumbs seasoned with salt, pepper, garlic and pimentón and sautéed chopped onions, perhaps with bits of chorizo, or tiny tastings of jamón. Add a little broth to the baking dish, cover, and roast.

PIMIENTOS: Spanish peppers are appreciated for their distinct, subtle, on-point flavors, not because they add heat. Flavors range from fruity, acidic, and slightly sweet to pungent.

PIQUILLOS are wood-roasted, sweet red peppers preserved without chemicals and sold in jars. The best are from Navarra and La Rioja, grown near the Ebro River. They are so delicious that noted restaurants throughout Spain are proud to serve them. Having a fresh, slightly sweet, smoky taste, fill them with *bonito del norte tuna*, capers, and chopped sweet onion for tapas, or with Spanish cheese, and fry in olive oil. Piquillos make a delicious side dish stuffed with cooked rice, chives, currants, and pine nuts, or as a coulis served with roasted quail (see recipe in this chapter).

ÑORAS are dried peppers that offer a slightly fruity taste. As explained in the previous Pantry section, after reconstituting in hot water—the meager meaty part is scraped out, pounded and combined with other ingredients such as nuts and EVOO to make sauces. Ñoras also are used to flavor stews. Sometimes I leave the skin on when I use them with garlic, as when frying bread to season romesco sauce.

CHORICEROS, a favorite of the Basques, are mild, slightly sweet/pungent in taste, and also require reconstitution in hot water. The pulp is added to all sorts of recipes including stews, red beans, and even spicy tomato sauce to serve with garbanzo, cabbage and sausage stew. These reconstituted peppers or the more convenient paste (available from Spanish food importers, see Resource Guide) is outstanding, and can be used for marmitako, a seafarer's stew. The classic Basque Vizcayan sauce is made from choricero pulp, cooked with fried chopped onions, and peeled tomatoes with garlic.

Spanish Sherry Insights: Expert on Spanish wines and gastronomy, author Gerry Dawes, suggests the following:

- *Manzanilla* or *fino* sherry for dishes such as gambas al ajillo (garlic shrimp) or paired with grilled shellfish and a wide variety of tapas.
- Dry *amontillados* (many amontillados are sweetened) for tapas and mushroom dishes.
- Sweetened amontillados, for asparagus, artichokes, and cheeses.
- Dry *olorosos* for mushroom dishes; to add to sautéed red peppers with garlic as an accompaniment to beef, pork, chicken, and game dishes; and with cheeses.
- Cream sherries with cheeses and nuts, or combine with orange juice and add to sliced strawberries.

The sauce is thickened with bread and flavored with a little pimentón. There are many versions of this historic Basque sauce. José Angel Iturbe, author of *La Salsa Vizcaína*, 2009 (essentially all about choricero sauce), explained that *salsa vizcaína*, choricero peppers combined with sweet red onions, is "to be cooked for 4-5 hours." Intriguing, right? You might want to grow this hard-to-find pepper yourself. See Resource Guide to order choricero seeds.

PADRÓN peppers, when in season, can be shipped to your door by a Spanish food importer. Roast them in coarse salt for tapas; however, as explained earlier, once in a while a padrón can be extremely hot, so watch out.

GUINDILLA peppers are mild, pungent, with a slightly fruity flavor and make their way to the United States, usually in jars.

RECIPES

TAPAS / PINTXOS

Gathering with family and friends to enjoy simple, fresh food epitomizes Spain's Mediterranean diet. Tapas and Basque pintxos are traditional in this way of life. Be sure to enjoy with Spanish wines.

When you offer something impromptu, tapas and pintxos presentations can be simple. Try for example, olives with herbs and a little Spanish cheese served with mini bread sticks (*picos de pan*) or slices of membrillo with Manchego, speared on toothpicks. A kind of sandwich, *bocadillos* are really good baguettes that can be filled with all kinds of tasty offerings like pate, cheese, jamón, or eggs. Vegetarian offerings work, too, such as zucchini with tomato sauce or mushrooms. If you splurge, Spanish food importers offer inspiring choices, such as jarred or canned seafood, including bonito del norte tuna,

> Pintxos, the Basque equivalent to tapas, obtained its tag from the wooden picks used to spear the food, but one can also find pintxos on slices of toasted or untoasted bread (*montaditos*) or on small plates.

> TIP: Manzanilla or queen olives stuffed with anchovies make a popular tapas/pintxos offering, and are available from Spanish food importers. See Resource Guide.

scallops in tomato and paprika sauce called *salsa gallega* from Galicia, and Cantabrian anchovies packed in extra-virgin olive oil. Mild white boquerones (anchovies packed in vinegar) can be speared with a pitted manzanilla olive and a guindilla pepper, making "Gilda" lollipop pintxos, named after Rita Hayworth, (see recipe below). When ingredients are skewered together, the presentation is known as a *banderilla*.

Olives, artisan seafood, cheeses, and Marcona almonds all from Spain are outstanding, as are breads and crisps. Galician bread from Lugo, *barra cantábrica*, is extra airy and made with authentic local yeast. *Tortas de aceite* crisps made with olive oil are habit-forming.

Gilda

(Serves 1)

Pickonus.com offers eco-friendly bamboo spears, perfect for pintxos.

Serving suggestions: place Gilda "lollipops" in a small bowl (one to a bowl) filled with a little tomato juice mixed with EVOO and a pinch of cayenne as dipping sauce. *Topa* is Basque for Cheers!

1 wooden appetizer spear
1 pickled guindilla pepper
1 manzanilla olive, pitted
1 boquerone anchovy filet
Optional: Add 1 small cornichon pickle, or 1 large caper.

Skewer ingredients on the spear and serve.

Pa Amb Tomàquet

(Serves 2)

This recipe must be made with great bread. Catalans, who invented pa amb tomàquet, often eat it for breakfast, maybe topped with a sliver of jamón. If you are vegetarian, do not fear. Pa amb tomàquet is excellent by itself.

Toast thin slices of artisan country-style bread under a broiler until each slice is light golden. Rub first with a peeled garlic clove and then with a halved, very ripe tomato, so that the pulp saturates the toasted bread. Anoint with EVOO, sprinkle with salt and serve.

Tapenade

(1½ cups)

Tapenade can be served with bread sticks for tapas, or enjoyed as a sandwich spread.

- 1¼ cups of black olives
- 3 tablespoons of capers
- 2 cloves of garlic
- Optional: 2 boquerones (anchovies), torn into pieces
- 6 tablespoons of EVOO
- 1 tablespoon of Pommery Moutard de Meaux, or another country-style mustard
- ⅓ teaspoon of minced fresh thyme leaves, pulled from the sprig
- 1 package of picos bread sticks (tiny Spanish bread sticks)

Pit olives and place in a food processor. Add the rest of the ingredients, except for the EVOO and thyme, and process for 10 seconds or less. Slowly add the EVOO; process several moments more. Then add the thyme just before processing is finished. Serve with picos bread sticks.

Fifty years ago, allergic reaction to gluten was virtually unheard of. Since then in the United States, an entire industry has developed around gluten-free foods, the value of which is expected to reach $33 billion by 2025. Currently three million Americans suffer from celiac disease, a severe gluten intolerance, and another eighteen million show symptoms. Master herbalist/nutritionist Donnie Yance, in a 2019 report posted on his blog, "Glyphosates, Not Gluten is the True Villain," pointed out that the problem with wheat, barley and rye is not gluten content, but rather how far we have drifted away from consuming pure, unadulterated food. Consider farming methods. GMO or not, most grains are grown in nutrient depleted soil, and worse, subjected to pesticides and herbicides including most prominently, glyphosate, which in 2015, the World Health Organization classified as a probable human carcinogen. The result is an alteration in the natural structure of the grain with effects that we are only now beginning to understand. By the time the grain is harvested, processed/packaged, warehoused and finally on store shelves, it will have been stripped of nutrients and become rancid. And then, of course, there is the finished product, including bread and other baked goods. Much of the time, they contain refined sugar, and health-bashing vegetable oils.

Roasted Marcona Almonds with Rosemary

(Makes 1½ cups)

There is always a bag of blanched Marcona almonds in my pantry. I roast and sprinkle crushed over sautéed/steamed vegetables, or whole, dusted with salt and herbs for guests. I'm still discovering new ways to cook with Marcona almonds, for their mellow, sweet flavor is unique among nuts.

> 1½ cups of unroasted blanched Marcona almonds
> 1 rosemary sprig
> 1½ teaspoons of salt
> EVOO

Blanched Marcona almonds can be purchased from Spanish food importers. Mince the rosemary. In a large fry pan, sauté the almonds, rosemary, and salt in EVOO. When almonds are golden, remove from pan and put in a bowl. Taste. Adjust salt, toss, and serve.

Antonia's *Tortilla Española*

(Serves 6-8)

For a classic tapas or brunch, enjoy this recipe contributed by Liz Stell, in memory of her mother, Antonia Perez Bruchhof, from La Coruña, Galicia. Thank you, Liz. If you are serving this as a tapas, cut into small squares.

> 1 tablespoon plus about 2 cups of EVOO
> 1 medium yellow onion, thinly sliced
> 6 medium waxy potatoes (about 2 pounds), peeled,
> quartered, and thinly sliced
> 8 large eggs
> Salt to taste

Heat 1 tablespoon EVOO in a large skillet over medium-high heat. Add onion and sauté, stirring occasionally until it begins to caramelize, which will take 10–12 minutes. Let cool slightly. Meanwhile, heat about ½ an inch of oil in a large skillet (cast iron preferred) over medium heat. When oil is hot, add potatoes and more oil if necessary until potatoes are completely covered, season with salt, and cook uncovered on low, lifting and turning, until potatoes are tender but have not taken on any color, about 20 minutes. Let cool slightly.

While potatoes are cooking, beat eggs and season with salt. Add caramelized onion. Diced ham could also be added. Transfer sautéed potatoes with a slotted spoon into egg mixture. (Save oil for later use.) Combine egg mixture, potatoes, and ¼ cup reserved oil in a large bowl and gently mix with a fork. Allow to sit for about 20 minutes.

In the same skillet used to cook the potatoes, heat 3 tablespoons of reserved oil over medium-low heat. Add egg/potato mixture, spreading potatoes evenly. Reduce to low heat and cook uncovered, lifting at edges and tilting skillet to let uncooked egg run underneath, until bottom and edges of tortilla are set but center is still wet, about 6-8 minutes.

Gently shake skillet so tortilla doesn't stick, then slide a spatula along the edges and underneath tortilla. Set a large plate on top of skillet. Swiftly invert tortilla onto plate. (Some egg may spill and it will be messy, but that's okay.) Add 1 teaspoon reserved oil to skillet, then slide tortilla back into skillet, cooked side up. Use spatula to reshape edges of tortilla. Cook uncovered until center is just set, about 2 minutes longer. The secret is to leave the eggs slightly undercooked to give the tortilla a custardy texture. Cut into small squares and serve at room temperature.

Celery Stalks Stuffed with Asturian Blue Cabrales Cheese, Apples, and Walnuts

(Serves 8)

Cabrales, the buttery tasting Asturian blue-streaked cheese, is wonderfully rich, and less biting than Roquefort. Combine softened Cabrales with roasted pine nuts and serve on toast, or try it as a filling for celery.

4 celery stalks, cut into 4 inch pieces. Save the leaves for garnish.
A generous half-cup of cheese
5 tablespoons of chopped roasted walnut pieces
⅓ apple, peeled, cored and chopped
2 tablespoons of apple cider
2 tablespoons of cream
1 tablespoon of chopped fresh chives

Let the cheese come to room temperature. Preheat oven to 350°F. Roast the walnuts for about 8 minutes, or until they turn light golden. Set some aside to use as a garnish. Blend the softened cheese with the cider and cream, then add most of the walnut pieces, as well as the chopped apple and chives. Stuff celery with the filling, arrange the celery leaves on a serving plate and top with the Cabrales-stuffed celery. Garnish with remaining toasted walnuts and serve.

Potato and Anchovy in Gem Lettuce Leaves
(Serves 8-12)

3 heads of gem lettuce, leaves separated, washed, and dried
1 pound of small heirloom potatoes
4 cloves of garlic, minced
¾ cup of EVOO
½ teaspoon of salt
8-10 boquerones (anchovies)
½ teaspoon of freshly ground white pepper
Chives, washed, dried, and snipped into pieces

Lightly boil or steam salted potatoes until just tender. Splash with EVOO, and mash chunky style with salt and garlic. If you need to rinse the anchovies, use spring or filtered water and pat dry. If you are using boquerones, break by hand and combine with the seasoned potatoes.

Add white pepper and chives. Adjust salt. Fill lettuce leaves with a little potato/anchovy mixture, arrange on a colorful plate, and garnish with a sprinkling of chopped chives.

Poached Chicken on Endive with Saffron Yogurt

(Serves 10 for tapas, or 3 for lunch or dinner)

The chef who inspired this recipe, Papa Serra Jr., teaches cooking in Barcelona and adds a final note of surprise—a sprinkling of bee pollen. Enzyme-rich bee pollen enhances immunity and helps crush food cravings, so it is an ideal weight-management food for women. Spanish bee pollen is known to be some of the best in the world.

Clean 3 halved chicken breasts with bone in and halve again. The poaching liquid consists of 4 cups water, ⅔ cup white wine, juice from ⅓ lemon, parsley, ½ stalk celery, ½ small carrot, ½ cleaned leek, bay leaf, garlic clove, black and white peppercorns, sea salt, and 4 tablespoons EVOO. In a medium pot, bring ingredients to a boil, except for chicken, and cook for 10 minutes. Reduce heat, add chicken pieces, and simmer until chicken is just done, about 30-35 minutes. Remove chicken and drizzle with EVOO, a pinch or two of salt, and a grinding of white pepper. When cool to the touch, remove bones and cut into smaller pieces.

For the balance of the recipe, you'll need endive leaves—I suggest 2 for each half chicken breast—1 small onion, chopped and sautéed until caramelized, a handful of sliced red grapes and toasted almond slivers, 2 pinches of fennel seeds and a pinch or two of Spanish bee pollen. For the yogurt sauce, mix 3 pinches of crushed saffron threads—steeped in 2 teaspoons of hot spring or filtered water for 5-10 minutes—with ½ cup or so of yogurt. In a large bowl, combine the chicken, caramelized onions, saffron yogurt sauce, fennel seeds, grapes, almond slivers, and lemon zest. Fill endive leaves and serve, but not before adding Serra's final note: Bee pollen is one of the most nutrient-dense foods available.

Dried Salt Cod Croquetas

(Serves 8)

1 pound of salt cod
1¼ pounds of small potatoes
1¼ cups of milk
4 shallots, chopped
2 cloves of garlic, minced
A few pinches of pimentón
Salt, ground white pepper to taste
A handful of flat-leaf parsley, cleaned, dried and chopped
Juice of ½ lemon
2 beaten eggs
Flour for dusting
3½ ounces of breadcrumbs
EVOO (enough for shallow frying)

Soak salt cod in water for 24–48 hours, skin side up. Drain and add fresh water 3–4 times to remove salt. Cod will reconstitute and become plump. Sample a small piece—it should not taste salty. Pat dry. Cook unpeeled potatoes in lightly salted boiling water for 20 minutes. When cool, drain, peel, and mash. Combine milk and shallots in a medium-size pan and bring to a simmer. Add reconstituted cod and a swirl of EVOO, and poach gently for 12 minutes. Remove cod and flake into a bowl, discarding any bones and skin. Gradually mix in mashed potatoes, parsley, garlic, lemon juice, white pepper, a few pinches of pimentón and beaten egg. Blend well. Adjust seasonings, then chill the entire mixture until firm. Shape into 18 balls. Flatten into cakes. Coat each croqueta with a dusting of flour, and then dip into second beaten egg and dust with breadcrumbs. Chill until ready to cook. Heat about ½ inch of EVOO in a large pan but don't let the oil smoke. Add croquetas and fry each side until golden. Drain and serve with tartar dip and wedges of lemon over mixed salad greens with olives.

Manchego Cheese Topped with Quince Membrillo

(Serves 10)

The following tapas can be made in a flash.

1¼ pound wedge of Manchego cheese, with the rind removed
1 container of quince membrillo paste

Cut the cheese into ¼ inch thick triangles. Arrange on a serving plate and top with thin slices of membrillo.

Garlic Shrimp Cazuela

(Serves 6)

Garlic shrimp, or *gambas al ajillo*, is often found in tapas bars. Serve right from the cazuela, or transfer to small plates.

¾ pound of small shrimp, shelled
½ dried chili pepper, seeds removed
⅓ teaspoon of cumin
3 tablespoons of garlic, minced
2 tablespoons of parsley, cleaned, dried and finely chopped
2 tablespoons of dry white wine
EVOO
Salt

Clean shrimp and dry. Put on a plate, sprinkle lightly with salt, and set aside for 10 minutes. In a cazuela, sauté garlic in EVOO. When the garlic begins to turn golden, add the shrimp, parsley, cumin and chili pepper. Cook and toss shrimp until they just turn opaque. Add the white wine and cook for a couple minutes more. Serve right in the cazuela.

Gazpacho

(Serves 6)

Whenever you make gazpacho, remember the quality of tomatoes rule. And don't think of gazpacho just for lunch. This life-extending soup makes a great summer breakfast. When serving gazpacho as a part of tapas, it's fun to use small shot glasses.

5 medium-sized, very flavorful, ripe tomatoes, coarsely chopped
1 medium-sized green pepper, deseeded, deribbed,
    and coarsely chopped
1 medium-sized sweet onion, coarsely chopped
1 medium-sized Kirby cucumber, peeled and coarsely chopped
2 teaspoons of garlic, chopped
1 cup of mild EVOO (hojiblanca, from Andalucia)
4 cups of cold water
¼ cup of white wine vinegar
2 tablespoons of sherry vinegar
3 teaspoons of salt
4 cups of coarsely chopped crustless, day-old country-style bread
Garnish: finely chopped green pepper, onions, and cucumber

Using a big bowl, combine chopped vegetables, garlic, and bread. Add the salt, cumin, sugar, tomato paste, and water. In a blender on high speed for a minute or two, blend a couple of cups of the mixture at a time, adding olive oil as you go. When finished, add vinegar, taste and adjust salt. Put into a bowl covered with plastic wrap and refrigerate for a couple of hours. Before serving, stir and then ladle into serving bowls or spoon into shot glasses and garnish.

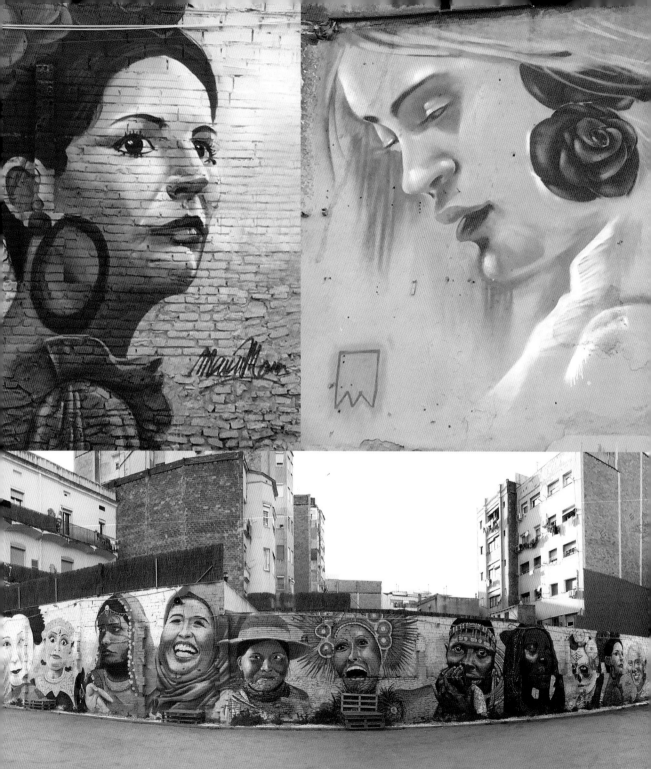

Barcelona street art mural, M'agraden les mares
I dones del món sencer, Manu Manu.

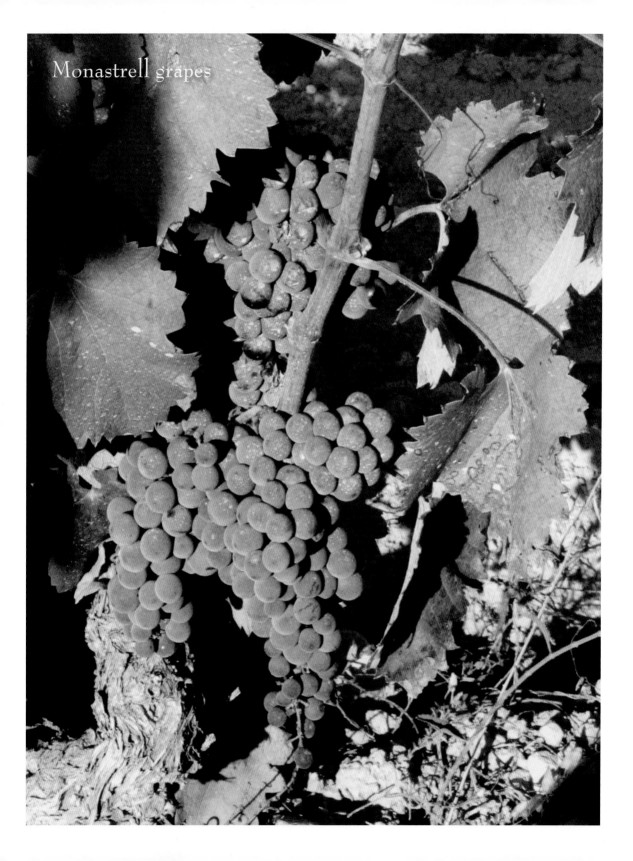

Monastrell grapes

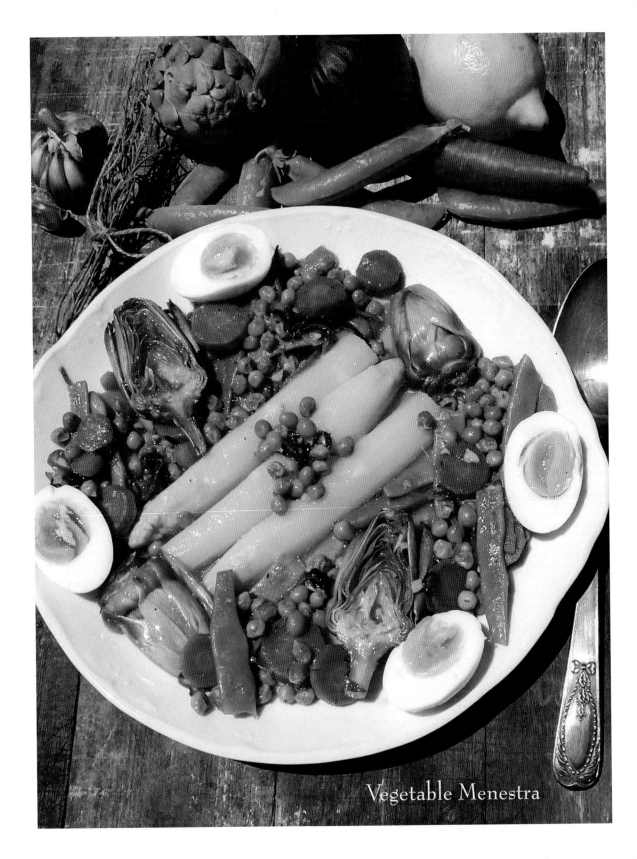

Vegetable Menestra

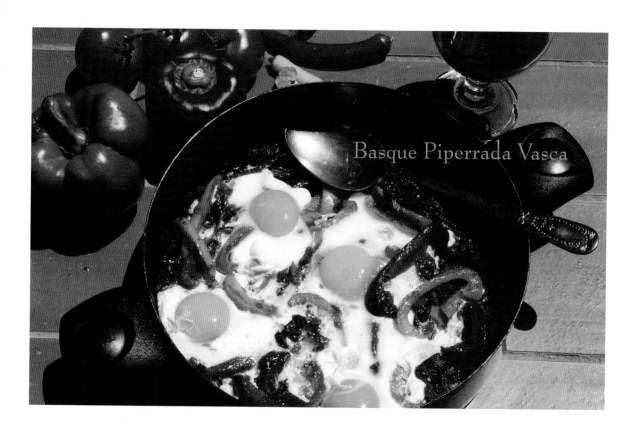

Basque Piperrada Vasca

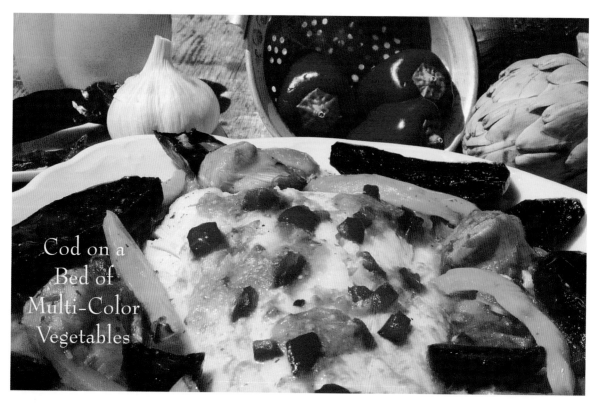

Cod on a
Bed of
Multi-Color
Vegetables

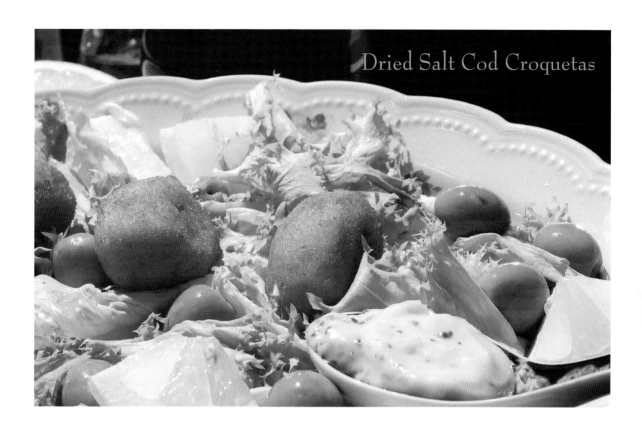
Dried Salt Cod Croquetas

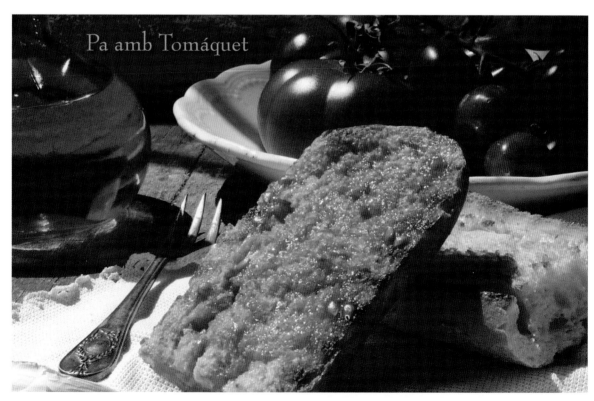
Pa amb Tomáquet

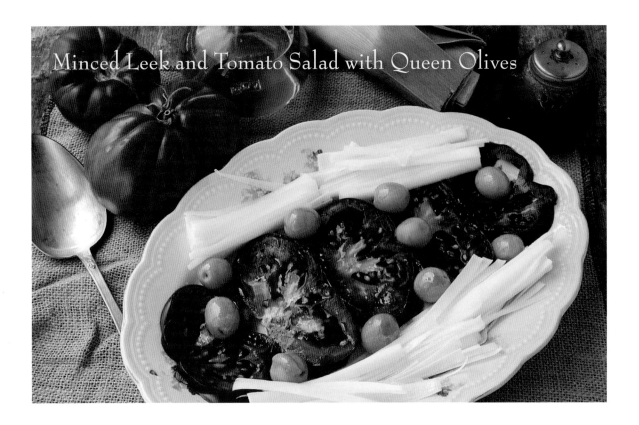

Minced Leek and Tomato Salad with Queen Olives

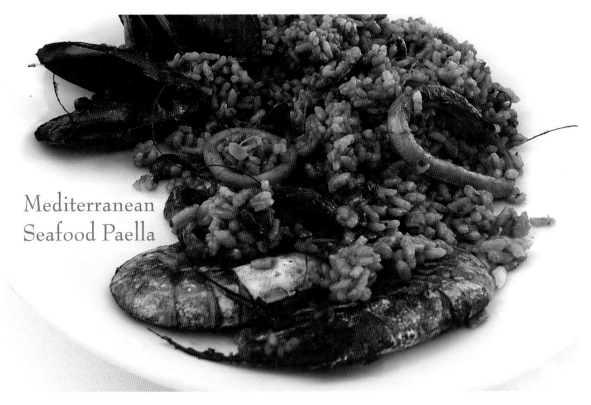

Mediterranean
Seafood Paella

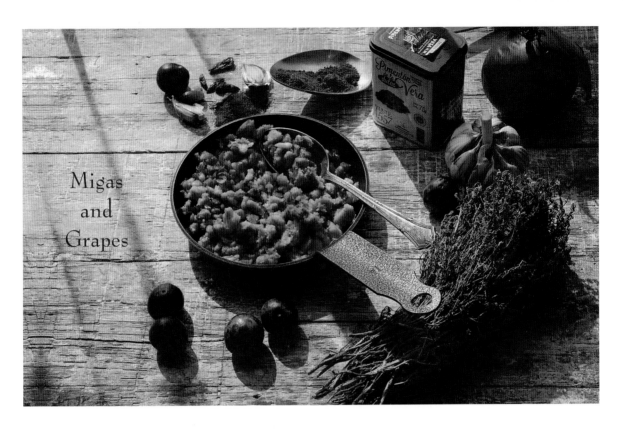

Migas
and
Grapes

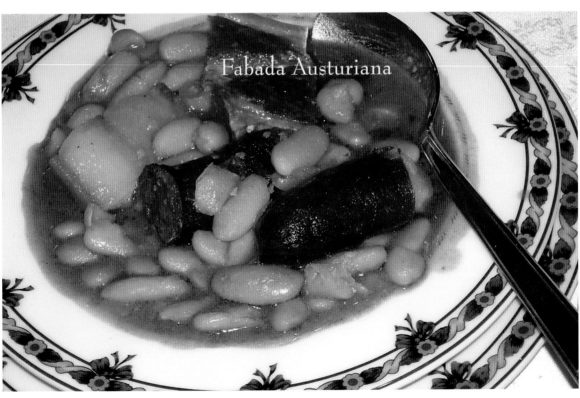

Fabada Austuriana

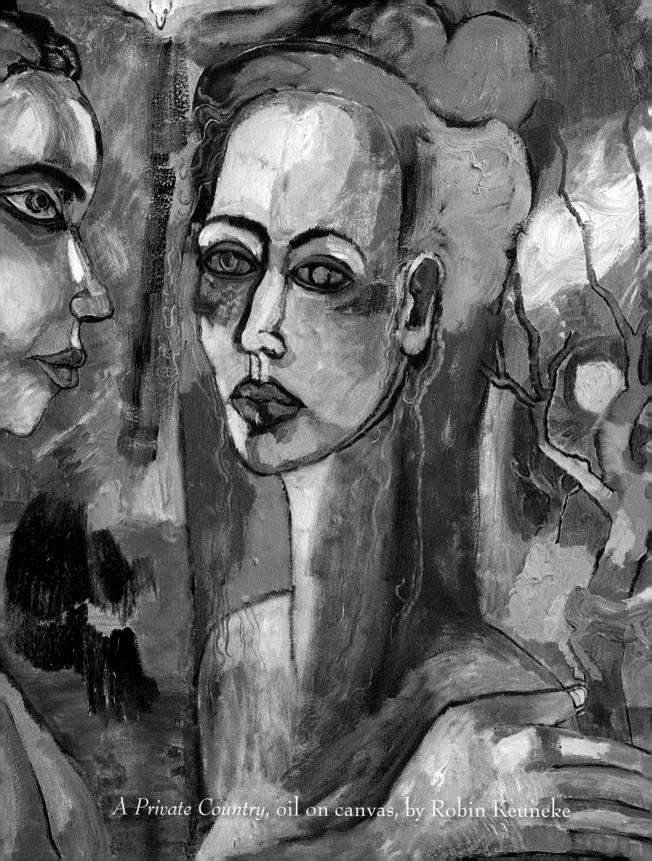

A Private Country, oil on canvas, by Robin Keuneke

BREAKFAST/BRUNCH

Basque *Piperrada Vasca* of Orange and Yellow Bell Peppers and Eggs

(Serves 4)

EVOO
Minced pancetta (optional)
1 cup of red, orange, and yellow bell peppers cut into thin strips
1 large yellow onion, sliced (about 1½ cups)
4 garlic cloves, minced
2 large tomatoes cut into bite-size pieces
6 large eggs, from cage-free hens
Salt, pepper

In a large skillet or a cazuela, sauté onion, half the garlic, and the peppers in EVOO for 15-20 minutes, seasoning with salt and pepper, and taking care to stir with a wooden spoon at intervals to prevent onions and peppers from burning. Remove. In the same pan slicked with plenty of EVOO, sauté remaining cloves of garlic (and pancetta) for about 5-7 minutes. Add tomatoes, season lightly with salt and a grinding of pepper. Continue sautéing until tomatoes soften. Stir in the peppers/onions. Break and arrange eggs over the mixture of tomatoes, peppers, and onions and salt lightly. Take care not to overcook. The yolks should be runny.

Migas and Grapes with Romaine Lettuce Leaves

(Serves 4)

In northern Spain, shepherds used to nibble these little treats while tending their flock. Migas are so good that citrus pickers still make them in communal pans. There are many ways to make migas—some with jamón, but our version is vegan. Migas are tasty, served with wine, as part of tapas, too.

> 1 pound of day-old dense country bread (do not remove crusts)
> 6 garlic cloves, crushed
> ½ teaspoon of sweet pimentón
>   and a couple of pinches of hot pimentón
> ¼ cup of EVOO
> Salt and pepper
> Romaine lettuce, washed and dried
> Red grapes

Cut the bread into strips, then into small bite-sized cubes, and place in a bowl. In a separate bowl, combine water with salt and pimentón. Lightly sprinkle the seasoned water throughout the bread and cover with a cloth, leaving for several hours or overnight. In a large pan, sauté garlic in EVOO for about 3 minutes, stirring the whole time. When the garlic is golden, remove from pan and discard. Add bread to EVOO, season with pimentón, and fry for about 20 to 30 minutes, breaking up into crumbs while you stir. The crumbs should turn crisp and golden and end up the size of garbanzo beans, but they'll remain soft on the inside. By the end of cooking, the oil will be soaked up by the crumbs—you will be stirring crumbs in a dry pan. Set aside to cool. Arrange by topping the romaine leaves with the migas and grapes.

Iberian Egg Salad Flavored with Pimentón and Garnished with Cornicabra Olives

(Serves 2)

The mayonnaise in this recipe should be an organic brand. Egg salad roll-ups make an easy, nourishing, and tasty lunch, especially accompanied by olives.

4 eggs from cage-free hens, hardboiled
1 stalk of celery, chopped
2 small mild onions, chopped
¼ cup of mayonnaise
1 teaspoon of pimentón
¼ teaspoon of salt
¼ teaspoon of ground pepper
Olives for garnish

Take care not to overboil eggs; yolks should be cooked until just done. In a medium-sized wooden bowl, chop eggs. Add mayonnaise, salt, pepper, pimentón, celery, and onions.

Herby Romaine Boats with Cheese and Peaches

(Serves 1)

Choose from Manchego, Roncal, or Idiazábal cheese. Crisp romaine leaves make the perfect vessel for interesting salads, so I devised this easy lunch that marries with fresh stone fruit—wonderful in summer when at their peak. If you crave something more substantial, add a little thinly sliced turkey or ham.

2 scallions cleaned, trimmed, and cut into diagonal pieces
1 tablespoon of rinsed, minced fresh basil or dill
Thin shaving of Manchego, Roncal or Idiazábal cheese
2 medium washed and dried crisp leaves of romaine lettuce
Salt and ground black pepper
1 fresh, ripe peach or nectarine
Your favorite vinagreta

Arrange the romaine leaves on a plate and season with salt and pepper. Add vinagreta, scallions, minced herbs, and top with thin shavings of cheese. Rinse, dry, slice the fruit, and serve together on the romaine leaves with the cheese and herbs.

Basque Mushroom Ragout with Egg Yolk Sauce

(Serves 4)

"Chairs should be set up at all universities, to prevent the loss of anything to do with the Basques. Such a move would benefit everyone. It is the only means we have of knowing what words are the oldest in Europe, perhaps the world."

– Alan H. Kelson de Montigyni,
Secretary, International Anthropology & Linguistic Circle, Philadelphia.

Select your favorite mushrooms. For this recipe, I chose shiitake, king trumpet, and maitake.

1¼ pounds of mixed mushrooms
2 cloves of garlic, minced
EVOO
Salt, pepper
4 egg yolks from cage-free hens (room temperature)
Optional: truffle oil

My preferred way to clean mushrooms is lightly with a damp clean cloth, and then dried with care. I do not use paper towels on my food, since the paper is likely to be treated with chemicals. Cut the larger mushrooms into chunks so that you have a medley of whole mushrooms and chunks of mushrooms. In a medium-size cazuela, sauté the garlic and mushrooms in EVOO for 10 minutes, seasoned with a little salt and pepper. Make sure you do not crowd the pan since the mushrooms must cook evenly. Turn gently, add more EVOO, a touch more salt and pepper, and continue sautéing for another 5-10 minutes. Add the yolks, and salt lightly. When yolks are warm to the touch but still runny, about a minute, remove the pan from the flame.

Wild Salmon Salad with Pimentón

(Serves 3)

In my kitchen, ingredients for this recipe always seem to be on hand, making it a lunch salad standby. Especially delicious when served with grapes.

1 six-ounce piece of cooked salmon
1 stalk of celery, chopped
1 small mild onion, chopped
1 teaspoon of sweet pimentón
3 tablespoons of good-quality health food store mayonnaise
Spanish sherry vinegar
Salt, ground white pepper
Broccoli sprouts

Mix salmon into bowl, separating with a fork. Add other ingredients, and finish with a spritz of sherry vinegar and a garnish of sprouts.

Optional: 1 boiled egg. I especially like to add an egg during winter, when vitamin D levels fall from lack of sunlight. Best to leave the yolk a bit runny; it adds richness and combines well with the mayonnaise.

Salad of Clementinas, Fennel, and Roncal Cheese, with Sherry Vinagreta

(Serves 6)

If you love fennel, add more than the recipe calls for. If you prefer avocado instead of cheese, have a go. With ingredients that are fresh, you can't lose.

4 peeled and segmented clementinas
1 fennel bulb—washed and thinly sliced
½ thinly sliced sweet onion
12 black olives, with pits
1 head of bibb lettuce, separated, rinsed and dried well,
    with outer leaves discarded
Ribbons of Roncal cheese—use a vegetable grater for slicing

Arrange lettuce leaves at the bottom of a platter. Combine all ingredients, except for the cheese and arrange artfully on top of the lettuce. Garnish with ribbons of Roncal.

CLEMENTINA VINAGRETA:
⅓ cup of EVOO
2 tablespoons of sherry vinegar
Juice from 2 clementinas
Sea salt and ground black pepper

Combine and spoon over salad.

SOUPS

Red Lentil Soup with Chorizo

(Serves 10)

1 cup of rinsed red lentils
2 large chopped yellow onions
2 quarts of organic chicken or vegetable stock
1 quart of filtered or spring water
¾ cup of minced carrots

1 shallot, peeled and chopped

3 cloves of garlic, crushed and minced

2 chorizos, diced

Several pinches of thyme

2 bay leaves

Several pinches of sweet pimentón

Pulp from 3 reconstituted choricero peppers,
    or 1½ tablespoons of choricero pepper pulp

Salt and pepper

EVOO

Using the method described at the beginning of this chapter, reconstitute the peppers. Then remove pulp with a spoon and set aside in a tiny bowl. In a heavy soup pot sauté chopped onions in a generous amount of EVOO. Add salt, 1 bay leaf, a little pepper and garlic. The onions will turn deep golden after about 35-40 minutes. During caramelizing, be sure to stir with wooden spatula or spoon, and when the onions just come to color add the chorizo. After 10 minutes more, add remaining ingredients. Stir. Add water and bring to a boil. Reduce heat to a low boil for the first hour, then reduce heat again and simmer for 1½ more hours, stirring at intervals, and taking care to skim the surface. In the last hour, add the choricero pepper pulp. Taste. Adjust seasonings by adding EVOO and, if necessary, more salt, pepper. Continue cooking for 30 minutes more.

Gabure: Vegetable Soup with Beans, Chestnuts, and Sausage

(Serves 6)

Though gabure is an ancient French recipe, I was introduced to this rich soup in Aragón, which borders France. The noodles in the version I had gave the dish distinctive Aragonese character. Janet Mendel offers another recipe in her *Cooking in Spain*.

TIP: Look for packaged organic Galician chestnuts. See Resource Guide.

Since there are many versions, make gabure your own. It can be cooked vegetarian style, or with pieces of lamb, chicken, or pork sausage, and ham or lamb bone. Even chicken bones can be used. Regardless, toward the end I like gabure with tiny noodles, which reminds me of Aragón.

Choose vegetables according to the season. In the fall, add chestnuts. Pick your favorite combination of herbs and spices to complement the meats, beans, and vegetables. In the spring, try a touch of fresh lemon juice at the end, and include a green such as chard.

INGREDIENTS:
Select vegetables and meat from each category, according to the season. Chop vegetables:

Summer/Spring: bok choy, chard, pole beans, shelled *fava* beans, peas, zucchini, small heirloom potatoes, patty pan or yellow squash; large peeled tomatoes, 1 pound of dried red lentils, 2 cups of precooked white or garbanzo beans; artisan lamb or pork sausages cut into bite-sized pieces.

Winter/Fall: parsnips, chestnuts, turnips, carrots, pumpkin, hard squash, yellow onion, potatoes, cabbage, cauliflower, leeks, celery root; 2 cups of precooked navy or garbanzo beans, artisan lamb, pork or duck sausage cut into bite-sized pieces.

THE METHOD: In a deep soup pot, begin by sautéing 1 large chopped yellow onion and 1 bay laurel leaf in EVOO. Season with thyme, salt, and pepper. Onions should be golden. If you are preparing the soup with meat bones, brown them along with the onions. In a separate large sauté pan add a glug of EVOO and sauté vegetables with a little chopped pancetta. Season with a touch more thyme and rosemary, along with salt and pepper. Do not add delicate vegetables, such as peas, until final stage of cooking. To the deep soup pot, with the caramelized onions, add 2-3 quarts of organic free-range chicken or vegetable stock. Add the sautéed vegetables and beans, along with pieces of meat, sausages, garlic, and herbs to the liquid. Season with salt and ground pepper, and one more bay *laurel* leaf. Bring to a boil and simmer uncovered for 1½ hours, stirring occasionally with a wooden spoon. Add the potatoes and chestnuts and continue to simmer for 40 minutes more. Build flavor by tasting, adjusting the seasonings along the way. Remove the foam. For noodles, precook and combine in the final 10 minutes of cooking, along with delicate vegetables such as peas.

Caldo Gallego or Bean Soup with Turnip Greens and Lacinato Kale

(Serves 6-8)

Caldo gallego, or Galician soup, is a rural dish that is sustaining enough to be dinner, especially when topped with migas or a slice of fried bread. If you prefer a vegan approach, eliminate the bones, cubed ham, etc. Smoky pimentón, caramelized onions, garlic, and good Spanish olive oil add robust flavor making this hearty dish soul-satisfying.

½ pound of dried Great Northern beans

1 pound of pork bones

1 beef bone

1 pound of mixed turnip greens and kale, cleaned, trimmed, and broken into pieces

1 trimmed and chopped leek

2 large onions, chopped

1 turnip, peeled and cut into chunks

6 cloves of garlic, crushed

1 pound of red potatoes, cut into small to medium cubes

⅓ cup of EVOO

1 teaspoon of salt, ground black and white pepper to taste

2 teaspoons of pimentón

3-4 pinches of dried thyme

1 sprig of fresh rosemary

3 bay leaves

A generous grinding or two of nutmeg

3 quarts of organic chicken bone broth
  or stock

Spring or filtered water

2 cups of diced ham or equal amount
  of vegan sausage

TIP: You may remember, I told you about the many benefits of bone broth. Studies show that bone broth encourages immunity, strong bones, and the formation of collagen for better hair, skin, and nails, so cook with bone broth often.

Rinse beans, cover with water, and soak overnight. The next day, drain and place in a large soup pot. Cover with a mixture of 3 parts chicken stock and 1 part water, or vegetable stock and water. Stock and water mixture should cover beans by about 4 inches.

Add the pork and beef bones, a sprig of rosemary, a splash of EVOO, 2 cloves garlic, 1 teaspoon of pimentón, and 1 bay leaf. Bring to a boil, lower heat, and simmer for 30 minutes, skimming foam off while beans cook. Add the thyme and mix with wooden paddle. Set aside.

In a large sauté pan, begin caramelizing the onions and potatoes in EVOO, with 2 more cloves of garlic, 1 bay leaf, seasoning with salt and pepper, and a second teaspoon of pimentón. This will take about 35 minutes. Aim for a light caramelization.

Add potatoes and onions to the pot of beans, and, if necessary, more water to ensure all ingredients are covered with liquid by at least 3 inches. Bring to a boil and cook gently for 40 minutes, uncovered, stirring at intervals with a wooden spoon, and skimming off foam. Add another pinch or two of dried thyme.

Meanwhile, separately sauté the turnip greens, kale and the remaining garlic in a generous splash of EVOO. After the greens begin to wilt, add the chopped leek. Season with salt, and a generous amount of black and white pepper, and sauté for 5 minutes more.

Add the greens and leek mixture to pot of beans, with the cubed ham or vegan sausage. Stir and continue cooking for 1 hour on medium, uncovered. As the soup cooks, add another splash of EVOO. If you like greens to be well done, cook longer. Remove the bones, taste and adjust seasonings, including the nutmeg, pepper, and perhaps a final dusting of pimentón. Top with a piece of bread fried in EVOO with a clove of garlic, or migas.

Lobster Soup

(Serves 4-6)

This recipe is given by Michelin-starred chef/restaurateur María José San Román. Her restaurant, Monastrell in Alicante on the Costa Blanca, is highly regarded in Spanish culinary circles. Thank you, chef María Jose San Román.

    2 quarts of spring water
    1 fennel bulb, finely diced
    1 small onion, diced
    1 teaspoon of salt
    ½ teaspoon of black pepper
    EVOO
    1 lobster
    1 pound of fresh clams
    ½ cup of white flour
    1 ripe tomato, diced
    2 good pinches of saffron powder
    1 bay leaf

Cook the lobster for one minute in boiling water. Remove and cool it down in ice water. Remove the meat from the shell and dice. In a large pot, fry the onion and fennel in EVOO until golden. Add the tomato and bay leaf and cook for 5 minutes. Mix in the flour, stir well, and pour the water in the pot with the saffron. Bring to a boil and add the lobster meat. Season with salt and pepper, cook 10 minutes more, and then add the clams. Cook until clams open and serve.

SALADS

Salad of Steamed Baby Purple Potatoes over Fennel, Sweet Onion, and Capers

(Serves 4)

The pleasing bite of sweet onion sets off lemony potatoes, herby fennel, and briny capers to perfection.

6 small purple potatoes, washed
Several pinches of saffron
1 cup of cleaned and sliced fennel
½ sweet onion, sliced
EVOO
½ teaspoon of grainy country-style mustard
½ lemon
Salt, black pepper
2 tablespoons of rinsed capers

Slice potatoes and place in a steamer basket. Season with a splash of EVOO, salt, and pepper. Steam until tender; may take 20 minutes. Toward the end, add the saffron threads by crushing in your fingers. After potatoes are tender (do not overcook) remove from steamer basket and set aside on a plate. Lightly anoint with a touch more EVOO and season with a delicate sprinkling of salt. As potatoes cool, combine the fennel and onions in a shallow bowl and season with more EVOO, plenty of lemon juice, a touch of mustard, and freshly ground black pepper. Add capers and place mixture on the steamed potatoes.

Rafa's Minced Leek and Tomato Salad with Manzanilla Olives

(Serves 4)

Rafa's, a pocket-sized seafood restaurant in the coastal town of Roses near the border of France, inspired this salad, which is meant to be enjoyed when summer tomatoes reach perfection. The olives provide a savory/salty element, so no need to use much salt, but do pick your sharpest knife. In my version of this salad, I use more leeks than Rafa; however I recommend that they be sliced thin.

½ leek, trimmed
1 large ripe tomato
8 Manzanilla olives
1 to 3 teaspoons of sherry or red wine vinegar
1 to 2 tablespoon of EVOO
2 teaspoons of lemon juice
Salt, ground black pepper

The inner section of the leek is used for this recipe, so remove outer leaves as well as the stalky parts at the top. Cut the inner section in half, lengthwise, and take care to rinse well. Dry and slice the leek paper-thin, and set aside. Slice tomato and arrange slices on plate in a circle and add the minced leeks to the center. Salt very lightly and add the vinegar and EVOO to taste. Finally, squeeze fresh lemon over everything, and surround with Manzanilla olives.

Evohe's Cured Organic Goat Cheese Salad with Roasted Pine Nuts and Membrillo Vinagreta

(Serves 4)

"From early times, Spanish food has been enriched by the different cultures that arrived in the area where the Basques and Iberians, believed by some historians to have been the original inhabitants of the peninsula, were already living. Cereals and peas moving westwards across the Mediterranean began feeding the Iberian across the Mediterranean and southern Atlantic coast and Celts in the north and northwest of the peninsula, where they would settle to raise animals and cultivate the land."

– María José Sevilla, *Delicioso, A History of Food in Spain*

This inventive recipe is created by Eva Espinet and Olga Moya, two home cooks living in Barcelona. For visitors to their city, these women offer a five-course home-cooked dinner (with wines) in a stylish flat, an experience that exemplifies the richness of their cultures more than any restaurant. Both are fluent in English, and their cooking uses the finest local products. As a teaser, Eva and Olga serve this salad with pa amb tomàquet. See Trip Advisor, Evohe Barcelona.

SALAD INGREDIENTS:

6 cups of salad greens, rinsed and dried

4 ounces of organic aged goat cheese, cut into thin slices

4 tablespoons of pine nuts

MEMBRILLO VINAGRETA:

2 tablespoons of quince membrillo paste

3 tablespoons of EVOO

1 tablespoon of Modena balsamic vinegar

1 teaspoon of country-style Dijon mustard

Salt, pepper

In a small sauté pan, heat 1 tablespoon of EVOO and carefully brown the pine nuts by gently stirring with a wooden spoon until lightly golden in color. Take care not to burn. Remove and set aside to cool. Combine vinagreta ingredients. The membrillo does not need to be finely pureed—it is quite good when it retains texture. Dress the salad greens with a drizzle of olive oil, salt and pepper. Toss lightly and add the roasted pine nuts and vinagreta. Immediately top with slices of cheese and, if you want, some additional slices of membrillo for color.

Mediterranean pine nuts, know in Spain as *piñones reales*, distinctive because of their elongated shape, have amazing health attributes and are better for us than regular pine nuts. By comparison, *piñones reales* contain more protein, have a higher concentration of balanced omega-3 to omega-6 fats, and are lower in calories.

Long Life Andorra Onion and Honey Salad

(Serves 6)

Grab your sharpest knife. Onions with potent anticancer compounds are waiting. Science confirms the fresher the onion, the more potent the protective compounds. This bold salad is a signature dish of the Andorrans, who have, on average, one of the longest life expectancies in the world.

3 onions, coarsely chopped
1 cup of black olives
2 tablespoons of chopped flat-leafed parsley
Salt, pepper
3 tablespoons of white wine vinegar
4 tablespoons of EVOO
1 tablespoon of honey

Remove pits from olives and set aside. Whisk the honey into the olive oil and vinegar and season with salt and pepper. Spoon the vinagreta over the chopped onions and marinate for one hour. Combine the pitted olives with the onions and vinagreta, garnish with parsley and serve.

Pipirrana Salad of Cucumber, Green Pepper, Sweet Onion, and Scallions

(Serves 4)

This salad is widely popular in southern Spain where the climate is *cálido*.

1 chopped cucumber
½ chopped green pepper
½ cup of chopped sweet onion
2 scallions cut into thin diagonal slices
6 tablespoons of flat-leaf parsley
2 cups of heirloom cherry tomatoes, halved
1 clove of crushed garlic
6 tablespoons of EVOO
4 tablespoons of sherry vinegar (or red wine)
12 pitted black olives
Salt, pepper
1 teaspoon of cumin
Lemon wedges, for garnish

Rub a salad bowl with the garlic. Discard garlic. Combine all ingredients except for the seasonings and lemon wedges into the bowl. Taste to ensure the right balance of EVOO and vinegar. If not, adjust. Add salt, pepper, and cumin. Toss ingredients. Taste one final time to adjust seasonings, garnish with lemon wedges and serve.

Bonito del Norte Tuna Salad
with Green Beans, Purple Onions, and Olives

(Serves 4)

Packed in olive oil, Bonito del Norte from the North of Spain is a world beyond ordinary tuna.

1 jar (approximately 1 cup) of Bonito del Norte tuna
1 pound of washed and trimmed green beans
1½ tablespoons red wine vinegar
EVOO
1 small purple onion cut chunky style
8 olives of your choice, pitted
3 cloves crushed garlic
2 pinches saffron
1 pinch cayenne pepper
4 tablespoons chopped fresh parsley, half for garnish
Juice from ½ lemon
Salt, pepper

Place beans in a steamer basket, salt lightly, and anoint with a little EVOO. Steam for about 7 minutes. Remove beans from basket and set aside on a plate. Meanwhile, heat a swirl of EVOO in a large sauté pan and sauté 2 cloves of garlic for 3-4 minutes. Add the steamed beans and season with pepper and a little more salt. Cook beans for 10 minutes or until tender. In the final minutes, crush the threads of saffron in your fingers, and sprinkle over the sautéed beans. Continue cooking for a few minutes more. Remove beans from pan onto a large plate and let cool. Drain tuna, and after beans cool a little, combine the tuna with the beans on the serving plate along with the remaining ingredients including 2 tablespoons of EVOO. Garnish with parsley.

> TIP: To increase weekly consumption of seafood, take a cue from top chefs and incorporate products from Spain.

Salad of Softened Pear over *Arugula* with Shaved Manchego and Pear Vinagreta

(Serves 3–4)

The contrast of sweet, juicy pear with the rustic bite of Manchego against spicy *arugula* makes a unique flavor story.

3 ripe pears
Several handfuls of cleaned fresh arugula
1/3 cup of shaved aged Manchego

FOR VINAGRETA:
2 tablespoons of pear balsamic vinegar
1 teaspoon of country-style mustard
4 tablespoons of EVOO
1 minced shallot
Salt and pepper

Preheat oven to 400°F. Slice pears in half and roast for 8–10 minutes. Remove from baking dish and set aside. Toss arugula in a bowl with salt and pepper. Spoon a little vinagreta on top of the greens and arrange on plates. Place half a roasted pear on top of each serving, add a light touch more of the vinagreta, top with Manchego shavings, and serve.

VEGETABLE DISHES

Navarran Mixed Vegetable *Menestra*

(Serves 6)

Adoring every type of vegetable since I can remember, this recipe speaks to me. And, yes, it does require a few pots and pans, but some things are worth the effort. After all, if chef Elena Arzak wants her final meal to be "all vegetables, cooked separately, and prepared just right," then I'm in the best company. Be sure, however, that the vegetables are not overcooked.

Options: After all the vegetables are combined, Serrano ham or slices of hardboiled egg can be added as garnish.

2 artichokes, cleaned, trimmed, split, and quartered
1 cup of shelled and cleaned peas
8 large trimmed brussels sprouts
1 large carrot, washed and cut as you like
    (can be julienned or thin slices)
EVOO
2 cups of chicken stock or bone broth, diluted with a cup
    of spring or filtered water, making 3 cups of liquid
4 cloves of crushed garlic
1 large peeled onion, thinly sliced
Salt, black pepper, white pepper
¾ cup serrano ham, sliced into strips

In a medium-sized pot, sauté 2 cloves of crushed garlic in 2 tablespoons of EVOO. Add the brussels sprouts and season with salt and black pepper. Continue sautéing for about 10 minutes, stirring with a wooden spoon. Add the chicken stock and water mixture and cover. Continue cooking until just tender, then remove the brussels sprouts from pan and set aside in a serving bowl.

In a medium-sized pan, sauté the onion, seasoned with salt, for about 20 minutes until golden, stirring gently at intervals to insure that the onion doesn't burn. Remove and place in the bowl with the brussels sprouts.

To the same pan used to sauté the onions, salt and sauté the artichokes in a splash of EVOO, with 2 cloves of crushed garlic for about 10 minutes, stirring gently with a wooden spoon. Then add the mixture of stock/water to barely submerge, and cook artichokes, covered, for about 10 minutes or until they are tender. In a small pan, sauté the carrots in a little EVOO, a couple pinches of salt, and a little freshly ground white pepper until just tender. As with all of the vegetables, take care and do not overcook. Remove the carrots and put them in the bowl with the brussels sprouts and onion. Add the peas to the pan that was used to sauté the carrots, spoon a little EVOO over them, season gently with salt and a little white pepper, and cook until just tender. Gently combine all vegetables and serve warm. Ham or sliced hard-boiled egg is added on top as a garnish.

Rutabagas in Saffron and Honey Sauce

(Serves 4)

This recipe follows the ancient Arabic and Sephardic traditions by combining saffron with honey.

    2 medium rutabagas cleaned and cut into large bite-sized chunks
    1½ tablespoons of honey
    3 pinches of saffron threads
    1¼ cups of chicken stock or bone broth
    Salt
    2 to 3 tablespoons of EVOO

In a small saucepan, combine rutabagas, chicken stock and salt, and bring to a gentle boil. After several minutes, reduce heat to simmer.

Add EVOO, stir with a wooden spoon and cover with a bamboo sushi mat, which maintains a steady, gentle heat. Cook for 25 minutes, stirring occasionally. When rutabagas are almost tender, add the honey and stir again, gently. Then crush the threads of saffron in your fingers over the rutabagas and combine with the wooden spoon. Cover with the bamboo mat and cook a few minutes more on low, until tender.

> TIP: A bamboo sushi mat is a useful addition to your global kitchen. When used to cover a pot (or pan) of cooking food, the mat allows the food to breathe while covered in this way.

Eggplant *Samfaina*

(Serves 10)

Samfaina is so filled with sunny Mediterranean flavor that I cannot resist including another version here. The recipe in Chapter Six has anchovies. The version below contains olives and cumin.

12 large Spanish olives, pitted
5 pounds of eggplant, cut into 1-inch cubes
5 cups of onions, chopped rustic style
2 cups of zucchini, cubed
1 cup of red bell pepper, chopped
4 tablespoons of garlic, minced
1 large can of chopped organic tomatoes, drained
3 tablespoons of flat-leaf parsley, cleaned, dried and chopped
EVOO
1 teaspoon of chopped fresh thyme leaves
1 sprig of fresh rosemary
Salt
¾ teaspoon of freshly ground black pepper
½ teaspoon of red pepper flakes

This recipe requires a touch less salt because olives are added at the end. Salt the cubed eggplant and set aside. In a large skillet, sauté onions, 1 tablespoon minced garlic, and a couple pinches of salt in EVOO for about 50 minutes, stirring with a wooden spoon. Onions should be deep golden.

Drain eggplant of water, wipe with clean dishtowel to remove the excess moisture, and add to the pan with the onions, along with the pepper, zucchini, and most of the remaining garlic. Season vegetables with a pinch of salt, and ground pepper. Add herbs and a little more EVOO. Cook uncovered for 10 minutes, continuing to stir gently. Add canned tomatoes, remaining garlic, and more EVOO. Keep stirring. Cover and continue to cook until vegetables are blended. Add cumin and pimentón, adjust pepper, and add olives. Cook for a few minutes more. Taste. If necessary, adjust salt. Serve.

Roasted Cauliflower with Olives

(Serves 6)

The flavors of golden roasted cauliflower, smoky pimentón, and briny olives are a pleasing change to predictable vegetable dishes.

> 1 head of cauliflower, washed and cut into slices
> 10 cloves of garlic, coarsely chopped
> 10 large Spanish olives, mixture of black and green (remove the pits)
> 4 to 6 tablespoons of EVOO
> 2 teaspoons of hot pimentón
> 4 tablespoons of flat-leaf parsley, cleaned, dried and chopped
> Salt, pepper

Preheat oven to 375°F. Add a glug of EVOO to coat the surface of a large baking dish, then arrange cauliflower and garlic. Add pimentón, a light application of salt and pepper, and roast covered for 20 minutes and after turning, another 20 minutes uncovered or until cauliflower turns golden. Add the olives and roast a few minutes more. Remove from oven, place on serving platter, garnish with the parsley, and serve.

Long Life *Trinxat*,
or Cabbage, Potato, and Bacon Pancake

(Serves 6 to 8)

This is another dish prepared by the long-living people in the tiny, mountainous country of Andorra. Catalan pa amb tomàquet often accompanies trinxat, along with the local specialty, grilled mountain trout.

½ head of green cabbage, cleaned, dried and finely chopped

4 thick slices of naturally preserved bacon from pigs
    that were pasture raised, and free of nitrates

1½ pounds of potatoes, cut into small cubes

8 cloves of chopped garlic

EVOO

Salt, pepper

Fry bacon until slightly crisp, but do not burn. Drain and set aside. In a covered pot, boil the potatoes and cabbage in an inch or so of salted water until just tender. Remove and mash together with half the garlic. Break apart most of the bacon and add to the mixture with 2 tablespoons of EVOO, seasoning with salt and pepper. The concoction should be slightly chunky. Meanwhile, coat a large sauté pan with EVOO, and gently fry the remaining chopped garlic for several minutes to infuse the oil and then discard the garlic. Using a large spoon, drop the mixture of potatoes, cabbage, and bacon into the oil and pat into smooth patties. Fry pancakes a few minutes on each side, until golden. You can skip this step and plate the trinxat without frying. Either way, garnish with remaining pieces of bacon and serve.

Trinxat is also popular in *la* Cerdanya, in the mountains of northern Catalunya. Remember, we spoke of the turnips from this region earlier when we toured *la* Boqueria? How good they are.

Roasted Parsnips, Green Beans, Cabbage, and Yellow Summer Squash Topped with Saffron Sofrito

(Serves 4)

TIP: To avoid exposure to aluminum, line roasting pans with lining paper—the parchment side is exposed to the food, while the aluminum liner is on the other side.

It is important to take care when roasting vegetables because they finish roasting at different times. Use tongs to carefully remove smaller vegetables, such as green beans, to set aside until the larger vegetables finish cooking.

3 parsnips, scrubbed and cut into chunks
2 yellow summer squash, halved lengthwise
½ savoy cabbage, cut into 4 sections
½ pound of very fresh green beans, with tips removed
¼ cup of EVOO
⅓ cup of organic chicken stock
2 teaspoons of dried rosemary powder
1 teaspoon of pimentón
3 cloves of peeled, crushed garlic
Salt, ground black pepper

Sofrito

1 large onion, 1 small tomato, a clove of garlic, pimentón, EVOO and saffron

Make the sofrito according to instructions in Chapter Four. For this recipe, make sure to crumble the saffron threads into the sofrito during the final couple of minutes of cooking.

For the vegetables, preheat oven to 425°F. Combine all of them in a large bowl with the EVOO, garlic, salt, pepper, rosemary and pimentón. Transfer to a medium-sized roasting pan. Add chicken broth to the periphery, cover and roast for 10 minutes. Reduce heat to 375°F, uncover and continue roasting until beans and the tips of the parsnips caramelize. At this stage remove the parsnips and beans. Turn over the cabbage sections and the halved squash, add a little more EVOO, a touch more salt, and continue to roast uncovered until the remaining vegetables are tender, about another 20–30 minutes. Remove from pan and combine with the rest of the vegetables on a serving platter with warm sofrito. Serve.

Green Beans with Anchovy Vinagreta

(Serves 4–6)

When summer green beans are their tender best, this recipe will be a favorite.

1½ pounds of green beans, cleaned and trimmed
1 clove of minced garlic

ANCHOVY VINAGRETA:
EVOO
1½ teaspoons of country-style mustard
2 tablespoons of red wine vinegar
2 to 3 cloves of peeled and minced garlic
1½ anchovy filets, crumbled
⅓ teaspoon of red pepper flakes
Salt and pepper

Preheat oven to 375°F. Combine green beans in bowl with a generous swirl of EVOO and season lightly with salt and one clove of minced garlic. Spread the beans on a Pyrex dish and roast 30 minutes or until tender. Combine the vinagreta ingredients in a small bowl. Taste and adjust seasonings. Spoon over the green beans and serve.

Centenarian Chard with Garlic

(Serves 4)

"Al atardecer de la vida te examinarán del amor," meaning in the twilight of your life, your last exam will be on love.

— Anonymous, etched into a stone at the hermitage in Córdoba, Spain

As I've said before, the long-living people of Aragón and Andorra eat chard often.

> 1 bunch of red or green chard, washed
> EVOO
> 6 to 8 cloves of peeled garlic
> Salt and pepper

Begin by crushing the cloves of garlic with a mortar and pestle, and leave in the mortar while trimming the chard. As explained earlier, when we do this, protective compounds in the garlic become more activated. To prepare the chard, trim the bottoms of the stems and any bruised sections at the ends of leaves as well. Rinse and dry. With a knife, remove the leaves from the stems and slice the stems lengthwise, producing long, thin pieces. Slice the leaves in half, then cut each one into diagonal pieces, sort of a large chiffonade. Heat up a pan with EVOO. When the oil is hot, add the garlic and sauté for a few minutes. Add the sliced stems and cook for 4 minutes. Salt lightly. Chard, which is high in minerals, seems to require less salt than other vegetables. Add the leaves and cook for 10-15 minutes more, salting lightly. Add ground pepper. When the chard is cooked to your satisfaction, remove from the pan and place into a shallow serving bowl. Delicate vegetables such as leafy greens continue to cook when we leave them in heated pans.

Haricots Verts with Roasted Orange Pepper and Anchovy Vinagreta

(Serves 4)

The anchovy vinagreta in this recipe is a variation on the one for Green Beans and Anchovy Vinagreta.

1 pound of haricots verts, cleaned
1 orange pepper
Salt
Freshly ground white pepper
EVOO

ANCHOVY VINAGRETA:
2 small anchovies, preserved in EVOO and crumbled
6 tablespoons of EVOO
2½ tablespoons of *Jerez* sherry vinegar
½ teaspoon of grated lemon zest
1 clove of garlic, minced
2 tablespoons of flat-leaf parsley, cleaned, dried and chopped
⅓ teaspoon of ground pepper

Begin by roasting the pepper. When cool, peel and slice into strips. Assemble dressing ingredients and set aside. Cook haricots verts in gently boiling salted water until just tender and drain. While still warm, toss into vinagreta with pepper strips and serve.

Turnips and Leeks in Chicken Broth

(Serves 4)

The simple foods and bright flavors of this dish make a cozy fall fare.

2 medium leeks, cleaned and sliced into large bite-sized pieces
½ pound of turnips, scrubbed and thickly sliced
EVOO
1 cup of chicken stock
4 to 6 garlic cloves
Salt and ground white pepper

In a large sauté pan, lightly brown garlic in EVOO. Add the turnips and sauté for several more minutes, seasoning with salt and ground pepper. After the turnips begin to soften, add the sliced leeks and continue sautéing for a few minutes more. Salt lightly. Separately, bring chicken stock to a boil and pour over the vegetables. Simmer until the leeks and turnips are just tender. Add a touch more olive oil and adjust salt and pepper.

Herbed Romanesco Broccoli

(Serves 4)

This radical-looking vegetable, in the cauliflower family, looks like it was sprayed fluorescent green. The flavor, well, it is a combination of the gentlest, tastiest broccoli and sweetest cauliflower under the sun.

1 head of Romanesco broccoli
EVOO
Dried herbs: rosemary and thyme
⅓ teaspoon of minced fresh garlic
Grated lemon peel, fresh or dried
Salt, ground white pepper, and red pepper flakes

Preheat oven to 375°F. Clean and dry Romanesco. Cut into half-inch slices—don't be concerned if ends crumble into florets. Coat the bottom of a Pyrex baking dish with EVOO and add the broccoli with the florets. Season lightly with the herbs—you want a subtle veil of flavor so the sweetness of the Romanesco won't be masked. Add the minced garlic, salt, white pepper, and red pepper flakes. Roast, covered with foil, for about 45 minutes. The slices should be tender but not overcooked. When done, remove from oven and add the grated lemon peel.

Catalan Spinach
with Toasted Pine Nuts and Currants
(Serves 2)

This version of *espinacas con pasas y piñones* is made with currants instead of raisins. See which you prefer. You may love them both.

    5 ounces of baby spinach, washed and dried
    1/3 cup of toasted pine nuts
    EVOO
    2 cloves of crushed garlic
    3 tablespoons of currants

Toast pine nuts in the oven or on the stovetop. If in the oven, place pine nuts in a ceramic or Pyrex dish and toast at 350°F for about 3 minutes, stirring a couple of times to ensure an even golden color. On the stovetop, sauté pine nuts in a little EVOO, stirring occasionally to ensure evenness of color. Either way, if done right, you will have pine nuts that are the color of a golden field of wheat. The taste? Like butter. In a medium pan, stirring constantly with a wooden spoon, sauté spinach in EVOO and garlic. After 3–4 minutes, the spinach will wilt. Season with salt and pepper, add the currants and continue sautéing. After 5 minutes, add the pine nuts and sauté for another 3 minutes. Plate and serve.

Baby Purple Potatoes
with Green and Red Bell Pepper

(Serves 4–6)

As reported in the cookbook *Arzak's Secrets*, it is affirming to know that chef Juan Mari loves these elongated, smallish amethyst delights as much as I do.

1½ pounds of baby purple potatoes, cleaned and sliced
½ green bell pepper, chopped
½ red bell pepper, chopped
4 cloves of garlic, chopped
EVOO
4 to 5 pinches of pimentón
Salt, ground black pepper
2 tablespoons of flat-leaf parsley, cleaned, dried and minced
Optional: 1 chorizo sausage, sliced

Place potatoes in a shallow pot and cover with water. Season with salt and a splash of EVOO. Bring to boil and cook until almost tender, taking care not to overcook. Drain and set aside. Meanwhile, in a large skillet, sauté chopped peppers and garlic in EVOO for 10 minutes, salting lightly. Add the cooked potatoes, a good sprinkling of salt, the pimentón, and a splash of EVOO. If you would like chorizo, this is the time to add it, but just be sure to use much less salt since chorizo is salty. Continue sautéing until potatoes begin to brown; stir frequently. Garnish with parsley and serve.

Roasted Endive

(Serves 4)

Occasionally, I like to roast vegetables on parchment-lined foil. It makes for quick cleanup, and I am happy that my food isn't touching aluminum.

6 Belgian endives, halved lengthwise
2 tablespoons of EVOO
2 tablespoons of orange blossom honey from Valencia
1 tablespoon of butter, melted
¾ teaspoon of coarse Spanish sea salt
½ teaspoon of ground black pepper

Mix honey, butter and EVOO in a small bowl. Preheat oven to 400°F. Arrange the halved endives, cut side up, in a baking dish. Drizzle olive oil/honey/butter mixture uniformly over endives, season with salt and black pepper, and roast for 15 minutes. Turn over and continue roasting until golden, which will take about 10-15 minutes more. Can be served immediately or at room temperature.

Catalan Tomato Petals

(Several dozen)

One of Carme Ruscalleda's recipes, from her *CR20: 20 Years of the Sant Pau*, inspired this. Thank you, Chef Ruscalleda. These petals are rich tomatoey treats to use as garnish for seafood dishes or as an ingredient in rice pilaf or pasta. They are also good for a tapas offering on toasted bread squares, rubbed with garlic, and anointed with EVOO.

3 large tomatoes
EVOO
Salt, pepper

Preheat oven to 225°F. Using tongs, place tomatoes in a pot of boiling water for 10 seconds. Remove, let cool. Skin should come off easily. Cut tomatoes in half, deseed, and trim meat into fanned out shape of rose petals. Place petals on a baking dish, and drizzle with EVOO, and season with salt and pepper. Roast for 1 hour.

Roasted Asparagus with Wild Mushrooms

(Serves 4)

Often, especially in the spring, I crave the cleansing, herby taste of asparagus, and the addition of wild mushrooms makes for a recipe that you will be proud to serve to friends.

> 18 to 20 asparagus spears, cleaned with bottoms trimmed
> 2 to 3 cups of mixed wild mushrooms, cleaned, trimmed and dried
> EVOO
> 3 to 4 cloves of minced garlic
> Salt and ground black pepper

Preheat oven to 400°F. Clean mushrooms as previously described in Basque Mushroom Ragout with Egg Yolk Sauce, slicing the larger ones in half. Put mushrooms in bowl with 2 tablespoons of EVOO, half the minced garlic, and season with salt and plenty of pepper. Arrange asparagus in baking dish. Add remaining garlic, a little more EVOO, and salt and pepper. Add mushrooms and toss together. Roast uncovered and after 10 minutes reduce temperature to 325°F and finish cooking for 10 minutes more.

Peas and Gem Lettuce Braised in Saffron Broth

(Serves 6)

Peas grown in the Maresme region of Catalunya are so good they are known as green caviar. Spring's first organic peas make a delicious substitute.

¾ cup of organic chicken or vegetable stock
3 cups of shelled peas
2 little gem lettuces
1 tablespoon of chopped shallots
3 pinches of saffron threads
Grated organic lemon rind
EVOO
Sea salt and ground black pepper

In a medium-sized pan, gently sauté shallots in EVOO, season with salt and pepper, and stir frequently. When shallots turn golden, crumble in the saffron threads and slowly pour in the stock, taking care to gently mix everything together. Add the peas and lettuce with more salt, pepper and EVOO. Increase heat, bring to a boil and simmer for 5 minutes. Finish with the grated lemon rind.

Roasted Pumpkin with Walnut Picada

(Serves 4)

During autumn, one sees all types of pumpkins and squash in the markets of the North, and many would be suitable for this dish. Chefs like to roast the orange-ribbed ones, but my favorite is *hokaido*, also known as kuri squash, especially the red variety, which is oh-so sweet, but not easy to find.

4 1½-inch thick slices of pumpkin or hard squash
EVOO
Salt and ground white pepper
1 teaspoon of freshly ground nutmeg

PICADA INGREDIENTS:
⅓ cup EVOO
10 lightly roasted walnuts
10 lightly roasted hazelnuts
2 cloves of garlic, minced
1 teaspoon of fresh parsley, cleaned and chopped
1 small slice of country-style bread, without crust
Salt and pepper

Preheat oven to 375°F. Arrange pumpkin/squash slices in a Pyrex or ceramic baking dish coated with EVOO. Drizzle more EVOO over the pumpkin/squash and season with ground nutmeg, sea salt, and white pepper. Roast the pumpkin for approximately 40 minutes until tender, turning once halfway through. In a separate pan, fry the slice of bread in a thin coating of EVOO. When browned, remove and combine with all of the picada ingredients in a large mortar and crush together with a pestle. You can use a food processor, but do not overprocess. The picada should be buttery but not puréed to smithereens. If the picada seems dry, simply add a little more EVOO. Serve the pumpkin/squash with picada over the top.

GRAINS AND PASTA

Arròs Negre

(Serves 4)

For many years now, squid ink has become on-trend for chefs, but the Catalans began cooking with it a long time ago, after which, recipes with squid ink spread along the Mediterranean coast of Spain and elsewhere.

SOFRITO:

¼ red bell pepper, chopped
¼ orange bell pepper, chopped
2 pinches of red pepper flakes

THE RICE:

2 cups of bomba or *Calasparra* rice
5 cups of fish stock
4 to 6 tablespoons of squid ink
⅓ cup of dry white wine
3 tablespoons of flat-leaf parsley, cleaned, dried and chopped
Salt and black pepper

In a medium-sized pot, make sofrito according to the ingredients and preparation given earlier in Chapter Four, but reduce the amounts of onion and tomato by half and sauté the bell peppers and onion together before adding the tomato. Season with pepper flakes towards the end. After sofrito is finished, if it sticks to the pot, add a teaspoon or two of water. Increase heat and gradually stir in half of the rice and then half of the fish stock. Separately dissolve the squid ink in a little of the remaining stock and add it to the pot along with the remaining rice and stock, and the wine. Season with salt and pepper and cook, uncovered, for 10 minutes on high, then reduce heat and cook another 10 minutes until liquid is absorbed and the rice is tender. Garnish each portion with chopped parsley and serve.

My Version of Pere Vilà's "*Rice Pelat*"
or Rice with Chicken, Shrimp, and Artichokes

(Serves 4-6)

Pere Vilà is a highly regarded Catalan composer. Included in his body of work is music for *sardanas*—the national dance of Catalunya, and he has written one in honor of seven-time Michelin star chef, Carme Ruscalleda. My recipe below takes its inspiration from a recipe by Pere Vilà, which I discovered in Ruscalleda's book, *CR20: 20 Years of Sant Pau.* I like Vilà's recipe because it demonstrates the flexibility of Catalan rice dishes, in that they sometimes include meat together with seafood and vegetables.

6 chicken thighs or legs, cut by the butcher into pieces

12 peeled and deveined shrimp

1 cup of bomba rice

2½ cups of spring or filtered water

12 pearl onions, peeled

1 medium-sized onion, chopped

½ cup of ripe, grated tomatoes

¾ cup of trimmed snow peas

2 artichokes, outer leaves removed and cut into fourths

EVOO

Salt, freshly ground white pepper

Several pinches of dried thyme

2 cloves of garlic

1 bay leaf

4 pinches of saffron threads

1 scallion, cleaned and diced

3 tablespoons of fresh parsley, cleaned, dried and chopped

Large green olives

Toast saffron and set aside. In an iron pot (around 6 quarts), brown the chicken pieces in EVOO, seasoning with salt, ground pepper, and a couple of pinches of thyme. Remove from pot. Add a little more EVOO to the pot and fry the artichokes with one clove of garlic and a few pinches of salt until lightly gilded. Set aside.

In the same pot, make a sofrito according to instructions in Chapter Four. Meanwhile, using a mortar and pestle, crush the remaining clove of garlic together with the parsley and toasted saffron. Dilute with a little water. Add the saffron and parsley mixture, the chicken and the artichokes to the sofrito with the rice. Add the water, a little salt, the bay leaf and a splash of EVOO. Bring to boil, reduce heat and cook for 8 minutes on medium, and then 10 minutes more on low. Rice will have absorbed most of the liquid at this point.

Separately brown the pearl onions until lightly golden in a small pan slicked with EVOO. Salt while cooking. Set pan with the onions aside. Drizzle the shrimp uniformly with a little EVOO and season lightly with thyme and salt.

Add snow peas and browned pearl onions to the pot. Arrange the shrimp around the edge and and bake in a preheated 350°F oven for 8 minutes, uncovered. Remove, allow to rest, and add a little more olive oil over the top. The snow peas should still be bright green. Serve garnished with chopped parsley, trimmed scallions, and olives.

Alicante Chicken and Vegetable Paella

(Serves 4)

This recipe is adapted from one by María José San Román, the distinguished chef and restaurateur from the province of Alicante, which Peter S. Feibleman described in *The Cooking of Spain and Portugal* as a region known for "a broad variety of foods around the central theme of rice." Paella is the most important dish there, and we are honored to have another recipe from this chef. I have chosen to substitute chicken for Black Turkey, which is easier to find in the States. Thank you, María José San Román.

FOR THE BROTH:

1 carrot

1 onion

1 leek

2 medium tomatoes

1 clove of garlic

1 small to medium size chicken

½ quart of spring or filtered water

FOR THE RICE:

1 cup of bomba rice

2½ cups broth

Dark chicken meat cut into pieces

About ⅓ pound seasonal vegetables
    (spring garlic, artichokes, green beans)

Picual EVOO

¼ teaspoon of ground saffron

2 pinches of sweet smoked paprika

Salt, pepper

Debone chicken. We will only use the dark meat in this dish, so save the rest for another recipe. Preheat oven to 425°F. In a pan, roast the carcass and bones with the onion, garlic, carrot, leek and tomatoes for 30 minutes, then transfer to a pressure cooker along with the water, and cook for 30 minutes more. Strain. This makes the broth.

In a pot, bring broth to a low boil, then remove about a ½ cup of it to a bowl and dilute the saffron. Cut the seasonal vegetables into thick brunoise slices. In a medium-sized paella pan, sauté the vegetables in EVOO. Remove, set aside and then sauté the chicken, lightly seasoned with salt. Add paprika, rice, saffron in broth and the remaining broth.

TIP: You might want to follow this paella with a little turrón, another specialty of Alicante. Turrón is nougat sweetened with honey and usually has pine nuts and walnuts, although a variety of types are available.

Bring to a boil and transfer to a 375°F oven until liquid is absorbed, about 15 minutes. Remove from oven, and top with the sautéed seasonal vegetables, with freshly ground pepper and sweet smoked paprika.

María José San Román's Wheat *Olleta* with Assorted Vegetables

(Serves 4)

This hearty vegan recipe, another offering from María José San Román, is what the chef goes to when fighting a cold. Thank you again, Chef. Her fortifying olleta is a soup/stew made from kamut and white beans with chard, turnips, green beans, fingerling potatoes, and artichokes. The flavor is deep with Cornicabra EVOO added right before serving.

¾ cup of kamut wheat, rinsed
½ cup of white beans
4 tablespoons of Cornicabra EVOO
2 cups of Swiss chard, cleaned, trimmed, and sliced
1 handful of green beans, washed and trimmed
1 artichoke, washed, trimmed and cut into 4 to 6 pieces
4 small fingerling potatoes
1 small turnip
1¾ quarts of water
4 pinches of saffron powder
¼ teaspoon of cumin
½ teaspoon of black pepper
1 teaspoon of salt

Soak the kamut and white beans separately overnight. Drain water and place beans in a pot with fresh water to cover. Bring to a boil and simmer for about 1 hour 45 minutes, uncovered. In another pot, combine the kamut with 1½ cups water and a pinch of salt. Bring to a boil and simmer covered for about 30 minutes. Coat the bottom of a large pot with EVOO, and gently sauté the vegetables, except for the chard. Add the white beans with the cooking liquid, if there is any left, along with the kamut, saffron, cumin, and water, seasoning with salt and pepper. Bring to boil and simmer uncovered for 1 hour. Add the Swiss chard and cook for 15 minutes more. Finish with the unheated Cornicabra EVOO.

Semi-Brown Calasparra Rice with Sherry-Marinated Pork Loin and Mushrooms

(Serves 4)

The spice rub adds flavor to the lean pork, and semi-brown Calasparra rice, mushrooms, laurel, rutabaga and sherry contribute to the rusticity of this pleasing dish. This rice is available from Spanish food importers. (See Resource Guide)

1 pound of boneless pork chops, trimmed of fat,
    and cut into large bite-sized pieces
EVOO
1 medium rutabaga, peeled and cubed into ½ inch pieces
1 large onion, chopped
½ pound of white button mushrooms, cleaned, and cut in half
4 cloves of garlic
½ cup of semi-brown Calasparra rice
1½ cups of chicken stock
2 bay leaves
3 tablespoons of dry *Oloroso* or another good Spanish sherry
Salt, pepper
Flat-leaf parsley, cleaned, dried and chopped

SPICE RUB:
2 tablespoons of EVOO
2 teaspoons of rosemary powder
1 teaspoon of dried thyme
2 teaspoons of garlic, minced
Salt and pepper

Prepare spice rub using a mortar and pestle. In a bowl, massage into pork, then cover and marinate in the refrigerator overnight. The next day, remove from the refrigerator 30 minutes before cooking. In a small pan, sauté the mushrooms in EVOO, seasoned with salt and pepper. When mushrooms brown, add 1 tablespoon of sherry and continue for 10 more minutes. Set aside.

In a large pan, sauté onion in EVOO for 15 minutes, stirring all the while, and season with a few pinches of salt. Add the rutabaga, pork, garlic, a little more EVOO and sauté for another 10 minutes, stirring occasionally. Meanwhile, in a medium-sized pot, heat the stock with a little EVOO and bring to a boil. Add the stock, rice, and 2 tablespoons of sherry to the pan with the pork, with a few pinches of salt and the bay leaves. Increase heat to high, stirring carefully. Once everything is softly boiling (this won't take long), reduce heat to a simmer and cook uncovered until rice is done, about 20 minutes. Since medium-grain rice absorbs more liquid than long-grain, you may need to add more water or broth as it cooks. Taste ingredients and adjust salt. Add the mushrooms, stir with a wooden paddle and remove from heat. Cover with a bamboo sushi mat and allow to rest for 10 minutes before serving so flavors will meld. Garnish with parsley.

BEANS AND LEGUMES

Did you know there are approximately 100 different kinds of beans in Spain? Many heirloom/regional types have no English translation.

Garbanzo Salad with Mahon Cheese, Pomegranate Seeds, and Empeltre Olives

(Serves 6)

The Harvard School of Public Health reported that women who consumed beans at least twice a week slashed breast cancer risk by 24 percent.

3 cups of cooked garbanzo beans

Seeds from half a pomegranate

½ small green pepper, finely chopped

½ medium cucumber, coarsely chopped

½ cup of sweet onion, minced

1 clove of garlic, minced

¾ cup of olives with pits removed

½ cup of Mahon cheese, shredded (Manchego if unavailable)

4 ounces of EVOO

2 ounces of Spanish red wine vinegar

½ cup of flat-leaf parsley, cleaned, dried and chopped

8 heirloom cherry tomatoes, halved

8 strips of piquillo pepper, roasted red or green pepper

½ teaspoon cumin

Salt, pepper

TIP: Empeltre olives are grown in Catalunya and have deep flavor without being bitter and are often served as table olives.

Roll the pomegranate on the table to loosen seeds. Cut in half, then halve again and turn each section inside out and push seeds out. Combine garbanzos, cucumbers and tomatoes in a medium-sized salad bowl, rubbed with a little crushed garlic. Add onions, chopped parsley, and pomegranate seeds along with the rest of the ingredients, including the garlic, vinegar and EVOO, but not the cheese. Add salt, cumin, and pepper. Taste and adjust seasonings. Marinate for 10 minutes before serving. Add cheese and toss through. Garnish with piquillo pepper strips and serve.

fabada asturiana, My Way

(Serves 6-8)

Though there are variations on *fabada asturiana*, this recipe is closest to the version I had in Oviedo, the capital of Asturias. As with many iconic Spanish recipes, *fabada asturiana* has humble origins, so whatever leftover sausages and pork could be had, well, it went into this peasant-style dish. Some claim that fabada is similar to French cassoulet, but I believe it is better. No other bean can be substituted for fabes. They are buttery in taste and hold together even when cooked for many hours, which is the requirement of this recipe. It is said that the success of fabada depends upon the quality of the foods.

You will note that this recipe (as compared to the others in this book) contains a nominal amount of EVOO. The richness comes from the pork products and buttery fabes. From the standpoint of health, *fabada asturiana* is composed of fiber and anticancer lignin-rich beans, which act to protect us in numerous ways.

1 pound of *fabes* beans
1 ham knucklebone or hock (where the foot of a pig attaches to the leg)
½ pound of *morcilla* or other artisan sausage
¼ pound of *chorizo de La Rioja o chorizo riojano*
3 ounce slab of lean cured bacon
6 cloves of garlic
1 onion, quartered
1 leek, cleaned, trimmed and split in half
2 bay leaves
1 tablespoon of bittersweet pimentón
3 pinches of saffron threads
EVOO
Salt and pepper

Place beans in a large bowl and soak overnight in plenty of water. Following day, clean the ham hock vigorously with a scrub brush and water. Place the hock in a pot, cover with water, and bring to a boil. Cook for 2 minutes, then remove with tongs, rinse in cold water and dry.

In a large cazuela, sauté the leek, onion, bacon and garlic in EVOO for 15 minutes, stirring with a wooden paddle. Add the beans, ham hock, sausages, bay leaves, saffron and pimentón and enough water to cover. Bring to boil, skimming fat and foam from the surface as it cooks. After 5 minutes reduce heat and gently simmer partially covered, continuing to defat the surface of the stew as it cooks. After beans are tender, about 2½ hours, set fabada aside to cool.

When ingredients are no longer steaming hot, remove the ham hock, leek, onion, bay leaves, bacon, and sausage. Put the hock, bacon, and sausages on a cutting board. Slice the ham from the hock, and cut the sausages and bacon into bite-sized pieces. Serve the beans in a large shallow soup bowl, and garnish each serving with a couple of slices of each type of sausage, some bacon, and a slice of ham.

Lentils over Grilled Cauliflower

(Serves 8)

This recipe can be enjoyed for those times you welcome tasty leftovers.

1 cup of lentils, rinsed
1 head of cauliflower, cleaned and cut vertically into 1-inch slices
4 cloves of crushed garlic
EVOO
Several pinches of saffron powder or crushed threads
1 bay leaf
¾ teaspoon of pimentón
¼ cup of fresh parsley, cleaned, dried and chopped
1 large ripe tomato, cut into wedges
12 Spanish olives, both green and black, pits removed
Salt and black pepper

Place lentils, bay leaf, a clove of garlic and a tablespoon of EVOO in a saucepan with water to cover. Bring to boil, reduce heat, cover with a bamboo mat, and cook until tender, about 25 minutes. Season with salt, pepper, and pimentón. Separately place the cauliflower in a large bowl with a splash of EVOO and season with salt and pepper. Mix well to ensure a uniform coating. In a large pan, sauté 1 clove of garlic and ⅓ of the sliced cauliflower in EVOO. You will do this in 3 batches. Add a pinch of saffron powder (or threads) and continue sautéing until very lightly browned, about 12-15 minutes. After the first batch of cauliflower is finished, remove and immediately repeat the process. When all the cauliflower has been cooked in this manner, place on a large serving platter and toss with parsley. Using a spoon with draining holes, scoop the lentils from the pot, and place on top of the cauliflower. Arrange tomato wedges and olives around the platter and serve.

Open-Face Tortilla with White Beans and Leeks

(Serves 4)

Inspired by Chef José Andrés from his book *Made in Spain*, this recipe offers a method for preparing a tortilla in batches that is most helpful.

½ cup dry navy beans
½ head of garlic, cloves crushed in a mortar and pestle
1 bay leaf
2 pinches of pimentón
EVOO
1 cup thinly sliced leeks (white parts only)
8 eggs
2 tablespoon flat-leaf parsley, cleaned, dried and chopped
Sea salt and ground black pepper

Rinse the beans and place them in a bowl. Cover with cold water and soak overnight. The next day, drain and place in a pot with 1½ quarts of water, the garlic, bay leaf, and 3 tablespoons EVOO. Bring to a boil and simmer until tender, about 1½ hours, all the time skimming the foam off the top. Add the pimentón, salt to taste and cook for another 10 minutes. Drain beans, remove bay leaf, and set aside.

Coat the bottom of a sauté pan with EVOO and bring to temperature without smoking. Spread half the beans in the pan and sauté on medium until lightly brown on one side, which should take just a few minutes. Uniformly add half of the sliced leeks and season with salt and black pepper. After another minute remove from pan. Repeat with the remaining beans and leeks.

To prepare the tortillas, first lightly whisk the eggs in a bowl and season with salt and black pepper. In a sauté pan, heat a tablespoon of EVOO and pour in a quarter of the whisked eggs. Working quickly with a spatula, run it around the edges of the eggs to keep them from sticking. It also helps if you shake the pan. Spread a quarter of the beans and leeks over the eggs and cook just until the eggs are warmed through. Eggs should be custardy and not overcooked. Repeat with the rest of the eggs and beans until you have 4 tortillas. Garnish with parsley and serve.

FISH AND SHELLFISH

Shrimp *Exprés* with Swiss Chard and Orange Peel
(Serves 2)

Serve with olives and a salad, and you are ready to watch a Pedro Almodóvar movie.

    8 ounces of shelled and deveined shrimp, rinsed and dried
    ½ orange or red bell pepper, sliced thin
    ⅓ sweet onion, thinly sliced

1 bunch of Swiss chard, rinsed, trimmed, leaves broken apart

3 cloves of garlic, crushed

3 pinches of saffron powder or threads

3 pinches of pimentón

2 teaspoons of *Jerez* sherry vinegar

EVOO

2 thin julienned strips of organic orange zest (avoid pith)

Salt, pepper

Slice stems of the chard into thin strips. Coat a skillet with EVOO and sauté onions and bell pepper for 10 minutes, seasoning lightly with salt and pepper. Add garlic and chard stems. Continue sautéing for 5 minutes, then add the rest of the chard along with a little more EVOO and saffron. Combine with a wooden spoon so that the oil and saffron meld into the vegetables. Season lightly with salt and pepper and continue sautéing. After 3 minutes, add a little more EVOO, then the shrimp and pimentón. Continue sautéing until shrimp is cooked through, another 7 or 8 minutes. Pepper and onions should be crisp. Stir in sherry vinegar and the orange peel and sauté for 3 minutes more. Remove from pan and serve.

Mussels Natural

(Serves 6)

Mussels offer the most nutrition over any other shellfish, being rich in healthy fats, vitamins, and immune-enhancing zinc and selenium. And they are inexpensive. Select ones that are firmly closed.

6 to 7 pounds of mussels, beards scraped off
    and washed in several changes of water

EVOO

¼ cup of fennel, chopped

¼ cup of onion, chopped

3 cloves of garlic, chopped

1 large ripe tomato
1 bay leaf
3 tablespoons of parsley, cleaned, dried and minced
¼ cup white wine
⅓ cup water
Salt, pepper

Prepare the tomato as when making sofrito by grating the pulp into a small bowl. In a large pan, sauté fennel, onion, garlic, and bay in EVOO. When onions turn golden, add the tomato and another splash of EVOO. Cook for several minutes, then add the cleaned mussels. Season lightly with salt—mussels contain sodium and other minerals so they don't need much—and pepper. Continue cooking over low heat for about 3 minutes, shaking the pan. Add the wine and water, and cook covered until mussels begin to open, about 4 minutes more. Keep shaking the pan and mix as they open. Serve in bowls garnished with minced parsley, and country-style bread. Or let cool and serve with aioli (recipe below).

Baked Cod in Red Sauce with Green Olives

(Serves 4)

Cod prepared with chunks of sweet yellow summer squash and savory sofrito is complemented by the flavors of rosemary, olives, and the heat of a little hot red chili. Regarding the use of salt, chefs know to salt lightly through every stage of cooking, especially for this recipe, since olives are added as a final step, and, of course, they are salty.

4 cod filets (about a pound total)
¾ pound of yellow summer squash, cut into ½ inch diagonal chunks
⅓ red bell pepper, cut into julienned strips

¼ cup of EVOO

1 teaspoon of manzanilla sherry

½ dried red chili pepper

1½ cups of sofrito

Salt, ground white pepper

¼ cup of flat-leaf parsley, cleaned, dried, and chopped

1 sprig of rosemary, rinsed and dried

3 cloves of garlic, minced

1 large shallot, sliced

Very generous handful of mixed olives, stone in

Make the sofrito according to the instructions in Chapter Four. Coat fish with a little EVOO and season with ground white pepper. In a medium pan sauté 1 clove of garlic and the shallot in EVOO. Add the squash, red pepper strips, sprig of rosemary and chili pepper. Season with a touch of salt, a grinding of white pepper, and stir with a wooden spatula. Continue until the squash turns golden, about 20 minutes.

Combine the sofrito and the squash mixture in a medium baking dish with a touch more EVOO. Remove pits and add olives. Salt the fish and in a separate pan, sauté in EVOO and the remaining garlic for 3–4 minutes. Turn the pieces and sauté for a couple more minutes and remove. Add the parsley to the mixture of squash, olives, and sofrito and arrange the fish on top. Drizzle with sherry and a touch of EVOO. If using a mister, combine equal parts sherry and EVOO, and very lightly spray on the cod.

To finish, place casserole uncovered in a 400°F oven until fish is just cooked through, about 5 minutes. It is better to remove earlier than later because after you test a piece of fish and it looks like it needs more time, you can put back into the oven for a few moments more. Garnish with olives and serve.

Quinoa Paella with Squid

(Serves 4)

The lightness of quinoa goes well with the slight chewishness of squid. And this dish is quick, so there is more time for play. How about a movie? Maybe *Ocho Apellidos Vascos*, aka *The Spanish Affair*? This very funny romantic comedy was filmed in the Basque country, in places not usually seen by tourists. The sequel, *Ocho Apellidos Catalanes*, was filmed in Catalunya and just as funny.

1½ cups of red quinoa, rinsed well
1 pound of squid rings and tentacles, rinsed and dried
1 large onion, cut into quarters, then thick slices
3 cups of chicken stock
Several pinches of saffron threads
2 cups of sliced broccoli crowns
Salt, ground white pepper
1½ teaspoons pimentón
4 cloves of garlic, crushed
½ teaspoon fresh lemon juice
Wedges of lemon for garnish
3 tablespoons flat-leafed parsley, cleaned, dried and chopped

Coat squid with EVOO, a quarter of crushed garlic, half of the pimentón, a grinding of white pepper, and a little salt. In a preheated 425°F oven, roast the squid on an iron grill pan for 8 minutes. Immediately remove and transfer to a plate so that it does not continue to cook.

In a saucepan, bring the chicken stock to a boil, reduce heat, stir in the rest of the pimentón, the another quarter of the crushed garlic, black pepper, and lemon juice and simmer for 30 minutes. Stir in crushed saffron.

In a large skillet or paella pan, sauté onion in EVOO until golden, seasoning with salt. Add remaining crushed garlic and continue sautéing for 5 minutes. Remove from pan. Add more EVOO to the pan, bring it to temperature without smoking and stir in the quinoa with a pinch or two of salt. After the quinoa begins to toast, a couple of minutes, slowly pour in the heated chicken stock. Bring to a boil, reduce heat, and simmer, covered, until liquid is absorbed, about 20 minutes. If there is a small amount of liquid left, do not worry because it will be absorbed in the oven. Add broccoli, and just before it turns bright green, the caramelized onion mixture and roasted squid. If there are drippings from the squid, mix into the paella, too, and finish cooking in a 350°F oven for 8 minutes. Garnish with parsley and wedges of lemon, and serve.

Roasted Cod over Potato and Leeks

(Serves 2)

I use the Spanish technique of "cooking to the side," as described below. This method can be used for anything you may want to slow-cook, such as long sautéed potatoes.

    2 6-ounce cod fillets (with skin, if available)
    1½ pounds of red potatoes, peeled and sliced
    1 cup of leeks (use the tender part), thoroughly cleaned and thinly diced
    4 cloves of garlic, minced
    EVOO
    ⅓ teaspoon of pimentón
    1 tablespoon of flat-leaf parsley, cleaned, dried and chopped
    Salt and white pepper

Using a medium-sized cazuela (or oven-proof dish), heat EVOO. Add potatoes and garlic and season with salt and pepper. Move potatoes and garlic to the periphery of the pan and cook on low for 50 minutes, stirring every ten minutes or so. After the potatoes are almost fully cooked, add the leeks to the center of the pan, and bring the potatoes from the edges and combine, adding a few pinches of salt, a dusting of pimentón, and a touch more of

TIP: Leeks and garlic are probiotic foods that boost gut health.

white pepper. Mix through the potatoes and leeks. Place the cod on top, drizzle with olive oil, salt lightly, add more white pepper, and a dusting of pimentón. Place cazuela in a 375°F oven covered with parchment-lined foil for 8 minutes. Remove foil and continue uncovered for 4 minutes more. Garnish with chopped parsley.

Basque Marmitako Tuna Stew
(Serves 4)

"A long time before the Swiss had formed their confederation, Iruracba; long before the English had won for themselves their Magna Carta; long before the North Americans and French had proclaimed their rights of man and the citizen; the Basques had organized a representative government, and their representatives met beneath the tree of Guernica. Thus they had government for the people, by the people, they had self-government."

– Alejo Peyret, French writer, from a conference published
in the *El Siglo* newspaper, November 13, 1879

Marmitako, or tuna and potato stew, has been cooked since the twelfth century by Basque seamen who went on expeditions to Newfoundland in search of whales.

A word about authentic ingredients: *Pimiento choricero* is the dried pepper typically used in this dish, but you might like the ease of pimiento choricero sauce, which is prepared from the pulp of the pepper (see Resource Guide under Spanish food importers). Or roast a red pepper and scrape off the flesh to use as a replacement.

¼ pound of very fresh tuna steak cut into cubes
1 pound of red potatoes
1 large shallot, minced
1 red pepper, finely diced

1 green pepper, finely diced

1 very large ripe tomato, cut into cubes

EVOO

2 small-medium onions, chopped

2 to 4 cloves of garlic, crushed

1 bay leaf

2 pinches of red pepper flakes

2 to 3 pinches of dried thyme

2½ tablespoons of pimiento choricero sauce, the flesh from
    1 roasted red pepper, or a reconstituted choricero pepper

3 tablespoons chopped flat-leaf parsley

1 cup of Txacoli Getaria, or another dry sparkling white wine

1½ cups of fish stock (See Appendix B)

Salt, pepper

For this recipe, try the Basque approach to cutting potatoes: "crack" them by twisting a knife into the potato, effectively halving it. In addition to creating rustic-looking pieces, this method releases more starch, which is helpful in making the sauce.

Using the cracking method, prepare the potatoes, taking care not to cut yourself. In a medium-sized enamel stew pot or cazuela, sauté onions in EVOO, taking care to stir the bits at the bottom so they don't burn. After 10 minutes, add the peppers, tomato, garlic, and a little more salt, and cook for 10 minutes more, stirring gently. Add potatoes, thyme, shallot, more salt and black pepper, mixing gently to combine and continue cooking for 30 minutes. Add the pepper paste, roasted red pepper flesh or break the reconstituted pimiento choricero into the mixture, and 5 minutes later, add the txacoli, fish stock, and bay leaf. Continue cooking uncovered for 30 minutes. Finally, gently mix in the cubed tuna and cook for 10 minutes more, adjusting salt, and adding half the chopped parsley. When you are ready to serve, garnish with the remaining parsley.

Basque Hake in Green Sauce with Clams

(Serves 4)

Basques love the combination of garlic, flat-leaf parsley and extra-virgin olive oil. The life-giving trio graces many recipes, and this particular one reaches back very early. Hake, or *merluza* as it is called by the Basques, was a fish that stone-age artists painted on cave walls and was cooked by the earliest Basque fishermen aboard their vessels. This recipe was inspired by Chef Dani López's restaurant Kokotxa in Donostia/San Sebastián.

2 pounds of hake, cleaned, dried and cut into 16 pieces
    (leave skin on for higher omega-3s and more flavor)
24 small littleneck clams, scrubbed and soaked in a bowl
    covered with water and salt for a few hours to remove excess sand
⅓ cup of EVOO
3 cloves of garlic, crushed
4 tablespoons of flat-leaf parsley, cleaned, dried and chopped
½ cup of dry white wine
½ cup of fish stock
Few pinches of flour
Salt and freshly ground white pepper

In a large, flat pan, sauté the garlic in EVOO. After a few minutes, add the flour, wine, and the fish stock, and season with salt and pepper. Bring to a boil, reduce heat and simmer until sauce thickens, stirring constantly. Add the fish, and continue covered for five minutes. Then turn the hake over, and add the clams and parsley. Cook for 3 more minutes, covered. Immediately take off flame so fish will be succulent. Serve in large shallow bowls, garnished with more chopped parsley.

Baked Oysters with Toasted Breadcrumbs, Dusted with Serrano Ham Powder

(Serves 4)

This recipe, which can be served as an entrée or a first course, was inspired by chef Elena Arzak, who developed the technique for creating Serrano ham powder in her Donostia/San Sebastián restaurant, Arzak, that she co-chefs with her father, Juan Mari. This father and daughter duo is *sortzeko eta asmatzeko*, which is Basque for creative and inventive.

    2 dozen fresh shucked oysters on half shell
    1 cup of breadcrumbs
    EVOO
    1 teaspoon of garlic, minced
    2 tablespoons of flat-leaf parsley, cleaned, dried and chopped
    2 thin slices of Serrano ham (approximately one ounce),
        torn into small pieces
    Salt, black pepper

Preheat oven to 225°F. Arrange ham on Pyrex dish and bake for approximately 1 hour until just crisp. Set aside to cool. Using a mini food processor grind into a fine powder. Now preheat oven to 425°F to bake the oysters. Meanwhile, in a large pan, sauté breadcrumbs and garlic in EVOO, seasoning with salt and pepper and stirring all the while until light golden, about 4 minutes. Take care not to burn. Place oysters on a baking dish. Lightly coat with EVOO, then breadcrumbs, and bake for 12 minutes. Plate the oysters (6 per person) and dust with Serrano ham powder. Garnish with parsley.

Cod on a Bed of Multicolor Vegetables with Two Sauces

(Serves 3-4)

The rainbow-colored vegetables surrounding the stark white of the cod reminds me a little of Parc Güell. This Barcelona modernist garden with boldly colored ceramic sculptures designed by Antoni Gaudí, is emblematic of Modernisme, which began in the nineteenth century when the region worked to restore its identity—and language—and set it apart from Castilian Spain. In no other part of the world did the art nouveau movement leave such a legacy as in Catalunya, especially Barcelona, thanks to the immense talent there, especially Antoni Gaudí.

You will need an olive oil mister for this recipe. See the beginning of this chapter.

1 pound of cod, preferably with skin on
3 artichoke hearts
8 small purple potatoes, peeled and cut into 3 slices
7 small orange, red, and yellow sweet peppers
4 cloves of garlic, minced
3 shallots, cut into slices
EVOO
Salt, white pepper
Manzanilla sherry
Tomatillo sauce (see Resource Guide)

THE TOMATO SAUCE:
2 pounds tomatoes, chopped
1 small yellow onion, chopped
EVOO
½ cup of chicken stock

1 bay leaf
Salt, pepper
2 cloves of garlic, crushed
a pinch or two of dried thyme

Prepare the fish by wiping lightly with a damp towel, pat dry, and place in a dish. Coat lightly with EVOO and cover with bamboo mat or plastic wrap. Set aside. In a medium-sized pot, sauté onion, bay leaf, thyme, and half of the garlic for 5 minutes, seasoned with salt. Add tomatoes and cook gently for 10 minutes until they break down—crush with wooden spoon to speed things along. Add chicken stock, a little more EVOO, and using an immersion blender, puree the contents of the pot. Continue cooking uncovered until it reduces to the consistency of tomato sauce, about 15 minutes. Taste, and adjust salt.

Cut peppers in half and in a medium pan, sauté slowly in EVOO with the remaining garlic and shallots, season with salt and pepper, and stir frequently with a wooden spoon to prevent burning. After 20–25 minutes, reduce heat and continue cooking peppers covered on low for 15–20 minutes more. Set aside. Arrange potato slices on a steamer basket in a small pot. Splash with EVOO and season with salt. Steam for 20 minutes or until al dente. Do not overcook.

Use the method described at the beginning of this chapter to trim the artichokes. Place hearts in a pot with water to cover, a little salt, and a splash of EVOO. Cover, bring to a boil, reduce heat and simmer for 15 minutes. Fill mister with 2 parts EVOO and 1 part sherry and spray the bottom of a large baking dish or a cazuela. Arrange sautéed peppers in the center, spreading out just a little. Place the cod on top of the peppers. The bright peppers should peek out from under the fish, making an artful border. Surround the fish and peppers with clusters of purple potato slices and artichoke hearts until the fish is surrounded by color. Spray the EVOO/sherry mixture lightly over everything. Do not saturate, just a couple of light mistings. Season potatoes lightly with salt. Dot the fish with small globs of tomatillo sauce, and then with the tomato sauce preparation. Bake uncovered in a 425°F oven for 12 minutes. Serve.

MEAT

Brandy-Roasted Red Peppers Stuffed with Beef

(Serves 8)

Peppers stuffed with rice and beef, even lamb or pork, is a homey recipe made throughout the Iberian Peninsula. A touch of Spanish brandy makes it distinctive.

¾ pounds of grass-fed beef, cut from shank
4 tablespoons finely chopped Serrano ham
4 red peppers
¾ cup of freshly cooked organic short-grain Calasparra rice
1 small onion
6 cloves of garlic
2 large shallots
¼ cup Torres five-year-old brandy or another fine brandy
EVOO
¼ cup of dried currants
1 sprig of thyme
1 sprig of rosemary
1 bay leaf
2 to 3 pinches of saffron threads
2 large, ripe tomatoes, halved
3 pinches of pimentón
2 pinches of cinnamon
Fresh ground nutmeg
Salt and ground black pepper
Flat-leaf parsley, cleaned, dried and chopped
⅓ cup grated Manchego cheese

In a large bowl, mix in a glug of EVOO to keep the cooked rice moist. Prepare red peppers for roasting by halving, deseeding and covering with a light application of EVOO. Place skin side down in baking dish, and roast in a 375°F oven for 15 minutes. Peppers should maintain their shape when done. Meanwhile, prepare meat by rinsing, drying, and cutting into even pieces, around ⅓ the size of your fist.

In a large baking dish, coated with EVOO, spread the cut meat, along with salt, halved tomatoes, herbs, the garlic, shallots, onion, and bay leaf. Arrange the meat, herbs, tomatoes, and aromatics so that they are not overlapping. Season with cinnamon, a few grindings of nutmeg, pepper, and more EVOO.

Cover with foil and place in a preheated 225°F oven for 1 hour, turning once. Add the brandy, combine with wooden paddle, and continue cooking for another 45 minutes, turning once or twice more. Remove from oven and place meat and roasted vegetables in a large bowl, along with the juices, and set aside to cool.

Cut the roasted tomato halves into smaller pieces over a separate smaller bowl (reserving juices in the bowl) and combine the tomatoes and juice into the cooked rice. Crush saffron threads in your fingers and gently mix into the rice with a drizzle of EVOO. Mince the meat and cut the shallots and onion into small bite-sized pieces, and add to the rice and tomato mixture with the currants, a few pinches of salt, 2 tablespoons chopped parsley, and the little pieces of jamón. Combine and moisten everything with more EVOO, and season with pepper.

> TIP: To make breadcrumbs, simply fry both sides of a slice of crustless, country-style bread in EVOO, half of a reconstituted ñora pepper, and a pinch of salt. When golden, drain on a clean dishtowel and crush to a fine consistency.

Place a sliver of garlic to the bottom of each roasted pepper half. Stuff each with equal parts of the meat and rice mixture and place in a baking dish coated with EVOO. Add a touch of brandy around the peppers to aromatize, and scatter grated Manchego over the top of each pepper. Cover with foil and cook for 30 minutes in a 350°F oven. Garnish with minced fresh parsley.

Lamb Meatballs with Currants and Queen Olives (Gordal)

(Serves 6)

I chose lean ground lamb for this recipe, but you can also use pork, chicken, or turkey. Queen olives have a slightly spicy flavor and silky texture, and add a sunny element to the sauce.

FOR THE MEATBALLS:

1½ pounds lean ground lamb, pork, chicken, or turkey

1 small onion, chopped

¼ red bell pepper, deseeded and chopped

3 large shallots, chopped

3 tablespoons of flat-leaf parsley, cleaned, dried and minced

⅓ teaspoon of cumin

2 teaspoons of dried rosemary

3 cloves of garlic, crushed

3 tablespoons of dried currants

1 egg, beaten

EVOO

Salt, pepper

Breadcrumbs made from 1 slice of crustless country-style bread, fried on both sides in EVOO, with 1 clove of crushed garlic, half a reconstituted ñora pepper and salt for seasoning. Crumble when cooled.

FOR THE SAUCE:

3 tomatoes

1 medium onion, chopped

4 cloves of garlic, crushed

⅓ cup of Rioja wine, or another bold Spanish red

½ cup of organic chicken bone broth

1 cup of Gordal olives, pits removed

1 teaspoon of sweet pimentón

3 pinches of saffron threads, crushed
2 sprigs of thyme
½ cup of flat-leaf parsley, cleaned, dried and roughly chopped

For the meatballs, begin by sautéing until tender, the onion, bell pepper, and shallots in a glug of EVOO, with salt and pepper for seasoning. Don't use too much salt because olives are added to the sauce at the end. Set aside. Moisten breadcrumbs with a touch of spring or filtered water. Make the meatballs by combining meat, sautéed chopped onions and peppers, minced parsley, beaten egg, and breadcrumbs with the cumin, rosemary, and currants. Form the mixture into 12–16 meatballs, cover with plastic wrap or foil, and place in refrigerator for 30 minutes to chill.

To make the sauce, start by dissolving saffron in ¼ cup hot water. In a large skillet or cazuela, sauté the chopped onion in EVOO for 10 minutes, seasoning lightly with salt. Add the garlic and continue for 5 minutes more. Cut the tomatoes in half, and using a metal grater, remove pulp into the onion/garlic mixture. Add more EVOO, the chicken broth, red wine, pimentón, pepper and a little more salt to season, and mix well with a wooden spoon. Add the sprigs of thyme. Bring to low boil, then reduce heat and simmer for 30 minutes, stirring frequently. Add the saffron, and 10 minutes later, the meatballs, and continue to simmer uncovered, defatting the sauce with a spoon. After 10 minutes, arrange the olives in the pan, cover, and continue to gently cook for 30 minutes more. Keep defatting. Remove from heat, and cover with a bamboo mat. Let flavors meld for 10 minutes before garnishing with the parsley and serving.

Loin of Pork Braised in *Garnacha Rosado* Wine from Navarra

(Serves 6–8)

1½ to 2 pounds of pork loin, boneless, lean, and center-cut
2 green bell peppers, cut into large chunks
1 large onion, cut into chunks

1 large tomato, cut into chunks
2 bay leaves
4 shallots, whole
6 cloves of garlic, crushed
EVOO
1 cup of *Garnacha rosado* wine from Navarra or a similar Spanish rosado
½ cup of water mixed with ½ cup organic chicken stock
2 tablespoons of dried rosemary
1 teaspoon of dried thyme
Salt and ground black pepper

Lightly rinse pork loin and pat dry. In a bowl, combine with 4 cloves of the crushed garlic, 3 tablespoons of EVOO, the rosemary, a light sprinkling of salt, and some pepper. Cover and refrigerate overnight. The next day, remove from refrigerator for about 20 minutes before cooking. In a large casserole or cazuela, sauté the peppers, onion, tomato, and shallots in EVOO until vegetables and aromatics begin to caramelize, about 15 minutes. As they cook, season with thyme, salt and pepper, and a bay leaf, and after about 20 minutes more, arrange the marinated pork loin over the mixture, with the remaining bay leaf and garlic. Pour the wine and water/chicken stock over the vegetables, and drizzle the pork with EVOO. After adding a few more pinches of thyme, cover, bring to a low boil, reduce heat and braise until pork is cooked through, around 25–35 minutes. Do not overcook.

Beef and Pearl Onion Stew with Picada

(Serves 4)

For me, picada occupies a special place in cooking. It thickens with more finesse than French floury roux. Best of all, picada provides another layer of flavor that is mysteriously lush and delicious, and can be applied as a finish to all sorts of stews.

1½ pound cut of grass-fed beef tenderloin, cut into cubes

¼ teaspoon of cinnamon

1 sprig of fresh rosemary

Dried thyme

10 pearl onions, peeled, whole

2 large tomatoes, pureed into pan with a grater

1 small yellow onion, sliced

2 cloves of garlic, crushed

1 bay leaf

EVOO

1 cup of flour

4 ounces of full-bodied red Spanish wine

Salt, pepper

PICADA:

18 almonds or hazelnuts, skinned, blanched, and roasted

½ slice of crustless country-style bread

   (Do not use sourdough, which will alter the flavor.)

¼ cup of flat-leaf parsley, cleaned, dried and chopped

2 cloves garlic, minced

EVOO

Salt

Prepare the bread to use in the making of the picada by browning both sides in very hot EVOO. After the bread turns golden, drain on a paper towel.

In a medium pan, sauté the pearl onions with one clove of crushed garlic, seasoning with salt and pepper. When onions have caramelized, remove from pan and set aside. In a large casserole or cazuela, sauté the pureed tomatoes and another clove of the crushed garlic in EVOO, with three pinches of dried thyme, and a few pinches of salt. After tomatoes have reduced, remove and set aside as well.

Put flour in a large bowl, seasoning with salt and pepper. Coat the cubed meat with EVOO and then the flour. Splash a little more EVOO into the casserole or cazuela, with another clove of crushed garlic, and heat oil until very hot. Add beef cubes, turning gently until all of the pieces are lightly browned. Add the pureed tomato, along with the wine and a splash of spring water and the cinnamon. Mix with a wooden spoon. Tie the rosemary and bay leaf together and add to the casserole. There should be enough liquid just to cover the meat, but not "drown it." Bring to boil, reduce heat and simmer uncovered. After 20 minutes add the caramelized pearl onions and bake in 325°F oven for 25 minutes.

Using a mortar and pestle, pound the 2 cloves of garlic with a pinch of salt into the nuts, and add small pieces of toasted bread, parsley and a little more EVOO as you work. When done correctly, the consistency of picada should almost be buttery. If necessary, finish with a food processor but take care not to overblend.

Finally, add picada to the stew and on the stovetop, cook for 5-7 minutes more, mixing gently with the wooden spoon. When finished remove the tied herbs, place into 4 shallow bowls, and serve.

POULTRY AND GAME

Whole Roasted Orange Chicken, in the Style of Ferran Adrià

(Serves 4-6)

It was once typical throughout Europe for chefs to guard culinary secrets from even their sous chefs, but as Raphael Minder tells us in a 2016 *New York Times* article "Chefs' Camaraderie Lifts Basque Cuisine," Basque chefs broke with this by initiating a philosophy that encourages the sharing of information between chefs. Nowadays, it is the norm and thankfully so for the home cook.

The recipe below was inspired by Chef Ferran Adrià. His roasted chicken in *The Family Meal* is indicative of the everyday cooking that this innovative chef may not be known for but understands only too well. After all, Adrià says his touchstone for flavor remains his mother's *tortilla española*. (Can you imagine cooking for Adrià when he was a little boy?)

Adrià tells home cooks in *The Family Meal*, that *pollo a l'ast*—made with lemon, black pepper, thyme, rosemary and bay—is a traditional Catalan dish. My version captures the practical method of roasting, shared by Adriá, ensuring a juicy, crisp chicken every time.

4 to 5 pound chicken, rinsed and dried
2 sprigs fresh thyme
½ teaspoon of fine dried thyme
Bay leaf
EVOO
3 tablespoons of Spanish white wine
1 organic orange, rinsed and dried
3 shallots
2 cloves of garlic
¼ teaspoon of salt
White pepper
1 tablespoon of orange juice

Zest half of the orange over a bowl, using the finest side of a grater taking care not to include the pith. Then quarter it. Trim the tips of the chicken wings with kitchen shears. Rub chicken inside and out with EVOO, doing the same with the orange zest and salt, and place in a roasting pan. Put the thyme sprigs, along with the shallots, garlic and 3 of the orange quarters inside the chicken. Season the exterior of the chicken with the dried thyme and roast, breast side down, uncovered, for 25 minutes in a 425°F oven. Turn chicken over and continue roasting until golden, about 35 minutes more. Remove and set aside.

To make the gravy, on the stovetop add the wine and juice from the remaining quartered orange and deglaze the drippings on the bottom of the roasting pan under medium heat, stirring with a wooden spoon until the gravy reduces, about 10 minutes.

Pilota Made with Spiced Turkey Sausage

(Serves 4)

Pilota means ball in Spanish, but Marimar Torres, in *The Spanish Table: The Cuisines and Wines of Spain*, recommends that the meat be formed into cylinders. I have adopted her idea and like it very much. For certain recipes such as this one, I remove the seasoned turkey from its sausage casing and work breadcrumbs, sautéed shallots, etc. into the meat. You can also shape the mixture into small meatballs and combine with vegetables and noodles to make a stew.

> 1 pound of seasoned (hot or mild) turkey sausage removed from its casing. Lamb is an excellent substitute.
> ¾ to 1 cup of breadcrumbs
> 2 eggs, beaten
> EVOO
> ¼ cup of dried black currants, reconstituted
> ¼ cup of pine nuts
> ¼ cup of flat-leaf parsley, cleaned, dried and roughly chopped
> ⅓ cup of shallots, chopped
> 4 cloves of garlic, minced
> 2 tablespoons of tomato paste
> 1 tablespoon of dried thyme
> ½ teaspoon of pimentón
> ½ teaspoon of cinnamon
> ½ teaspoon nutmeg, freshly ground
> ½ teaspoon salt
> Salt and ground black pepper

In a small pan, sauté the shallots seasoned with salt in EVOO until caramelized. Set aside. Moisten breadcrumbs in a small bowl with a little water (or dry vermouth) and while mixing, season with pimentón, ¼ teaspoon of thyme, and a little salt. Crumbs should be lightly moist but not soggy. In another small bowl reconstitute the currants with a small amount of boiling water until they are plump, about 10 minutes, then drain off the water. And in a third small bowl, beat eggs with a fork and season with salt. In a large bowl, combine the turkey sausage with the tomato paste, a splash of EVOO, and the garlic, taking care to keep meat loosely workable. Add shallots, parsley, breadcrumbs, currants, pine nuts and eggs along with cinnamon, nutmeg, and ample ground black pepper. Mix lightly but well, shape into 2 cylinders, and transfer to a cazuela or ovenproof dish coated with EVOO. Bake covered in a 400°F oven for 40 minutes.

Nada's Quail with Piquillo Pepper Coulis

(Serves 4)

In *Homage to Catalonia* (1937), George Orwell wrote that people living in the countryside trapped quail in nets at night by making noises like female quail. And yes. The males come a running. Today, farm-raised quail is the norm.

4 quail
Salt, pepper, thyme, and rosemary
2 cloves of garlic, crushed
EVOO
1 to 2 tablespoons of fresh lime juice

PIQUILLO PEPPER COULIS:
1 cup of piquillo peppers from Navarra, drained
4 tablespoons of EVOO
2 pinches of salt
¼ cup of onions, chopped and sautéed in EVOO
1 clove of garlic
2 tablespoons of sherry vinegar
2 tablespoons of organic chicken stock, or water

Split 4 quail in half, rinse, and pat dry. Place in a baking dish and season uniformly with salt, pepper, herbs, and crushed garlic. Mix and drizzle equal parts of EVOO and lime juice over the quail and roast in a preheated 375°F oven uncovered for 25 minutes. For the coulis, combine and puree all ingredients in a small food processor. To serve, spoon the coulis in a narrow, artful swirl pattern to the side of a white plate, and place the quail next to it.

Lemony Chicken Stew with Shallots and Eggplant
(Serves 6)

If you like chardonnay, enjoy this recipe with a glass of Galician Godello. You may never drink chardonnay again.

    3 to 3½ pound chicken, cleaned, dried and cut into pieces
    1 teaspoon of dried thyme
    8 large shallots
    2 Japanese eggplants, cleaned, dried and trimmed
    5 to 6 cloves of garlic
    1 bay leaf
    Salt, pepper
    ⅓ teaspoon of pimentón
    ½ lemon
    1 sprig of fresh rosemary
    ¾ cup of chicken stock
    ½ cup of Godello wine (or a good Spanish white)
    EVOO

Slice eggplants in half lengthwise, score the flesh with diagonal knife cuts, sprinkle with salt, and place in a platter while the water draws out. After 20 minutes, wipe with a clean dishtowel. Prepare the garlic rub by pureeing 2 cloves of crushed garlic with 4 tablespoons of EVOO in a mortar, with the juice from most of half of a lemon. Place eggplants, cut side up, on a baking dish with parchment-lined foil, and rub on the garlic mixture. Cook uncovered for 30 minutes. After eggplants are roasted, remove and set aside.

Mix 2 more cloves of crushed garlic with 4 tablespoons of EVOO. Rub onto the chicken, and season with half of the dried thyme and pepper. Let marinate for 10 minutes. In a large ovenproof pan or cazuela, sauté the shallots in EVOO, seasoning with salt, until they begin to turn golden. Add chicken to the pan, after evenly seasoning with salt, the pimentón, and the rest of the thyme and the bay leaf. Brown the chicken on all sides, taking care to also turn the shallots. Add the stock, sprig of rosemary, and wine and, what's left of the lemon juice, sprinkle over the chicken.

Cook in a 400°F oven for 30 minutes. Uncover and baste. Reduce heat to 325°F. (Depending on your oven, it will take 5-10 minutes for the actual temperature to lower, so in reality you will only be cooking at this lower temperature for the final 15 minutes or so.) Cut the roasted eggplant into large bite-sized pieces and place around the chicken. Finish cooking, uncovered, for 25 minutes more. Serve the shallots along with the chicken and eggplant.

SAUCES

Allioli a la Catalana

(Makes 1 cup; best used the day you make it)

Allioli, Catalan for aioli, is a garlicky, fresh-tasting sauce that is outstanding with fish, shrimp, roasted potatoes, chicken, and so much more. Try allioli with flaked fish, capers, and herbs wrapped in radicchio, or stuffed into piquillo peppers for tapas. When you make it, remember it's all in how slowly you add the olive oil. To accomplish this, it is best to use a little glass dispenser that allows you to add drips of the oil, slowly. For authenticity, look for Catalan Arbequina extra-virgin olive oil.

    2 to 3 cloves of garlic, crushed
    1 cup of Catalan Arbequina EVOO
    Salt

TIP: Allioli is delicious with cooked seafood such as lobster or shrimp, roasted chicken, and as a dip for artichokes.

Ingredients should be room temperature. To reduce sharp taste, cut garlic lengthwise and discard the little green parts of each clove. Using a mortar and pestle, grind garlic with salt to make a paste. Slowly add the EVOO and blend using the pestle in a circular motion until an emulsion forms. This will take some time, during which you must continue mixing with the pestle. When a thick sauce that adheres to the side of the mortar is obtained, taste and adjust salt.

Allioli with Egg

(Makes 1 cup and can be refrigerated for several days)

Garlic can be roasted to give a more mellow taste, but roasted or raw, if you are like me, you will love this sauce.

    2 to 6 small cloves of garlic, crushed
    1 cup of EVOO
    Salt
    Yolks of two eggs from cage-free hens

Grind the salt and garlic in a mortar. Add egg yolks to the mixture and blend. Very slowly add the EVOO as in the previous recipe until an emulsion forms.

Salsa Romesco a la Catalana

(Makes about 2 cups of sauce and can be refrigerated up to one week)

It seems like nutrition researchers have rediscovered the benefits of nuts, and the cooking of Iberia offers an abundance of recipes with this super healthy food. Zesty, smoky romesco—yet another Catalan invention—can be served with grilled vegetables, fish, and more. This recipe was developed in Tarragona on the Mediterranean coast by fishermen when they were out to sea.

The ingredients listed for romesco can be adjusted with practice. If the sauce is too runny, add a little more bread; if too thick, add a splash more vinegar or EVOO. Taste and build flavor as you go.

Make sure to use a fruity bold olive oil for romesco, and if you wipe the almonds with a damp cloth after roasting, it will make removing the skins easier. Romesco is usually made with a dried ñora pepper, reconstituted in water, but if one uses roasted red pepper, the sauce is delicious too.

> TIP: This recipe can use a whole head of garlic, but in that case, it must be roasted first in a 350°F oven for 30 minutes.

1 ñora (or 1 choricero bell pepper)
4 ripe tomatoes
1 head of garlic
1 glass of olive oil
¼ cup of almonds
1 slice of stale bread (or fried bread)
Parsley [optional]

Place tomato and red pepper halves, skin side up, in baking dish, coated with EVOO and seasoned with salt and pepper. Roast in a preheated 375°F oven and after 20 minutes, remove from oven and set aside covered with foil. This loosens the skin so that you will be better able to remove it. In the same oven, roast the nuts until they begin to turn golden. This won't take long. After the vegetables are cool enough to handle, remove the skins and deseed the tomato.

Pulverize nuts in a food processor or a mortar and pestle. Combine all of the ingredients including a glug of EVOO, and mix until coarse, not smooth. Taste and adjust vinegar, olive oil, salt, pepper, and pimentón.

DESSERT

Galician Almond Cake

(Serves 6)

This recipe is my version of the traditional single layer cake made in Santiago de Compostela.

¼ pound of almonds, skins off, blanched
¾ cup of sugar
Confectionery sugar for dusting
4 eggs, yolks separated
Zest of ½ lemon and ½ orange
¼ teaspoon of vanilla extract
2 pinches salt
Butter for greasing one 8-inch diameter cake or springform pan

Preheat oven to 350°F. Using a food processor, grind the almonds until fine. In a bowl, combine sugar, citrus zest, vanilla extract, salt, and egg yolks. Blend well. Add the almonds. In a separate bowl, beat the egg whites until they peak and fold into the mixture. Transfer to the buttered pan and bake for 45 minutes or until a knife comes out clean. Remove and cool. Dust with confectionery sugar.

Asturian-Style Rice Pudding

(Serves 8)

This rice pudding showcases the dairy in Asturias, which is superb. We should do no less by ensuring that the milk and cream for this recipe are the very best available, meaning organic and from pasture-fed cattle.

1 cup of bomba rice
5 cups of milk
1 cup of heavy cream
1½ cups of sugar
½ vanilla bean
1 stick of cinnamon
½ teaspoon of salt

In a medium-sized pot, combine rice, milk, cream, cinnamon stick, vanilla bean and salt, and bring to a boil. Remove cinnamon stick and vanilla bean, and reduce heat and simmer until the rice is tender, about 45 minutes, stirring frequently. Add the sugar, bring back to a boil, reduce heat and simmer uncovered for two hours, stirring at regular intervals. Spoon into dessert cups and sprinkle a little powdered cinnamon on top.

Mediterranean-Style Orange Rice Pudding with Meringue

(Serves 6-8)

My warm gratitude to Isabel Bertomeu for this recipe. The meringue provides a lightness that you will love.

½ cup bomba rice
Pinch of salt
3 cups of 2 percent milk
2 egg yolks, beaten
½ cup of golden raisins
1 tablespoon of brandy
Grated rind of one orange

MERINGUE:
2 egg whites
2 tablespoons of powdered sugar
¼ teaspoon of vanilla

Combine rice, milk and salt in a small pot and bring to a boil. Reduce heat and simmer until rice is tender, about 20 minutes. Remove from heat and quickly stir the yolks, raisins, sugar, brandy, and orange rind. Transfer pudding to an ovenproof dish. Beat the egg whites until stiff. Fold in powdered sugar and vanilla, and spread over the pudding. Bake in a 300°F oven until meringue is set and the peaks brown, about 15 minutes. Serve hot or cold.

Fig and Toasted Pine Nut Pinwheel Cookies

(Makes two dozen cookies)

Did you know that for hundreds of years, figs were considered medicine in the treatment of a variety of ailments, from skin conditions to coughs? Present-day research has come full circle, confirming that figs are a good source of antioxidants, protective compounds such as lectins, and fiber.

1 pound of dried figs
¼ cup of pine nuts, lightly toasted
¼ cup of sugar
¼ cup of spring or filtered water
2 tablespoons of anisette
1 cup of brown sugar
½ cup of softened butter
¼ teaspoon of salt
2 eggs
2 cups of flour
1 teaspoon of cinnamon

Cut figs in half and scoop out the meat. In a small pot, combine the figs, sugar, and water. Bring to a boil and simmer until mixture thickens. Add the anisette. Set aside and let cool. Beat eggs in a medium-size bowl. Add brown sugar, butter, salt, flour, and cinnamon. Fold in pine nuts. Roll dough out on a floured surface until about ¼ inch thick. Spread filling uniformly so it is flat and then roll up. Refrigerate for one hour. After the dough is chilled, slice cookies ¼ inch thick. Arrange on a buttered baking pan and bake in a preheated 375°F for 10-15 minutes or until golden.

Spanish Goat Cheese with Honey and Rosewater

(Serves 4)

The Arab people began the use of culinary rosewater in Spain. For this recipe we combine rosewater with a touch of honey.

Capricho de cabra cheese, or another similar soft fresh goat's milk cheese
  (plan on ¼ pound of cheese per person)
3 tablespoons of shelled and crushed pistachios

FOR THE SYRUP:
1½ tablespoons of culinary rosewater
2 tablespoons of water
1½ tablespoons of honey

Combine all ingredients for the rosewater syrup and taste. If you wish, adjust by adding more rosewater or honey. Place a small serving of cheese on each dessert saucer and spoon a little rosewater syrup on top. Garnish with crushed pistachios.

Watermelon Ice Slush with Flowers

(Servings vary)

Carme Ruscalleda inspired this recipe with her own for Watermelon Ice Slush, Jam, and Cake from *100 Easy Recipes to Cook at Home: Carme Ruscalleda's Mediterranean Cuisine*. Edible flowers are packed with anticancer, antioxidant-rich carotenoids.

½ of a small watermelon, rind removed
Packaged edible flowers, rinsed and dried

1½ tablespoons culinary rosewater

2 tablespoons water

1½ tablespoons lavender honey

Cut watermelon into large chunks and freeze. Make the rosewater syrup using the method described in the previous recipe. Using a grater with large holes, scrape the frozen watermelon against it, and begin layering in tall glasses. After a layer of watermelon ice, place an edible flower, and then drizzle with rosewater. Cover with a subsequent layer of watermelon ice and repeat with another flower, then rosewater syrup, and repeat until glasses are filled. Serve immediately.

Roasted Apricots with Gran Torres Orange Liqueur

(Serves 4)

When summer apricots are at their peak, this makes an elegant completion to dinner.

4 apricots, pits removed and cut in half

4 tablespoons of almonds, slivered

Butter, for greasing baking dish

4 tablespoons of mild-tasting honey

4 pinches of nutmeg, freshly grated

4 tablespoons of Gran Torres orange liqueur,
    or another excellent-quality brand

Preheat oven to 375°F. Arrange apricots, cut side up, in a buttered baking dish. Spoon equal amounts of the orange liqueur on each apricot half, followed with honey and a little freshly grated nutmeg. Bake for 12 minutes, add almonds, and bake 3–4 minutes more. Almonds should be browned but not burned. If desired, serve each brandied apricot with a small scoop of frozen vanilla yogurt or ice cream.

Pa amb Oli i Xocolata,
with Vanilla Ice Cream and a Dollop of Hot Fudge

(Serves 2)

Children will love toasted bread topped with melted chocolate for an after-school snack. As for adults, well, Ferran Adrià's crew at El Bulli, ate pa amb oli i xocolata for dessert. I relate, especially with a scoop of vanilla ice cream and hot fudge on the side.

2½ ounces of 72 percent chocolate
2 thin slices of country-style bread
1½ tablespoons EVOO
1 to 2 pinches of coarse salt or flakes
Organic vanilla ice cream
Hot fudge

Preheat the oven to 325°F. Place the bread on a baking sheet and taking care not to burn, toast both sides on the highest rack until light golden. Remove from oven and using a hand grater, coarsely grate chocolate over the slices of toasted bread and put back into the oven for a minute or so until the chocolate melts. Transfer each piece of toast to a shallow bowl. Drizzle with EVOO and a sprinkle of salt. Serve with a small scoop of ice cream and hot fudge.

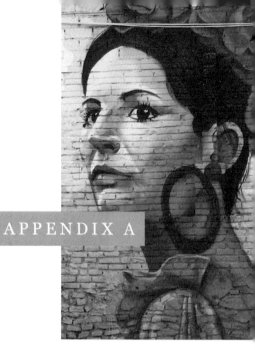

APPENDIX A

Cheese Chart

A variety of cheeses in Spain are produced and made from cow, sheep, or goat milk that are Protected Designations of Origin.

Protected Designation of Origin Cheeses

CHEESE	REGION
Afuega'L Pitu	Asturias
Arzua-Ulloa	Galicia
Cabrales	Asturias
Cebreiro	Galicia
Gamonedo/Gamoneu	Asturias
Idiazabal	Basque Country and Navarre

Mahon-Menorca	Menorca (Balearic Islands)
Picon-Bejes Treviso	Cantabria
Castellano	Castilla y Leon
Camerano	La Rioja
Casin	Asturias
L'Alt Urgell i *la* Cerdanya	Catalunya
Queso de la Serena	Extremadura
Murcia	Murcia
Murcia al Vino	Murcia
Valdeon	Castilla y Leon
Queso Flor de Guia/ Queso de Media Flor de Guia/ Queso de Guia	Canary Islands
Ibores	Extremadura
Los Beyos	Asturias and Cantabria
Maiorero	Canary Islands
Manchego	Castilla-La Mancha
Nata de Cantabria	Cantabria
Palmero/De La Palma	Canary Islands
Tetilla	Galicia
Zamorano	Castilla y Leon
Quesucos de Liebana	Cantabria
Roncal	Navarre
San Simon Da Costa	Galicia
Torta del Casar	Extremadura

Source: https://www.mapa.gob.es/es/alimentacion/temas/calidad-diferenciada/dop-igp/

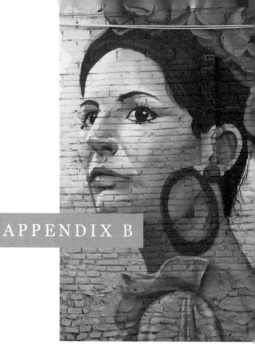

Thyme, Rosemary, and *Tomillo* Soup, a Home Remedy

The discovery of *El Sidrón* cave in Asturias, circa 46,000 BC, revealed remnants of the herbs yarrow (astringent) and chamomile (anti-inflammatory) on the dental remains of the cave's inhabitants, the Neanderthals. Researchers concluded that these prehistoric people had the advanced ability to select specific plants that they knew would be effective for self-medication.

During medieval times, Spanish monks grew an extensive variety of herbs for healing and culinary purposes in their monastery gardens. Remnants of these gardens can still be seen in many Spanish monasteries today.

In the 1500s, herbs were commonly used in Catalunya for cooking and for medicine, as documented in *Llibre del Coch*. The author, Robert de Nola, chef to Ferdinand, King of Naples, wrote of specific medicinal benefits associated with herbs found in many of the recipes. Published in 1520, it was the first cookbook printed in the Catalan language and was subsequently translated into Castilian five years later.

The medicinal properties of many herbs routinely used by healers in ancient times are validated by modern scientific research today. An example is rosemary, the herb for remembrance, which was confirmed by the "Short-term Study on the Effects of Rosemary on Cognitive Function in an Elderly Population," published by *The Journal of Medical Food* in 2012.

Rosemary and to a greater extent, thyme, are pillars of Spanish cooking. Knowing that these herbs have been used historically as medicine in Spain since very early times made me yearn to discover more.

So I consulted with Donald R. Yance, MH, CN, master herbalist, clinical nutritionist, and author of two comprehensive books on health, including his most recent *Adaptogens in Medical Herbalism: Elite Herbs and Natural Compounds for Mastering Stress, Aging and Chronic Disease.* Yance is aware of the singularly important place herbs hold in the historical context of traditional medicine. Specific to *The Iberian Table*, Yance believes "not enough has been done regarding the important place herbs hold within the Mediterranean Diet."

Yance points out that "rosemary and thyme are both amazing healing herbs that have a rich history of traditional usage and recently have been backed by an explosion of modern scientific research validating their historic use as health promoting foods. In the twelfth century, the great Spanish Jewish philosopher,

> TIP: Susan Lord-Williams's medieval-spanishchef.com is a fascinating blog about ancient recipes and the medicinal properties of herbs. Many recipes have been translated directly from *Llibre del Coch.*

> According to the *Swiss Times*, global demand for extract of thyme is expected to grow significantly through 2028; and according to *The Trusted Chronicle*, the rosemary extract market will be worth over $1 billion by then.

Maimonides, was said to have prescribed these herbs to his patients to treat a variety of ailments, including thyme for coughs and rosemary for circulation and brain health. Both rosemary and thyme have been shown to enhance cognition and neurological function, enhance circulation and cardiovascular health and even possess anti-cancer, anti-inflammatory, redox-anti-oxidative, and anti-microbial properties. Combined with an olive oil-rich diet, these common herbs have diverse health-promoting, age-retarding benefits."

For those interested in learning more about the traditional and scientific benefits of rosemary and thyme, and other herbs, I have included Donald R. Yance's books in the Bibliography, and his blog in the Resource Guide.

Chef Xavier Arrey Verges'
Tomillo Soup

Traditional Catalan tomillo soup (origin unknown except to say it reaches back many generations) is actually an herbal infusion meant to be healing for colds and flu. Infusions are an effective way to obtain the benefits of herbs, something that I learned years ago.

The first time I had tomillo was in Hotel Carlemany's Restaurant Índigo in Girona, which is centrally located in a historic area of great beauty.

I caught a chill on the flight over and to make matters worse, the weather was cold and rainy by the time we arrived at the hotel. It was lunchtime, but all I wanted was a bowl of soup. Asking for a recommendation, chef Xavier suggested tomillo. The soup arrived with four very small, flavorful pork meatballs in an aromatic thyme broth that, just by the look and smell, had the promise of something fortifying. My appetite was stirred, too. The soup was so delicious that I eagerly finished every drop along with the rustic cheese toast that came with it.

As the afternoon progressed, I felt increasingly better, and by the end of the day, no more cold.

A culinary note: Chef Xavier apprenticed under Jaume Subirós, whom I wrote about earlier. Chef Subirós's Restaurant El Motel is about a 30-minute drive north from Hotel Carlemany, so if you ever find yourself in Girona, I suggest you book reservations for Sunday lunch. The cooking is so exceptional that the French drive across the border through the Pyrenees to dine there.

Catalan Tomillo Soup

¼ ounce dried thyme
2½ quarts of spring or filtered water
2 organic chicken breasts, meat removed from bones
3 large yellow onions, cut into chunks
Cloves of fresh garlic, halved
EVOO
Unrefined gray salt

In a large pot over medium heat, sauté the onions in EVOO, salting lightly. As the onions caramelize, clean viscera from chicken breast bones, cut into pieces and add to the pot. Season with more salt, and continue to sauté until lightly browned. Add half the water and bring to boil. Reduce heat and simmer, removing the foam. After 35 minutes, remove from heat and when cool, remove any fat that accumulates on the surface of the broth. (Making this broth takes time, so you might want to cook it the day before.)

In a clean pot, combine the defatted broth, the rest of the water, thyme, and salt to taste. Bring to a boil, then remove from heat, cover, and let infuse for 5 minutes. Then strain the broth and serve in bowls rubbed with garlic, with a little more EVOO and dried thyme.

Below are serving options that Chef Xavier recommends:

- Serve with toasted, warm rustic bread drizzled with EVOO and garnished with finely chopped jamón Ibérico or grated mature Parmesan.

- Rub the inside of each serving bowl with a piece of fresh crushed garlic. Add one raw organic egg and thin slices of raw mushrooms. Pour the boiling soup into the bowl and serve.

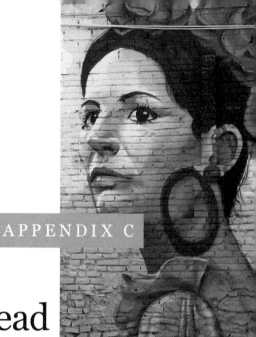

The Benefits of Fish Head Broth, and Recipes for *Caldo de pescado*, and Rice with Scallops and Shrimp

In the Iberian kitchen, nothing goes to waste. Fish bones and heads are combined to make stock as a base for all kinds of seafood dishes, from sauces, stews, soups, and rice, to noodle dishes and more, including, sometimes, adding essence to allioli. Chef Carme Ruscalleda, for example, makes a quick version with sherry. First, she juliennes leeks, onions, carrots, and celery, and sautés the mixture in EVOO with garlic and salt until the vegetables and aromatics caramelize. Then she adds dry sherry and the head and tail of a hake, along with thyme and

Fish Broth, Nutritional Gold The eyes of fish and shrimp contain EPA and DHA, hard to obtain omega-3 derivatives, which stimulate brain cells and help to prevent memory decline. EPA and DHA also help lower cholesterol, prevent hypertension, increase stamina, and help produce serotonin, which aids in the prevention of depression. And consumption of fish eyes has been shown by research to mitigate deterioration of eyesight. Iodine-rich fish bones, cartilage, and fat contain an abundance of omega-3 fatty acids, vitamin A, zinc, and calcium, and are sources of anti-breast cancer iodine.

TIP: If you are having a whole fish filleted, ask that the head and carcass be packaged separately. Or call ahead and ask for 3-4 pounds of these fish parts. When preparing fresh shrimp, do not discard the heads—or shells, for that matter—for they can be put into the stockpot as well.

bay laurel. The sautéing continues for a few minutes more, after which boiling water is added and the broth is allowed to simmer for 15 minutes. At the end, salt is adjusted, and the broth is strained.

Why cook with the head and tail—and bones—of fish? Because not only does it add flavor, it is incredibly life-giving, too. When I studied macrobiotics, I came to know that broth from fish was considered a healing food for people with cancer. Broth prepared with these parts, especially the head, offers hard-to-obtain omega-3 fats that stimulate immunity and brain cell activity, lower harmful cholesterol, help prevent hypertension, alleviate depression (by boosting serotonin) and help shield against macular degeneration. And this is only the beginning. Gel from the bones and heads of fish is a particularly rich source of iodine, a trace mineral all but missing from our food supply that is crucial in the prevention of breast cancer. Tissue levels of iodine have been found to be low in women with the disease. In addition, iodine supports thyroid function, bone formation, and is a basic building block for hormone production. We can conclude that broth made from the head, tail and bones of fish has a place in *The Iberian Table* kitchen, so let's do some cooking with it.

According to Chef Alice Waters in her classic *Chez Panisse Cooking*, "flat fish are particularly high in gelatin and give the broth structure." She recommends using light-skinned fish such as sole, halibut, and Pacific rockfish, and even cod and bass, but not "oily fleshed fish" including salmon and tuna. Waters points out that the shells of lobster and shrimp can be added to the stockpot, but only at the final 15 minutes to preserve their fresh taste. I also learned this same advice from a Thai friend, who makes seafood broth from fish and shrimp heads every week for her young children. She uses this broth for all kinds of recipes, especially noodles, which her children love.

Caldo de pescado

(makes about 3 quarts)

Call ahead and ask the fishmonger to set aside 4 pounds of fish heads and carcasses.

Discard entrails, blood, and fins—their strong taste will ruin the broth. Rinse the fish head and carcass under running water and put in a large stockpot with 2 tablespoons of EVOO. Add 3 trimmed scallions, a celery stalk, large yellow onion, trimmed leek and half of fennel bulb, all chopped, as well as 1 carrot, 4 cloves garlic, several sprigs of parsley and thyme, 3 white and 4 black peppercorns, 1 bay leaf, 6 cups of spring or filtered water, 1 cup of clam juice, and a few pinches of salt. Bring to a boil, cover and simmer for one hour. Remove from burner and infuse for 30 minutes. During this time, you can add wedges of lemon or saffron (diluted in a little hot water) or a few more sprigs of thyme. Strain and use for recipes such as Rice with Scallops and Shrimp, below.

Options: Begin the broth by first sautéing the chopped vegetables and garlic in EVOO, and after they become translucent, add the remaining ingredients. Choose from the following to add to your broth when you begin cooking:

> 1 medium frying pepper—for the sauté
> 1 peeled and deseeded tomato—for the sauté
> 6-12 mussels, scrubbed
> 1 small whiting
> 1 cup dry Spanish white or *Jerez* sherry wine

Rice with Scallops and Shrimp

(serves 6)

1 large red pepper

½ large yellow onion, diced

½ green pepper, diced

3 tablespoons of parsley, cleaned, dried and finely chopped

1 teaspoon of fresh thyme, minced

3 cups of fish head broth

1 cup of bomba rice

¼ cup of EVOO

¼ teaspoon of red pepper flakes

¾ pound of medium-size shrimp, peeled and deveined

¾ pound of scallops, rinsed

1 bay leaf

Salt

Freshly ground white pepper

Halve the red pepper, and roast cut-side down in a 375°F oven until the skin begins to char. This will take about 25 minutes. Remove the pepper from oven and place in a shallow bowl with a plate over the top and set aside. Put a glug of EVOO in a large sauté pan. When it reaches temperature, sauté onions until caramelized, then add the diced green pepper, garlic, parsley, thyme, scallops, and shrimp. Stir and season lightly with salt and white pepper, and continue to sauté until scallops and shrimp turn opaque. Remove seafood with a slotted spoon and set aside.

TIP: As mentioned earlier, for a vermouth and EVOO spray to add flavor to any seafood dish, in a bottle with a sprayer combine 1 part Spanish vermouth with 2 parts EVOO. Spray lightly over seafood right before you place into the oven.

In a medium-sized pot, bring seafood stock to a low boil. Add bomba rice, salt lightly, cover, bring back to a boil, reduce heat and simmer until all the liquid is absorbed, about 10-15 minutes. Set cooked rice aside. Remove skin from the halved pepper and cut into strips. In a Pyrex baking dish, combine the rice, pepper strips, and shrimp and scallops. Sprinkle with minced parsley and place in a 325°F oven for 10 minutes. Can be served with aioli.

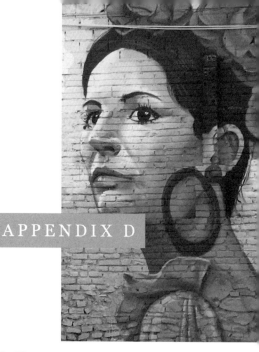

A Week of Menus, Additional Lunch Ideas and a Recipe

"Spain produces what is probably the highest quality and most expensive canned food in the world, and many tapas bars rely on it. Though much of it is good and interesting, for the most part I don't get it, since Spain also produces among the highest quality fresh food in the world. This is as true in Barcelona—which has farms within its city limits—as it is elsewhere in the country."

—Mark Bittman, "Five Catalan Stars with Small Plates and Long Menus."
New York Times, June 3, 2007

Mealtimes in Spain are very different from the United States. And snacking seems to go on all day. So how do the Spanish stay so slim? Let's just say they know there is a connection between moderate servings and good health.

Regarding mealtimes, upon awakening, say from 7—9 a.m., it is typical for the Spanish to have coffee—*café con leche,* most likely—with a small cookie or pastry. Then around 11 a.m., breakfast is taken, which might include a slice of tortilla or a small sandwich made with a little tuna, anchovy, or cheese, anointed with a touch of olive oil. Lunch, around 2 p.m., is often the most elaborate meal of the day. Then, after work, people usually meet at a tapas bar to grab a snack with a glass of wine or a beer. The evening meal typically is eaten around 9:00 to 10:00 p.m., and in most cases it is simple. However, if dinner is a family, friends, or business affair of several courses sometimes lasting until midnight, lunch would be modest.

Regarding breakfast, whether it be the early or the late one, once you get used to strong coffee mixed with an equal amount of very hot milk, well, in my experience there is no going back.

Café con Leche

Make a half cup of very strong coffee. Brew it on the stove, or use an espresso maker and then transfer into a cup or mug. Meanwhile, pour a half cup of milk in a small pot and heat until almost scalded. Immediately pour the hot milk over the coffee. If desired, sweeten to taste. Stevia works instead of sugar. Call me a Philistine, but in this case, I prefer coconut nondairy creamer over milk. No matter what you prefer, café con leche is *muy bueno*.

———•———

Before the menus, a word about organization. I'm sure it's evident, but cooking extra food saves time. For example, my recipes for soup or stews are always for several servings, as is *tortilla española*, which keeps well overnight at room temperature covered with a bamboo mat right on your kitchen counter.

The Spanish Mediterranean diet is "plant-forward" eating at its best. Once you get a feel for the ingredients of Spain, menu planning will become second nature.

Menu One

Breakfast

Café con leche, coffee or tea including green or chamomile

Catalan Pa Amb Tomàquet (p. 180) alone or with your choice of cheese, tuna, jamón, or sardine

Lunch

Antonia's *Tortilla Española* (pp. 182–183)

Lettuce, arugula, and sliced tomatoes with *A Su Gusto Vinagreta* (p. 52)

Did you know that eggs are an excellent source of protective sulfur? The liver needs high levels of this mineral to support what is known by nutrition scientists as phase II detoxification, which breaks down harmful toxins in the body. Sulfur is also integral in preventing certain cells from leading to cancer and other serious illness. And it also supports healthy skin, tendons, and ligaments.

Dinner

Gazpacho (p. 188)

Rice Pelat, or Rice with Chicken, Shrimp, and Artichokes (pp. 224–225), garnished with olives

Dessert: A piece of seasonal fruit with Caña de Cabra cheese

Menu Two

Breakfast

Café con leche, coffee, or tea

Huevos Rotos, or Fried Potatoes with Broken Egg (p. 307)

Lunch

Bonito de Norte Tuna with Quick Saffron Mayonnaise (p. 334)

Slice of rustic-style whole grain bread, toasted and drizzled with olive oil

A little Spanish cheese with a piece of fresh seasonal fruit or grapes

Dinner

Alicante Chicken and Vegetable Paella (pp. 225–226)

Elena Arzak's Gem Lettuce (p. 154)

Dessert: Manchego Cheese Topped with Quince Membrillo (p. 187)

Menu Three

Breakfast

Café con leche, coffee, or tea

Saffron-Strawberry Smoothie (p. 330)

Lunch

Red Lentil Soup with Chorizo (pp. 194–195)

Anchovy Toast (p. 311)

Dinner

Quinoa Paella with Squid (pp. 238–239)

Steamed asparagus with lemon wedge and olive oil

Salad of Clementinas, Fennel, and Roncal Cheese, with Sherry Vinagreta (pp. 193–194)

Dessert: Roasted Apricots with Gran Torres Orange Liqueur (p. 265)

Menu Four

Breakfast

Café con leche, coffee, or tea

Multigrain toast with tomato slices and virgin olive oil

Lunch

Gabure: Vegetable Soup with Beans, Chestnuts, and Sausage
(pp. 195–197)

Catalan Spinach with Toasted Pine Nuts and Currants (p. 217)

Dinner

Celery Stalks Stuffed with Asturian Blue Cabrales Cheese, Apples,
and Walnuts (pp. 183–184)

Carme Ruscalleda's Irresistible Ibérico Ham Croquettes (p. 150)

Herbed Romanesco Broccoli (pp. 216–217)

Dessert: A small piece of 70 percent dark chocolate with a handful
of hazelnuts

Menu Five

Breakfast

Café con leche, coffee, or tea

Toasted rustic bread, drizzled with olive oil and garnished with grated
mature Parmesan

Lunch

Navarran Mixed Vegetable Menestra (pp. 207–208)

Roasted Marcona almonds, with grapes

Dinner

Green Beans with Anchovy Vinagreta (p. 213)

Roasted Cod Over Potatoes and Leeks (pp. 239–240)

Dessert: Peaches Poached in Rosado Wine Topped with Frozen Yogurt
(p. 128)

Menu Six

Breakfast
Café con leche, coffee, or tea
A piece of seasonal fruit
Fig and Toasted Pine Nut Pinwheel Cookies (p. 263)

Lunch
Wild Salmon Salad with Pimentón (p. 193)
Fresh grapes with a handful of walnuts

Dinner
Orange Salad with Spanish Cheese, Olives, and Sweet Onion (p. 124)
Alicante Chicken and Vegetable Paella (pp. 225–226)
Dessert: Slow-Roasted Figs (p. 128)

Menu Seven

Breakfast
Café con leche, coffee, or tea
Majorcan Farmer's Breakfast Salad (p. 69)

Lunch
Lentils over Grilled Cauliflower (pp. 232–233)
Salad with mixed fresh greens, tomatoes, sliced sweet onion, and one hardboiled egg, with *A Su Gusto Vinagreta* (p. 52)

Dinner

Evohe's Cured Organic Goat Cheese Salad with Roasted Pine Nuts and Membrillo Vinagreta (pp. 202–203)

Slow-Roasted Lamb Shoulder (p. 55)

Baked Kabocha Squash Topped with Sofrito (p. 61)

Dessert: Mediterranean-Style Orange Rice Pudding with Meringue (p. 262)

More Ideas for Lunch

When I began *The Iberian Table*, people constantly asked, "What do you eat for lunch?" They still do. Perhaps because lunch is often solo, revealing what I liked to eat was a way for people to get to the heart of the Spanish Mediterranean diet. Lunch is direct. It speaks to one's habits, favorite foods, and the like.

And so, I hope you enjoy the lunch menus below, including my latest obsession, at the end.

- Salad of Softened Pear Over Arugula with Shaved Manchego and Pear Vinagreta (p. 206), with a modest handful of toasted pecans
- Garbanzo Salad with Mahon Cheese, Pomegranate Seeds, and Empeltre Olives (pp. 229–230)
- Quinoa Paella with Squid (pp. 238–239)
- Open-Face Tortilla with White Beans and Leeks (pp. 233–234)
- Basque Piperrada Vasca of Orange and Yellow Bell Peppers and Eggs (p. 189)

A splurge-worthy note: Spain's gourmet tinned fish and seafood, called *latas*, are like nothing you can imagine. Canning is usually done the day after fish and seafood are caught or harvested. Ingredients for canning are of the highest quality, e.g., actual ink from squid, extra-virgin olive oil, or gentle brine to simulate the sea. Latas are served with pride in gourmet tapas bars and restaurants throughout Spain. Known by leading chefs all over the world, Spain's tinned fish and seafood is of dazzling quality, so cost is not a bargain. For quick lunch indulgences, you might want to keep a few of these prizes on hand. Be it cod in tomato sauce, mackerel, sardines, mussels, clams, squid, anchovies, or scallops, tinned seafood and fish from Spain delight.

- Lunch sandwich made with Catalan Pa Amb Tomàquet (p. 180) and Tapenade (p. 181)
- Steamed baby carrots and kale, topped with Hazelnut Picada Sauce (pp. 251–252)
- A handful of Roasted Marcona Almonds with Rosemary (p. 182), a piece of seasonal fruit, and your choice of Spanish cheese
- Samfaina with Anchovies (p. 100)
- Romesco Sauce (pp. 102–103) with steamed or roasted leeks
- Shrimp *Exprés* with Swiss Chard and Orange Peel (pp. 234–235)
- Spanish tinned fish or seafood, on a melon slice with a wedge of lemon
- María José San Román's Wheat *Olleta* with Assorted Vegetables (p. 227)
- Piquillo Pepper Coulis (pp. 255–256) over salmon or shrimp burger
- Herby Romaine Boats with Cheese and Peaches (p. 191)
- Steamed asparagus with Allioli a la Catalana (pp. 257–258)

And finally,

- Eggs Over Mushrooms: My lunch version of Basque Mushroom Ragout with Egg Yolk Sauce (p. 192) is perfect for one or two. I especially love sliced, cleaned and dried shiitakes, trumpets, and maitakes. Just button mushrooms are delicious, too. Sauté mushrooms in butter, olive oil, and a minced clove of garlic. Season with salt, and very generous grindings of pepper. Cook until tender. Top with one or two sunny-side eggs. Leave yolks runny.

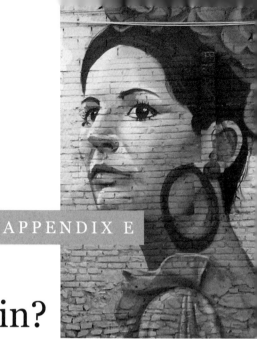

Why the North of Spain?

"The Basque Country, it is widely accepted, is perhaps the best place to eat in Europe, where the quality flowing out of modernist kitchens is equaled by the pleasures found in San Sebastián's weathered pintxo bars."

> – How Spain's Tiny San Sebastián became a Global Force in the Food World,
> *Thegentlemansjournal.com*, June 2, 2022

"Spanish chefs grace the pages of international gastronomic magazines, and some food critics believe they have replaced their French counterparts at the vanguard of culinary innovation."

> – Victoria Burnett, *Spain's Top Chefs Clash Over Ingredients and Culinary Innovation,*
> *New York Times*, June 1, 2008

The *Iberian Table*, which examines the Mediterranean diet of Spain, is more than an extension of my previous books written in support of healthy food and cooking. It is a reflection of my feelings about a place that goes to the heart of what I have been writing about for decades.

This place is the north of the country, a region that author Jenny Chandler describes as the gastronomic heartland of Spain. The centrifugal power of the food movement found today throughout Spain began here and came to be a global force. The late Catalan chef Santi Santamaría, who lived and worked in the North, embraced seasonal produce, lavish use of olive oil, sustainably caught fish, and additive-free cooking, all building blocks of the Mediterranean diet. Railing against the junk food culture, healthful foods meant everything to this chef. In 1994, Santi' restaurant in Barcelona, Racó de Can Fabes, was the first in Spain to receive three Michelin stars. He was eventually inspired by the presentations of the inventive Basque chef, Juan Mari Arzak, from San Sebastián, the small Northern coastal town that came to be distinguished as having more Michelin stars than any other city in the world, except for Kyoto. It wasn't long before the North came to boast the preponderance of three-starred restaurants in Spain, including those of the father daughter duo, Juan Mari and Elena Arzak, Eneko Atxa, Martín Berasategui, Jordi Cruz, the Roca brothers, Ferrán Adrià, and Carme Ruscalleda. Shaping this northern movement is El Motel, the popular name for the historic restaurant at Hotel Empordà in Figueres. This sanctuary of Catalan cuisine was founded in 1961 by chef Josep Mercader, described by Adrià as "the father of modern Spanish cooking." Today El Motel is run by Mercader's son-in-law, chef Jaume Subiròs. Some things are kept the same at El Motel, like the menu cover created especially for the restaurant by a 17-year-old Salvador Dalí, who dined regularly there, as did Josep Pla, political essayist, memoirist, novelist, and gastronome.

By focusing on the North, I am in no way diminishing the excellent gastronomy that can be found elsewhere in Spain. For this, chefs María José San Román and Quique Dacosta, both with celebrated restaurants in Alicante come readily to mind. There are many others. But it should not go unnoticed that in 2022, the World's 50 Best Restaurants group in announcing its annual winners, distinguished Barcelona's Disfrutar as number three on the list, with several other restaurants of the North included in the first twenty.

This book examining the Spanish Mediterranean diet is fueled by a region that captures my writerly interest. By focusing on the North, I am able to detail basic health precepts and culinary traditions that bring the diet to life. The variety of vegetable dishes alone in Chandler's gastronomic heartland, drives me to know and report more, such as the recent study done by EAE Business School in Barcelona finding that the North spent more than any other region on fruits and vegetables.

For me, though something special is happening in the North, this region remains reflective of a country whose people are drawn to healthy foods and cooking in an innate way. Because of this inclination towards well-being, the Spanish are blessed with long life. To look at other regions of Spain could be in my future, but during this time when a new vision for health is needed more than ever, my focus on the North is a good way to begin.

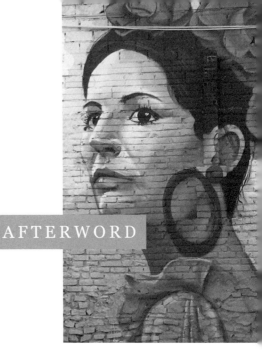

Lampreys, Thrips, Desmans, and Sea Anemones

"During the last Ice Age, the Iberian Peninsula served as a biological refuge for a large number of species, and its vascular flora, numbering about 7000 species, is the richest in Europe."

– Javier Tardío, Manuel Pardo de Santayana, and Ramón Morales.
"Ethnobotanical Review of Wild Edible Plants in Spain,"
Botanical Journal of the Linnean Society, 152, no. 1 (August 2016):27–71.

Recipes in northern Spain are so ancient their origins are sometimes untraceable. No doubt mushrooms were roasted over bonfires by cave dwellers there, and are still gathered in the same ferny forests that they frequented, continuing to teem with hare and venison. There is dark amber mountain honey, wild berries and nuts. The buds of cardoons are quite tasty, and can be found in the late summer meadows of Navarre and Aragón. I imagine early humans collecting them to feast upon. Sea anemones, showing rainbow colors, shimmer in shallow pools of sunlight—some of the oldest creatures on earth. They still taste as pristine as the Costa Brava waters from whence they come. Oils are pressed from wild olives in this land. Recipes are flavored pungently, while at the same time subtly, for cooks there know what we are tasting is larger than what we think, for it is nature itself.

If food is nature, then this region has no equal. The Atlantic Ocean, Cantabrian Sea, Bay of Biscay, the Mediterranean Sea, and several ranges of mountains with rivers and streams, all give form to a gastronomy so abundant, and enigmatic, one yearns to know more. To know, for instance, about the earliest evidence of direct pollination on the planet recently discovered in the North in the form of a thrip, the miniscule first pollen-carrying insect found in a block of amber tree resin 100 million years old.

Or, if you are like me, you will want to know that ten million years ago, after the extinction of dinosaurs, when the first bats, horses, and whales came into being, a hand-sized creature called a desman could be found in the Catalan Pyrenees, an outcrop of land older than the Alps. Last in an evolutionary line, these furry little beings have retractable platypus-like snouts and webbed feet, and can still be found in streams that rush through the Pyrenees, hungrily searching their own food.

Or you may want to know about the biblical bearded lammergeier vulture, the rarest bird of prey in Europe. The Pyrenees is home to these wildly beautiful creatures, the largest flying birds on earth having wingspans up to ten feet with brain power exceeding that of ravens. Wily birds, they burrow into the soil to turn their white bibs blood-red in order to better terrify; so cunning they know the exact angle at which to smash their prey against the stone of the granite mountains to better obtain the marrow. According to mythology, lammergeiers are strong enough to pick up a child or a baby lamb.

Sometimes young lammergeiers make their way west to the Picos de Europas. Due to its elevated height and close proximity to the sea, this mountain range bequeaths flora and fauna so astonishing that it rivals any other on earth. Bordering Cantabria, Asturias, and Castilla y Leon, its climate is biodiverse. In the southern part, one may spot a family of Cantabrian brown bears, and in elevated regions, with the sea as background, young chamois climbing precipitous peaks with grace. In summers that might be dusted by occasional snow, reptiles of various species, patterns, and colors can be seen. Salamanders, newts, snakes, and lizards hide in rocky crevices, burrow into stream beds, or sun themselves on cliffs overlooking the sea, taking the grandeur of their kingdom for granted. One particular variety of lizard, with emerald body, and wise eyes set in its helmet-like turquoise head, waits patiently for dragonflies, a species of insect 300 million years old. The largest lizards in mainland Spain also wait in the Picos de Europa, but not to dine on dragonflies. Even snakes are wary of these giant creatures.

To know that in summer, as one heads deeper into the valleys with snow-capped peaks in the distance, meadows rush with the scent of carnations. Huge swathes of wild purple orchids blanket the meadows, the source of the perfume. Morning will bring a day teeming with all sorts of butterflies; they thrive in the grasslands bordering these forests and travel in throngs of vivid colors and patterns. Meadows lush with pink pyramidal orchids emit a spicy scent, suggesting cloves. And when night falls, these orchids gleam in the moonlight as though specks of velvet. To think that all of these wild orchids existed with dinosaurs in the valleys of the Picos, millions of years ago, speaks to the origins of earth.

Or to know that off the coast of Galicia, Cíes Islands, an archipelago of three islands, remains a marine and botanist's treasure, smelling of pine and honeysuckle, mingling with the sea. Forests and mountainous coastline provide sanctuary to the many birds that migrate there. Their calls echo across waters. Recently, a blue whale, the largest creature on earth—some as long as 100 feet—was sighted off the northern coast of Galicia, playing with dolphins and smaller whales in waters like paradise. Since the fifteenth century, octopus has been trapped in these waters, cooked in copper pots on the beach, and served on wooden platters.

You will certainly want to know that it is the rivers of Galicia that provide habitat to one of the earliest creatures on earth: the eel-like lamprey, which for centuries was regarded as a food fit for royals. With a tail at one end and a parasitic mouth at the other, this primitive creature has inhabited the rivers of Galicia for more than 500 million years, long before dinosaurs ever set foot on earth. And for at least a thousand years, from January through April, along Galicia's Miño River, the tribal-like tradition of cooking *lampreia* in clay cazuelas continues to this day.

This land, where people have been cooking for a very long time, has yet to show me everything. Guided by rivers where lampreys have flourished since time immemorial, by tides of oceans and windswept seas, by berry-strewn paths winding through prehistoric mountains, by secrets revealed in ancient forests with tender plants that thrust through mossy soil every spring, I am still driven to know more. If you are like me, you will want to know it. As the artist-poet Juan Muñoz wrote, "Our most beautiful days we have not yet seen."

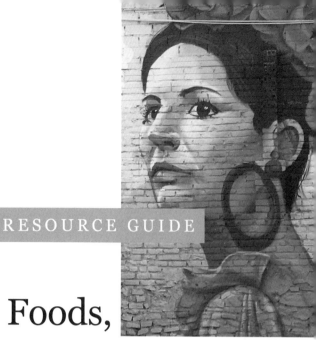

Imported Spanish Foods, a Few Final Recipes, Books, Culture, and More

"He didn't smoke . . . and he instinctively looked after his health in very precise ways. The unconscious plays a key role in the preservation and destruction of health. Man is born to conserve as well as to destroy. That's why those who think conservers don't have fun are sorely mistaken."

– Josep Pla (1897-1981) *Life Embitters*
Archipelago Books

One of the challenges in writing—actually finishing—this book was deciding when to stop reporting new findings that continuously emerge from this fascinating country. Not only about nutrition, but also the land. How could I, for instance, close this manuscript without including news of the discovery of a human jawbone, dating back 2.4 million years ago, that was unearthed in the North and believed to be the earliest evidence of humans found anywhere in Europe?

But end the book, I must.

And so, I hope you enjoy this guide, which contains some of my favorite resources for food, culture, travel, and health.

> As Josep Pla said,
> look after your health with care,
> Robin

theiberiantable.com

My blog/site features cooking demos, new recipes and occasional interviews with nutritionists and chefs, as well as breaking reports on health related to *The Iberian Table*. I can't wait to see you there.

A Brief Overview of Green Markets in Northern Spain

In *The Iberian Table*, we explore Barcelona's Mercat de Sant Josep de *la* Boqueria; however, there are other green markets you won't want to miss. A roundup, below:

Mercat de Santa Caterina, Barcelona

Mercat del Lleó, Girona. This market's Open Gastronomic Classroom occasionally features famed chef Joan Roca of Michelin-starred El Celler de Can Roca. Chef Roca features foods from the market's stalls to cook a seasonal menu.

Mercado de Abastos, Santiago de Compostela, Galicia

La Bretxa, San Sebastián

Mercado de la Ribera, Bilbao

Mercado de la Esperenza, Santander, Cantabria

Mercado de Cangas de Onís, Cangas de Onís, Asturias

Mercado de Sahagún, León

Medicinal Herbal Market: Tuesdays in Oviedo where medicinal herbs can be explored.

During summer in the Pyrenees, village markets are usually held on Saturdays in town squares.

The Health Benefits of Artisan Cheese: Markets throughout Spain offer a wide variety of artisan cheese. Asturias produces around forty to fifty different kinds. When we regularly eat artisan cheese, the body's production of immune-enhancing gut microbiome is supported. Because cheese is the richest source of Vitamin K2 (menaquinone) in the Western diet, and since low levels of K2 are correlated with increased risk for blood clots and heart disease, a little cheese eaten daily can benefit the heart and keep arteries flexible. Intake of vitamin K2 may also be a factor in creating bone health and preventing type 2 diabetes.

Spanish Food Importers

United States

Culinary Collective:
Gourmet Foods from Small-Scale Producers

Based in Lynwood, Washington, the Culinary Collective is an importer of cultural Spanish and Peruvian foods from small-scale producers. The Collective's own Matiz line, including *Sofrito de paella* and Aneto broths are among my favorites. Look on the Collective's site for Blanxart Dark Chocolate with Marcona Almonds and straightforward recipes created by nutritionist/chef Christine Weiss that inspire.

culinarycollective.com
Instagram: @culinary_collective

Despaña Brand Foods and Tapas Café

Since 1971, Despaña has been selling Spanish foods wholesale and direct to consumer, including a variety of fine extra-virgin olive oils and artisan seafood, artisan cheese, jamón, sausages, turrón, cuts of ibérico pork, and sliced ibérico jamoń. Specialty tapas items including lobster pâté, artichokes stuffed with seafood and piquillo peppers with cod. When in New York, visit Despaña Foods and Café in SOHO for lunch or tapas.

despanabrandfoods.com
Instagram: @despananyc

Despaña Vinos y Mas

Vinos Y Mas is stocked with Spanish wine. Popular weekly wine tastings illuminate.

Despanafinewines.com
Instagram: @despanavinos

Donostia Foods

This online specialty store overviews the gastronomic paradise of Donostia/San Sebastián and Spain as a whole, including elegant and simple recipes. Their Cantabrian anchovies are a do not miss, as are their tinned *Mussels en escabeche*, which arrived sauced and ready to serve. Donostia offers razor clams in brine, small squid in olive oil, queen olives stuffed with blue cheese, and *sardinas picantonas* (sardines in spicy tomato sauce). Basics are offered, too, such as fine extra-virgin olive oils and Bonito del Norte Tuna. The French Basque spice pimiento de Espelette is on hand. Happy eating, or as the Basques say "On egin."

donostiafoods.com
@donostiafoods

Marti Buckley's *Basque Country: A Culinary Journey Through a Food Lover's Paradise* (Artisan Books, 2018) brings to life authentic Basque cooking and daily routine. More on Ms. Buckley later.

La Tienda, Traditional Spanish Foods and Products

La Tienda Tapas Bar and Market in Williamsburg, Virginia remains a regional destination. Their online store is very popular, too, with favorites including organic Can Solivera extra-virgin olive oil from wild Arbequina olive trees, assorted D.O. certified cheese, artisan seafood, *bomba* and semi-brown Calasparra rice, and many types of gourmet beans, most with D.O. certification including Asturian fabes and mammoth Judion. Specialty foods made in small batches and then frozen, such as croquetas, are also available, as well as La Tienda breads. Some arrive frozen ready to bake. An assortment of cazuelas are also offered. Flash sales are regularly held. Hard-to-find items are stocked, such as chufa (tiger) nuts. Gift boxes delight and La Tienda's recipes are outstanding. Don Harris (1936–2024), founder, is the author of *The Heart of Spain*, a book of cultural essays focused on the food, people, and country that he loves so much.

latienda.com
@latienda_us

Cazuela Shallot-Turkey Thighs in Red Wine Pan Sauce

Use 9½ inch cazuela. Thinly slice a handful of peeled shallots. Set aside. Using a small pot, heat 1/3 cup of red Spanish table wine with an equal amount of free-range chicken stock and one bay leaf. Bring to boil, immediately turn down, and simmer for 15 minutes. Preheat oven to 425°. Clean and dry two turkey thighs. Rub lightly with EVOO and season with salt, ground black and white pepper, Penzeys garlic powder (it is always fresh tasting; almost sweet) and a sprinkle of all-purpose seasoning, such as Instant Gourmet. Finish with dried thyme and rosemary. Coat bottom of cazuela with EVOO; add shallots and two peeled large cloves of fresh garlic. Sauté on medium-high 7 minutes.

Add turkey and cook until both sides are just browned, about 5–6 minutes per side. Immediately add wine/stock, bring to low boil, then simmer covered for 25–30 minutes. Take a piece of foil to cover hot cazuela—take care not to burn your fingers. Place the covered cazuela in preheated oven, and roast for 10 minutes. Reduce heat to 350°, uncover, and roast for about 25 minutes, until turkey skin looks glazed, and crisp at the edges.

If you find yourself in the North, do not miss the modern Basque fare of Arzak, in Donostia-San Sebastián (Alcalde J. Elosegi, Hiribidea, 273, 20015) nor the modern Mediterranean cuisine of Moments and Blanc in Barcelona. (Mandarin Oriental Hotel, Passeig de Gràcia, 38-40, 08007.)

Additional Spanish Food Importers in the US, Canada, UK, and Australia:

A Southern Season

201 S. Estes Drive
University Mall
Chapel Hill, NC 27514

southernseason.com
@southernseason

Yaya Imports

530 Boulder Court #105
Pleasanton, CA 94566

Yayaimports.com

Catalan Gourmet

113 Broadway, Suite 1614
New York, NY 10011

Catalangourmet.com
@catalangourmet

Beaune Imports

Callol i Serrats 1847 L'Escala anchovies are available here.

Beauneimports.com
@beauneimports

Zingerman's

422 Detroit St.
Ann Arbor, MI 43104

zingermans.com
@zingmailorder

La Española Meats, Inc.

25020 Doble Ave.
Harbor City, CA 90710

Rice, chorizo, pimentón, and more

laespanolameats.com
@laespanolameats

Market Hall Foods

5655 College Avenue, Suite 201
Oakland, CA 94618

Markethallfoods.com
@markethallfoods

Horchata de chufa, a nonalcoholic, slightly sweet, chilled drink composed of ground tiger nuts, almonds, sesame seeds, barley, and rice, is the unofficial drink of Valencia.

The Spanish Table

181 San Pablo Avenue
Berkeley, CA 94702

800 Redwood Hwy 123
Mill Valley, CA 94941

130 Clement Street
San Francisco, CA 94118

Wine, including sherry, and vermouth, cava,
beer, foods and cookware from Spain
spanishtable.com
@spanishtable

TIP: Wanting to cook with less meat but don't know how, check out *New York Times* writer, Mark Bittman, author of more than 30 books including the series, "How to Cook Everything."
http://courses.markbittman.com

Canada

Pasquale Bros.

16 Goodrich Road.
Etobicoke, ON M8Z 4Z8
pasqualebros.com
@pasqualebros

Bayley & Sage

There are many locations throughout London; for the complete list, visit its blog/site.

> bayley-sage.co.uk
> @bayleyandsage

Brindisa

9b Weir Road
London SW12 0LT
United Kingdom

> brindisa.com
> @brindisaspanishfoods

"The true food of Spain is not all about the tapas," says founder Monika Linton, and author of *Brindisa: The True Food of Spain*. Abundant in recipes, Linton's book is a personal favorite.

Iberíca

Iberíca has locations in London, Manchester, Leeds, and Glasgow. Each has a separate email address and phone number available on the website.

> ibericarestaurants.com
> @ibericarestaurants

R. Garcia and Sons

248-250 Portobello Road
London W11 1LL
United Kingdom

> rgarciaandsons.com

María José Sevilla, a food writer/author and broadcaster who lives and works in London. Her book *Delicioso: A History of Food in Spain* (Reaktion Books 2019) helps us understand how Greek, Roman, Jewish and Middle Eastern influences have all left their mark on Spanish gastronomy.

Mariajosesevilla.com

Chandos Deli

Chandos has locations in Bristol, Bath, and Exeter. Information is available on its website.

chandosdeli.com
Bristol: @chandos.whiteladies
Bath: @chandosdelibath
Exeter: @chandosdeliexeter

Define Food and Wine

Chester Road, Sandiway
Cheshire CW8 2NH
United Kingdom

definefoodandwine.com
@definefoodandwine

Australia

Delicado Foods & Wines

134 Blues Point Road
McMahons Point, NSW
Australia

delicado.com.au
@delicado_foods

Casa Iberíca Deli

Multiple locations in Melbourne.

casaibericadeli.com.au
@casa_iberica

Mercado

No. 4 Ash Street
Sydney 2000
Australia

mercadorestaurant.com.au
@mercadorestaurant

Huevos Rotos, or Fried Potatoes with Broken Eggs

This recipe makes a tasty and nutritious last-minute dinner, hearty breakfast, or weekend brunch. Figure one thinly sliced Yukon Gold per person. Chopped onion, one or two eggs per person, extra-virgin olive oil, fresh minced garlic, salt, pepper, pimentón, cayenne pepper, and red pepper flakes. Coat a sauté pan with olive oil. Add potatoes, garlic and onion. Season with salt and pepper. Sauté on medium heat for 20 minutes until just brown. Turning a couple of times, season with pimentón and sauté 5 minutes more. Add the eggs, cook sunny-side up until just done. Serve the potatoes and eggs, with the yolk intact. Break yolk with tip of knife before eating.

Organizations, Educational Resources, Cooking Schools, and Tours

Mediterranean Diet Foundation

This global resource in Barcelona covers research findings regarding the Mediterranean diet and disseminates information in several languages about health, diet, cultures, cooking, and agricultural methods to the world. This site remains one of my favorite resources.

dietamediterranea.com

Culinary Reads

- *Catalan Food, Culture and Flavors from the Mediterranean*, by Chef Daniel Olivella;
- *Etxebarri*, by Juan Pablo Cardenal and John Sarabia (Etxebarri is a Michelin-starred restaurant outside Bilbao, renowned for grill cooking);
- *Arzak & Arzak*, a book for professional chefs reflecting the work of the Basque father-daughter duo, Juan Mari and Elena;
- *Cúrate: Authentic Spanish Food from an American Kitchen*, by Katie Button. Chef Button was schooled in the kitchen of El Bulli;
- *Taste of the Camino, 30 Authentic Recipes Along The French Way*, by Yosmar Monique Martinez, Gormand World Cookbook Award.

Don't Miss

- *Jaialdi: A Celebration of Basque Culture*, by Nancy Zubiri.

Foundation Alícia: A Defining Food and Nutrition Center, and A Book for Chefs

Foundation Alícia, located in San Fruitós de Barges, Catalunya, is under the strategic leadership of Chef Ferran Adrià. Alícia is composed of researchers, chefs and educators. In addition to humanitarian projects that include preparing menus for the elderly, the foundation works to develop culinary initiatives for the business sector and is known for extensive organic vegetable and stone fruit gardens open to the public. Alícia's *Chef's Guide to Gelling, Thickening, and Emulsifying Agents* (CRC Press), demystifies thickening agents such as agar-agar, kudzu, gelatin, guar gum etc. Techniques are revealed.

alicia.cat

Foods and Wines from Spain

Discover the ultimate digital newsletter that takes you on a journey through the vibrant world of Spanish wines and foods. Delight in a curated collection of articles, interviews, reports and captivating photography that encapsulate the essence of Spain's culinary treasures. Immerse yourself in the rich tapestry of flavors as you explore book reviews and engaging commentaries on the latest gastronomic and wine events and prestigious awards. Indulge your taste buds with tantalizing recipes from renowned chefs that will leave you craving for more. Uncover the secrets of Spanish cuisine with mesmerizing video demos, including the delectable Vegetarian Oven-baked Rice. Embark on unforgettable gastronomic wine routes across every enchanting region of Spain. Join us and experience the irresistible allure of Spanish wines and foods.

Instagram: @spainfoodwine

The Natural Gourmet Institute: Program taught at the Institute of Culinary Education, New York City

In 2019 the Natural Gourmet's long-standing health and culinary arts curriculum was absorbed into the Institute of Culinary Education. Founded in 1977 by Anne Marie Colbin Ph.D, the Natural Gourmet was America's first plant-based nutrition-focused culinary school, offering chef's training and classes for home cooks. More than 2,600 people from thirty-three countries graduated from the Natural Gourmet over its forty-year history. I taught a workshop there on women's health. Carrying forward the tradition, in addition to professional chef's training and classes for home cooks, ICE also offers multiday immersion and two-week programs.

www.ice.edu

Oldways: Inspiring Healthy Cooking Through Traditional Cultures

This Boston-based food and nutrition nonprofit is dedicated to improving public health through traditional diets. In 1993, together with the Harvard School of Public Health and the World Health Organization, the late visionary and founder of Oldways, K. Dunn Gifford, introduced the Mediterranean Diet Pyramid over twenty years ago, when I was writing *Total Breast Health: The Power Food Solution for Protection and Wellness*. I remember conversations with Dunn about the benefits of olive oil during a time when it was not widely available. He honored my book by welcoming me to reprint the Oldways Mediterranean diet food pyramid. Today, Oldways continues to report the science behind the Mediterranean diet and through the leadership of its current director, Sara Baer-Sinnot, the organization expands understanding of the diet and spearheads initiatives such as the Chef's Collaborative, which supports local and sustainable food in America's restaurants.

oldwayspt.org
Instagram: @oldways_pt

Chef Alice Waters' Edible Schoolyard Project

Chef, writer, and founder/owner of Chez Panisse restaurant in Berkeley, California, Alice Waters has done more than any other American chef to champion the Mediterranean diet. Ms. Waters remains dedicated to improving the diet of young people through her Edible Schoolyard Project. Through this initiative, students learn to grow and cook their own food. Schools with gardening and cooking programs, food banks, and government agencies are encouraged to join the Edible Schoolyard's network, which offers program development and curriculum support. Alice Waters' cookbooks, available on Amazon, are among my favorites.

edibleschoolyard.org
Instagram: @edibleschoolyard

Anchovy Toast
Inspired by Alice Waters' Recipe

Toast narrow slices of country-style bread. After nicely browned, rub with garlic, top with an anchovy, and finish with olive oil. Serve slightly warm. Ms. Waters' anchovies are from L'Escala Spain on the northern end of the Costa Brava, a region we will discuss in a moment.

Nancy Harmon Jenkins

Jenkins has traveled the world experiencing traditional food and cultures, and has written articles and cookbooks on these subjects. She has also led tours, including to Catalunya and the Basque country. Pertinent to *The Iberian Table*, among her publications are: *The Mediterranean Diet Cookbook, The Essential Mediterranean, The New Mediterranean Diet Cookbook,* and *Virgin Territory: Exploring The World of Olive Oil.*

nancyharmonjenkins.com

Sara Jenkins

Cookbook author, and chef/owner of Nina June restaurant in Camden, Maine, this daughter of Nancy Harmon Jenkins wrote *Olives and Oranges: Recipes and Flavor Secrets from Italy, Spain, Cyprus and Beyond*. If you are in Camden, her Mediterranean-style restaurant serves up the freshest food that Maine offers, including theme dinners such as "One Night in the Basque Country," with chef Lauren Radel.

Ninajunerestaurant.com

Paula Wolfert

Author of nine distinguished cookbooks including five about the Mediterranean, *The Cooking of South-west France*, which melds Spanish and French elements, remains one of my favorites. The more recent *Unforgettable, The Bold Flavors of Paula Wolfert's Renegade Life* begins with Wolfert's Brooklyn childhood and traces her adventures in the Mediterranean. For those who aren't familiar with Wolfert's work, *Unforgettable* acts as an introduction to one of the most influential culinary voices of our time.

Paula-wolfert.com

La Española Health

This website covers the many benefits of extra-virgin olive oil and interviews guests, including researchers and scholars. The leader of the PREDIMED study, Dr. Ramón Estruch, is a frequent and honored guest. In addition to interviews, La Española offers recipes, meal plans, news, and opinion columns.

laespanolasalud.com

Gourmet Cooking Classes in the Basque Region: Escuela de Cocina Luis Irizar

Luis Irizar, one of the founding fathers of avant-garde cooking, remains a lightning rod for the best French and Basque cuisine, offering classes in Donostia/San Sebastián at his legendary Escuela de Cocina Luis Irizar. Group sessions in English can be arranged.

escuelairizar.com

World Central Kitchen

In 2010, World Central Kitchen, headquarters in Washington, DC, was founded by chef José Andrés in response to the earthquake in Haiti. Since its inception, WCK has expanded into a global network of chefs. At the onset of the war in Ukraine, in Przemyśl—a Polish city near the border of Ukraine that received tens of thousands of refugees every day—WCK cooked 100,000 meals daily.

worldcentralkitchen.org
Instagram: @wckitchen

Chef Andrés' Book on Vegetable Cookery: *Vegetables Unleashed: A Cookbook*, is a do not miss.

The World's Healthiest Foods: George Mateljan Foundation

A thorough resource for students of nutrition, health bloggers, and home cooks, the Mateljan Foundation remains dedicated to optimizing longevity by presenting thorough information covering health-promoting superfoods, spices, and nutrient-dense cooking.

whfoods.org
@whfoodsdotcom

Support Breast Cancer Prevention Partners

Intent on making change, Breast Cancer Prevention Partners works to prevent cancer by eliminating our exposure to toxic chemicals and radiation.

bcpp.org
@bcppartners

Les Dames d'Escoffier International

This association of women has achieved success in the fields of food, fine beverages, and hospitality, and is dedicated to assisting committed students who wish to enter the culinary world through mentorships, scholarships, etc. The late and great Julia Child was a member.

ldei.org
@lesdamesintl

Cheese from Spain

cheesefromspain.com

Wiki Spanish Food

wikispanishfood.com

Olive Oil from Spain

oliveoilfromspain.com

Wines and Wineries

Though distinguished wine regions can be found throughout Spain and Portugal, my overview touches upon the viniculture of Northern Spain. For a comprehensive view, refer to *The Wines of Northern Spain: From Galicia to the Pyrenees and Rioja to the Basque Country*, by Sarah Jane Evans (Oxford, 2018).

Upon my first trip to Spain, I found the wines exceptional. For one thing, no more headaches. Even the table wines seemed more pure.

Vinologue's Enotourism Recommends Young, Low Alcohol Wines

"Spain as a whole has been shifting to fresher, less alcoholic wines that showcase the exceptional locales," say Miquel Hudin and Elia Varela Serra, authors of vinologue.com, a guide offering detailed information on planning tours to wine regions in the North. *Priorat: A Regional Guide to Enotourism in Catalonia Including 104 Producers and 315 Wines* is available on the Vinologue site and Amazon. Hudin and Varela also cover the wines of Montsant and Empordà. Guides contain profiles of wineries, GPS coordinates, full-color photos, maps, and tasting notes for hundreds of wines.

> vinologue.com
> @vinologue

Today, Garnacha is used as a base to blend some of the world's most delicious wines. On the debut of the *vinos aragoneses* in the 12th century, Garnacha spread by way of the crown of Aragón to the rest of Spain, Southern France, and Sardinia. I find it interesting that Sardinia's Cannonau wine, reported to have more antioxidants than any other wine, is believed to be a contributing factor in the long lives of Sardinians.

Does Wine Improve Health?

Some researchers say that moderate intake of red wine as part of the Mediterranean diet offers natural antioxidant properties that may help in the prevention of cardiovascular disease, type 2 diabetes and, according to a 2022 study by Spanish researchers, may slow cognitive decline as well.

> wineinmoderation.eu and
> wineinformationcouncil.eu

Spain's Organic Vineyards

Spain's total hectares of organic vineyards surpasses Italy and France combined, with Navarra the largest. Spanish Organic Wines, an association of small- and medium-sized family-run wineries, encompasses thirty-five members, including wineries in ten Autonomous Communities belonging to eighteen Denominations of Origin.

> spanishorganicwines.com

Catalunya: Wine and Gastronomic Tourism

Discover the wine/cava regions of Catalunya, including Priorat, Penedés, Montsant, Empordà, and Alella.

> Catalunya.com
> @catalunyaexperience

Wines from Spain

This website presents current information regarding wine, sherry, and cava regions, as well as the history of Spanish wine and wineries, including organic winemaking. Wine terms, innovations, and interviews with authors and vintners complete this blog/site.

> winesfromspainusa.com
> @winesfromspain

Bodega Torres Winery in Penedés, and La Vinoteca Torres, Barcelona

Tucked between the mountains and the Mediterranean Sea in sunny Catalunya, Bodega Torres, one of Spain's most distinguished wine exporters and leading supplier to the Spanish national market, can be discovered. Torres, which began in 1870, has been awarded first place several times in the UK's *Drinks International* as the most admired wine brand. It is a fourth-generation family-owned winery that includes organic wines, led by Mireia Torres. Located in Penedés, Torres offers an educational visitors' center, which sheds light on the history of winemaking. Cooking classes are taught at the Torres restaurant, Mas

Rabell, by Chef Sergi Millet. La Vinoteca Torres, a restaurant and wine bar on Barcelona's Paseo de Gracia, presents a variety of Torres wines by the glass.

torres.es
@familiatorreswines
lavinotecatorres.com
@vinotecatorres
masiamasrabell.com

The Wines of Priorat, in the Province of Tarragona

The grape vines of Priorat grow on ancient terraced cliffs, less than twenty miles from the Mediterranean Sea. The region's beauty and early wine-making skills must have drawn the Romans who settled there during the first century AD. Records show the Romans praised the wine as some of the best in the empire. In 1262, Carthusian monks grew grapes in Priorat. Today, the area yields some of Spain's finest reds. Garnacha Tinta has long been classic, but vineyards are mostly planted with Cariñena grapes. Wines produced in this Catalan region are a blend of both, complementing full-flavored fare such as wild game, sausages with peppers, and so on.

doqpriorat.org
@d.o.q.priorat

Codorníu Organic Cava, and Josep Puig's Celebrated Art Nouveau Headquarters

Codorníu Cuvée Original Brut Ecológico is made from grapes grown in the organic vineyards of Penedés. Codorníu Raventós, the oldest business in Spain and one of the oldest in the world, has more than 450 years of experience producing wines. Codorníu brought cava to light in the 1800s. During this time, Codorníu commissioned the architect Josep Puig i Cadafalch to design its headquarters, which has become an international historic art nouveau treasure. The building in northeast Penedés offers tours.

codorniuraventos.com

Province of Girona: Empordà-Costa Brava, One of The Oldest Winemaking Regions in the World

The gastronomy in the Catalan province of Girona, in part prepared by chefs with restaurants possessing a combined total of twenty Michelin stars, is so outstanding that local wine producers must strive to offer wines that match the quality of the region's cooking. Organic and biodynamic grape growing is popular with these young vintners. Despite the excellence of the wines, due to several setbacks, Empordà's wine story has been held back. However during the past two decades there has been a renaissance. Ancient paths from the town of Figueres north to the French border define. Grapevines were cultivated in this region where the Pyrenees tumble into valleys to finally meld with the Mediterranean since the Greeks arrived on the coast of Ampurias in the sixth century BC. Fresh-tasting rosés from Cariñena and Garnacha tinta grapes are tradition. Wines also include white Garnacha, Macabeo, Syrah, and Tempranillo. Wineries, small or large, can be toured in Girona province, including Castillo Perelada, an impressive inland vintner that set up shop in a medieval fortress.

visitemporda.com
perelada.com

Asturias, Spain's Hidden Treasure, and Low Alcohol *Sidra*, Made from Apples

Did you know that the natural paradise of Asturias—with snow-capped Picos de Europa in the distance—was a nation and a kingdom, centuries before Ferdinand and Isabella unified Spain? Don't miss touring this hidden treasure. Maybe you also did not know that the national drink, low-alcohol *sidra*, made from indigenous crabapples, dates back about sixty years before Christ? In October and November, sidra mills offer tastings, or "espichas," served from the barrel.

turismoasturias.es/en/gastronomia/sidra
turismoasturias.es

Archaeologist-Led Expeditions of Catalunya's Wine Regions

Former postdoctoral fellow at the University of Barcelona and *National Geographic* expeditions expert, Killian Driscoll, PhD, brings a passion for the Stone Age and prehistory to his customized wine/gastronomy tours of the Catalan regions. Dr. Driscoll also offers a walking tour of Barcelona that will be mentioned later.

artobatours.com
@artobatours

A Taste of Barcelona: The History of Catalan Cooking and Eating, by H. Rosi Song and Anna Riera, overviews the region's rich cooking history.

La Rioja: Three Regions Producing World-Class Wines

Located in northcentral Spain, La Rioja is considered by many to be Spain's most prestigious wine region. Divided into three large areas consisting of more than 65,000 hectares of vineyards, each region is composed of distinctive soil and climate, producing wines having individual character. Rioja Alavesa, north of the Ebro river in the Basque country, yields some of the most sought after tempranillos in the world. Framed by Cantabrian mountains to the north, Alavesa wines are a result of Atlantic and Mediterranean climates. With over 200 wineries and considered one of the top destinations for wine in the world, Rioja Alavesa, Rioja Alta, and Rioja Oriental can be toured through the site below.

Cellartours.com

La Rioja, the First Winemaking Region in Spain to Receive the Prestigious *Denominación de Origen* Certification

Wines have been produced in La Rioja since the eleventh century. In the Ebro valley, La Rioja was the first wine region in Spain to be granted the honored Denominación de Origen. Known throughout the world, it is aged in oak and made from grapes grown in the autonomous communities of La Rioja, Navarra, and the Basque province of Álava.

riojawine.com
@riojawineuk

Basque Txacoli Wine

Txakolí (choo-co-li) means "farm wine" in Basque. Known outside the region as chocolí, the drink is white, dry, and slightly bubbly with the subtle taste of minerals. Complementing seafood, sliced sausages, or Idiazábal cheese with rustic grace, this fresh-tasting wine is meant to be drunk young. In 1990, Txakolí de Getaria-Getariako Txakolina was granted Denomination of Origin status. Txakolí is produced in all three Basque regions—Álava, Vizcaya, and Gipuzkoa.

> Getariakotxakolina.com
> @txakoli_aizpurua

Galicia's Wine Story

In the northwest corner of Spain hugging the Atlantic coast, is Galicia. Lush vegetation, rainfall, and humidity defines. With its Celtic feel, Galicia is a spectacle of mountains, sky, cliffs, rocky inlets, forests and the sparkling Atlantic. Enjoy the Rias Baixas region, where can be found the elegant, crisp DO Albariños as well as other regions where DO wines also can be found, including Ribeiro, Ribeira Sacra, Valdeorras, Os viños da terra, and Monterrei. Red Mencia from Riberia Sacra is full and fruity, and springs from soil rich in slate. Godello, from the mountains of Valdeorras can't be overlooked. Experience all these wines and breathtaking locales firsthand.

> Riasbaixaswines.com
> proguias.es
> Vinepair.com

Galicia's Playa de las Catedrales beach—serenity straddled by majestic stone arches so awe-inspiring it is known as nature's cathedral. The water there is said to be holy. This dramatic spot is fully revealed when the tide is low, so return to the main beach before the tide returns. Book your visit with the Galician government beforehand.

Travel, Cooking, and Conservation

Eat Northern Spain: Gastronomic Tours in Areas of Natural Beauty Led by a Native

This family-owned tour company with forever roots in Spain, founded by Elías González, offers luxury accommodations in Cantabria, Asturias, Galicia, and Castilla y León. Tours are personalized. Only twelve a year are arranged, and each is individually tailored. Elías González, who was born in the North, personally leads tours. Experiences and settings are "off the well-traveled path." YouTube overviews ENS's culinary highlights and locales. Meet Elías there.

eatnorthernspain.com @eatnspain

Lauren Aloise and James Blick: Touring, and Spanish Sabores Blog

Devour Tours is an award-winning tour company created and led by Lauren Aloise, a transplanted American who has lived in Spain since 2009. Along with her co-founder, James Blick, Lauren began Devour in 2012 to connect "curious travelers with small family-run local food businesses, and introduce them to the gastronomy and history of local areas." Devour Tours Online Cooking Classes and YouTube's "Spanish Feasts from the Devour Kitchens" transport you to Spain. The Devour Digital Cookbook, with more than fifty recipes from Barcelona, Seville, San Sebastián, Madrid and Lisbon, makes these culinary hotspots accessible. Lauren's The Spanish Food Club Facebook is lively. Her Spanish Sabores Cooking Blog provides a weekly recipe at no cost, and Sabores "Fifty Top Tapas Recipes" is also free. James Blick's YouTube "Spain Revealed" is enlightening.

Devourtours.com
Spanishsabores.com
@devourtours

Full Throttle Nature: Mallorca

For unsurpassed nature and diverse cuisine, discover the Balearic island of Mallorca. Swim in turquoise waters, hike along rugged shoreline, cycle through ancient villages past olive groves toward the mountains of Tramuntana. Vistas offer spectacular views of the Mediterranean. There are cooking classes, too. Don't miss Palma's Gastronomic Mercat 1930.

mallorca.com

Customized Adventure, Led by Wine and Gastronomy Authority Gerry Dawes

Gerry Dawes, author, blogger, photographer and expert on Spanish wine and food, has traveled the roads of Spain for forty years. Galician wines are his passion. Experience these wines and breathtaking locales firsthand. Gerry organizes and leads trips for small groups, including chefs. His blog, distinguished as one of the "Top Fifty Gastronomy Blogs" of 2019, is filled with anecdotes, history and lore. His book, an illuminating read, *Sunset in a Glass: Adventures of a Food Warrior in Spain*, published in 2021, has a foreword written by José Andrés. Gerry received Spain's prestigious *Premio Nacional de Gastronomía* 2003 (National Gastronomy Award). His articles have been published in *The New York Times, Food & Wine, Martha Stewart Living, The Chicago Tribune* and *Departures.*

gerrydawesspain.com

Gerry Kerkhoff's Spanish Fiestas Tours

Kerkhoff's blog with photos and articles sheds historic light, including "Walking the Camino de Santiago." Gerry's ebook, *Spanish Mediterranean Diet Recipes: Healthy Recipes from the Kitchens of Spain,* offers historic context, authentic recipes, and homey tips. Suggestions such as adding a little red wine to lentil soup or crushing saffron with a touch of salt are practical. *Pamplona Travel Guide*, available on amazon.com, also illuminates.

spanish-fiestas.com

Tour the Basque Country

Tourism Euskadi covers one of the most culturally-rich and beautiful regions on the planet. Through their site, this organization presents information and visuals covering Donostia/San Sebastián, Bilbao, and lesser-known Basque villages and towns.

tourism.euskadi.eus/en
@visiteuskadi

Day Trip: Galicia Mystic Tours

Explore the provinces of Galicia with family-owned Mystic Tours. Major cities, or wine regions are options. English-speaking Vincente and Rose Marie guide you to some of the most vividly beautiful places in Spain. Private transportation. Travel the picturesque coast of the Rías Baixas. Or tour bodegas to sample world-class wines. Based in Pontevedra, the couple customize tours to culturally-rich cities including Lugo, Santiago del Compostela, and Vigo. Explore coastal towns. Come to understand the Celtic history, and remarkable plant life of verdant Galicia. At the southern-most tip, the Celtic ruins of Castro de Santa Tecla captivate. Galicia Mystic Tours can be accessed through the site below.

Toursofgalicia.net

Island Paradise: Galicia's *Islas* Cíes

Cíes, an archipelago off the coast of Galicia, is composed of three islands, known as "the islands of the gods." Unspoiled beaches, marine caves, and translucent waters define. There are no hotels, but campgrounds are free. Bikes and cars are not allowed. Campers carry their garbage with them to the mainland. Visitors to the islands must reserve their place on the ferry.

campingislascies.com
buceoislascies.es
@buceoislascies

A Worldwide Destination for Prehistory Seekers;
Kayak Adventure, and Some of Spain's Best Anchovies

Costa Brava's northern end, Cabo de Creus, hugs the Mediterranean and is punctuated with sea caves, known as *calas*. Surrounded by cliffs, the inlets are perfect for kayaking. South of Cabo de Creus, on a cliff overlooking the Mediterranean embedded in a secluded mountain setting, a mysterious structure of stone was constructed five thousand years ago. Somehow humans carried huge slabs, forming walls and a roof to create the dolmen, Creu d'en Cobertella. What type of ritual was this cult-like place used for? Don't miss this top destination that the world's prehistory seekers flock to. For lunch, some of the best anchovies in Spain can be found in L'Escala, a half hour away.

creativecatalonia.com

Oceana: Supporting Ocean Conservation
and the Mediterranean Sea

Though the world's bodies of water have capacity to feed one billion people a day, antibiotics and mercury are an increasing threat. Founded in 2001, Oceana was created to make our oceans more abundant by winning policy victories in the countries that govern much of the world's marine life. Oceana maintains international offices focusing on conservation. The Mediterranean Sea has recently become part of their mission.

Oceana.org
@oceana

The Ocean Cleanup: Ridding the Seas of Plastic

Led by the Dutch inventor Boyan Slat, "The Ocean Cleanup" began when fifteen-year-old Slat went scuba diving off the coast of Greece and noticed there was more plastic in the water than fish. Today, Slat and his group have created technologies to gather and remove plastic from oceans and prevent the flow of plastic pollution into the world's oceans by way of the rivers.

theoceancleanup.com
@theoceancleanup

Synthetic fabrics, including stretchy Pilates wear, are harming marine life. During machine washing, these garments break down, leaving microfibers to be flushed into water treatment plants where they are transferred into streams, rivers, lakes, and oceans to be consumed by fish and other marine life, after which the artificial fibers become embedded in their tissue.

Eliminate Plastic Bags

Spearheaded by two Indonesian teens who managed to get plastic bags banned in Bali, this initiative is now worldwide. With over twenty-five global locations involving young people, the founders continue spreading their message about the toxic effect plastics have on sea creatures, humans, and the planet.

byebyeplasticbags.org
@byebyeplasticbags

4 Ocean: Proceeds Clean Oceans and Coastlines

To support this endeavor, purchase cloth shopping bags, permanent water bottles, collapsible straws, and memorial bracelets from the site below.

This organization pulls one pound of trash from coastlines and oceans for each product sold.

4ocean.com
@4ocean

Pink Pangea

Pink Pangea, an online community created by women, covers travel-related topics including safety, restaurants, accommodations, and more.

pinkpangea.com
@pinkpangea

CNBC's "10 Best Hotel Restaurants Around the World" includes El Motel at Hotel Empordà in Figueres. Food writer/author Colman Andrews describes El Motel as "the cradle of modern Catalan cuisine." Led by the inventive Chef Jaume Subirós, the menu of this long-established restaurant just a little north of Barcelona is abundant in plant foods, mushrooms and other seasonal specialties, including wild game. October 2013.
@elmotel and @jaumesubiros

Iberian Wildlife Tours

For wildlife tours of the Pyrenees and Picos de Europa, contact guides below.

Jeffclarkeecology.co.uk
Iberianwildlife.com
@teresa-farino-trips

Snowboarding and Skiing: The Pyrenees of Aragón

In the Tena Valley of Huesca, one finds the fastest slope in Aragón, descending three hundred meters from the top of Tres Hombres peak. One can ski other slopes in the region that are not as extreme.

onthesnow.com/aragon/ski-resorts.html
turismodearagon.com/en/

Hidden Spain: Discover the Beauty of Aragón

To the north of Huesca, still in the Pyrenees, Ordesa and Monte Perdido National Parks, known as the Grand Canyon of Europe, draw hikers during summer and fall to their high-altitude, narrow passes. One can spot more than three hundred different species of birds there. The abundance and genera of wildflowers are also remarkable and include assorted orchids. Heading lower, Romanesque churches and castles provide insight into ancient times. Farther south in Zaragoza, a dozen powerful paintings by master Francisco de Goya can be viewed. Medieval villages dot the landscape. In Teruel, exotic Mudéjar architecture reigns.

turismodearagon.com/en/

A Centuries Old Tradition: Walking the Camino de Santiago

This pilgrimage is about five hundred miles in length and winds through the Pyrenees to Santiago de Compostela. Walking the Camino began during the Middle Ages; religious people were drawn from throughout Europe to make their way to the Cathedral of Santiago de Compostela in Galicia, to attend Mass. Walking the Camino remains popular today, providing a respite from daily life to connect with nature. If one walks fourteen miles a day, the Camino takes about thirty-five days.

santiago-compostela.net
caminoways.com

Tourist Offices of Spain

With offices throughout the world including Miami, Chicago, Los Angeles, and New York, the resource below is abundant in material to plan lodging as well as gastronomic, sporting, and cultural activities.

spain.info

Andalucía: The Olive Oil Workshop, Organized by Olive Oil Taster Alexis Kerner

Andalucía is known to produce many of the best olive oils in Spain, and is home to the Olive Oil Workshop, founded by American Alexis Kerner, who has lived in Andalusia for over twelve years. After moving to Spain, Kerner's activities in olive oil production led to her being distinguished as a Professional Olive Oil Taster by both the University of Jaen and the International Olive Oil Council. Kerner leads her workshop in Andalucía through education. Join her to explore a local market while she discusses the benefits of Spain's Mediterranean diet.

Theoliveoilworkshop.com

Interested in the cooking of southern Spain? José Pizarro's *Andalusia: Recipes from Seville and Beyond* delights. (Hardie Grant Books, 2019).

Travel Agencies: Whenever possible, seek local travel agencies in Spain. That way you will find places of interest off well-traveled roads and support Spanish business at the same time.

Botanical Medicine, Natural Foods, and More

A growing body of evidence shows that the Mediterranean diet, rich in healthy fats and fiber, is the best diet for prevention of disease. When one's diet is optimal, botanical medicine can be effective. Lifestyle can help protect, too. Maintain a positive approach to life. Don't be sedentary. And remember, sleep is a significant protector of health.

Are *siestas* part of Spain's long-life paradigm? When we have adequate sleep, including naps, Alzheimer's plaque is eliminated from the brain. Find out more in *Why We Sleep: Unlocking the Power of Sleep and Dreams*, by Matthew Walker, PhD.

Udo Erasmus, PhD, Best-Selling Author and Health Pioneer; Books and a Recipe for Saffron Smoothie

"One of the most recognized experts around the world is Udo Erasmus... he created a very specific product that is recommended by people all over the world."

– Anthony Robbins, Motivational speaker and author

"Essential dietary fats are the least understood and most overlooked nutrient" says Udo Erasmus, PhD, author and expert on fats and oils. He continues to help countless people realize the crucial place that dietary fats hold in human health. Before his bestseller *Fats That Heal, Fats That Kill: The Complete Guide to Fats, Oils, Cholesterol and Human Health*, nutritionists were promoting fat-free foods. In addition to educating people on essential dietary fats, Erasmus pioneered production of flax and other oils by developing methods of pressing fresh nuts and seeds, advancing the health of millions along the way. Udo has lectured in more than thirty countries and has given thousands of radio interviews in the US and in Canada. His most recent book *Totally Sexy Health: The 8 Key Parts Designed by Nature*, provides autobiographical glimpses into one of the foremost health experts of our time. Udo consults and speaks on key global issues, including the environment. Courses with nutritional advice described on his blog/site, inspire. Through the site below, discover Udo's 3•6•9 Blend oil.

> udoschoice.com
> udoerasmus.com
> totalsexyhealth.com
> @udoschoiceofficial

Donald R. Yance, MH RN, Books, Mederi Centre for Natural Healing, and Natura Health Supplements

Author of *Herbal Medicine, Healing & Cancer: A Comprehensive Program for Prevention and Treatment*, Donald Yance, master herbalist and clinical nutritionist, has over three decades of successful practice. Yance's second book *Adaptogens in Medical Herbalism: Elite Herbs* and *Natural Compounds for Mastering Stress, Aging, and Chronic Disease* (Healing Arts Press, 2013) provides authoritative information on advanced nutrition of our day. The Mederi Center for Natural Healing, founded and led by Yance, offers personalized patient care. Mederi Academy advances educational programs for professionals. Yance pioneered the development of medical herbalism, so the professional supplement line that he created, Natura Health Products, was founded upon his unique expertise. Vital Adapt Tonic is an adaptogenic formula that supports the body's ability to mitigate physical and mental stress. Yance created Vital Adapt 30 years ago. In addition to being a leading health authority and nutrition author, Yance is an accomplished musician and an excellent natural foods chef. Look for his recipes, and articles through his blog.

medericenter.org
naturahealthproducts.com
donnieyance.com

Saffron-Strawberry Smoothie

The medieval *Llibre de Sent Soví* documents recipes with almond milk, which is the basis for this smoothie. To begin, crush a pinch of saffron into 2 tablespoons of warmed spring or filtered water. Threads won't completely dissolve. Combine saffron water and threads into a glass of unsweetened almond milk. Stir. Add 1 scoop of Natura Health Product's Beyond Whey (promotes immune and digestive health) along with 1 tablespoon collagen powder, 2 teaspoons of crushed chia seeds, 2 teaspoons of Udo's 3•6•9 Blend, and 1 tablespoon of Spanish honey. Stir. Add a small handful of minced strawberries, blend, and drink.

Tori Hudson, N.D.

Dr. Tori Hudson, medical director of A Woman's Time Clinic in Seattle, has been in practice for more than thirty-four years. The author of *Women's Encyclopedia of Natural Medicine: Alternative Therapies and Integrative Medicine for Total Health and Wellness* (McGraw-Hill, 2008), Hudson graduated from the National College of Naturopathic Medicine and has served the college as medical director and academic dean. She is now adjunct clinical professor at NUNM, Southwest College of Naturopathic Medicine, and Bastyr University. Dr. Hudson offers an information-packed blog covering many topics, including breast cancer prevention, pregnancy, and more.

drtorihudson.com

500 Acres of New England Wilderness: Sage Mountain and Botanical Sanctuary

Founded by master herbalist and author Rosemary Gladstar, Sage Mountain Retreat Center and Nature Preserve in East Barre, Vermont, remains New England's foremost learning center. Online and printed courses are available.

www.sagemountain.com
herbs@rosemarygladstar.com

In 2023, the World Health Organization expressed support for traditional medicine including homeopathy and herbal medicine pointing out that 70-80 percent of the world's population relies on traditional medicine for much of their primary health care needs.

Willner Chemists: The Oldest and Largest Natural Pharmacy in North America

Willner, founded in 1911, has staff pharmacists available to answer questions. Through its educational website and print newsletter, supplements are profiled and studies overviewed. Archives of radio interviews with doctors and other experts can be accessed through Willner's site. Helpful topics are covered such as herbs that help mitigate migraines. Willner ships almost anywhere.

dongoldberg.com
willner.com
@willnerchemists

Gary Kracoff, RPh,

Gary is a registered pharmacist with a doctorate in naturopathic medicine, who provides in depth consultative services. Lecturer and educator, Gary's guiding philosophy is to treat the person as a whole and not chase symptoms.

Johnson Compounding and Wellness
577 Main Street
Waltham, MA 02452
781-893-3870

Combat Fatigue: Metagenics Licorice Plus Adrenal Support

Exercise, a nutrient-dense diet, adequate sleep, and stress reduction all play a part in creating health. One of my favorite Metagenic products, Licorice Plus, has been found to normalize cortisol levels during stressful times.

metagenics.com

Periodontal Health: Dental Herb Company

Gum hygiene is linked to heart health and also cancer prevention. Since 1996, Dental Herb Company offers a 100 percent natural antimicrobial approach to gum care and oral hygiene. Under The Gums Irrigant and Tooth and Gum Tonic (mouthwash) are favorites. Dental Herb Company, located in New Hampshire, ships nationwide.

dentalherb.com
@dentalherbcompany

Adopt a Dog. Extend Your Life. Do you know that dog owners live longer lives? A 2017 study profiled in *Scientific Reports* found that people who have dogs had a reduced risk for cardiovascular disease, enjoyed better overall health, and live longer.

Whiskers Holistic Pet Care, A Manhattan Favorite

Whiskers, Manhattan's first natural pet store since 1988, remains a local favorite. The staff is knowledgeable and their supplement line for dogs and cats is excellent. Liquid DMG (dimethylglycine) helps pets recover from sickness by boosting immunity. Ultimate Canine and Feline Digest soothes all kinds of digestive upsets. Products are also available online or can be ordered by phone. Whiskers has stores in Manhattan and Queens. Nationwide shipping.

1800whiskers.com
@instaphilpfk

Gluten-Free: Gillian's Bread Crumbs

Family-owned and operated Gillian's Gluten-Free Italian Bread Crumbs has home-style taste. Gillian combines seasonings including smoky paprika and thyme, so the bread crumbs are ideal for Spanish-style recipes, such as stuffed squid, bell peppers with ground meat and rice, or Spanish-style meatloaf.

gilliansfoodsglutenfree.com
@gilliansfoods

Sir Kensington's Mayonnaise Hits Different

Store-bought mayonnaise is listed as a staple in Ferran Adrià's book *The Family Meal*, so it's good enough for me—but it must be first rate. Sir Kensington's Organic non-GMO Mayonnaise contains no artificial ingredients, and the eggs are from chickens that roam free. My tuna recipe, made with Sir Kensington's mayonnaise, follows.

sirkensingtons.com
@sirkensingtons

Bonito del Norte Tuna
with Quick Saffron Mayonnaise

Crumble 4 pinches of saffron threads into 2 tablespoons of warm water, stir, and leave for 10 minutes. Meanwhile, in a medium-sized bowl, combine 2 small minced shallots (seasoned lightly with salt and ground white pepper) along with a cup of Sir Kensington's Organic Mayonnaise. Blend the saffron water into the mayo, season with a little white pepper, and marinate for 15 minutes. Place a jar of crumbled Bonito del Norte tuna into a bowl, flake with a fork, add 2 tablespoons of finely minced mild sweet onion and 2 teaspoons of rinsed and dried capers. Toss, add the saffron mayonnaise, and serve.

Susun Weed is an Extraordinary Teacher with an encyclopedic knowledge of herbs and women's health. She appears on television and radio, including National Public Radio. Ms. Weed's six herbal medicine books focus on topics including childbearing, breast health and menopause. She is a contributor to *Routledge International Encyclopedia of Women's Studies* as well as popular magazines, including *Sagewoman*. Discover her site below for information on her bookstore, workshops, and correspondence courses. *Abundantly Well: Seven Medicines* is her newest book. I have all of them.

www.susunweed.com

Garden Hack: Organic Non-GMO Choricero and Gernika Pepper Seeds

Secret Seed Cartel, owned by preservationists committed to sharing heirloom and endangered seeds in Ohio, specializes in rare seeds such as heirloom tomato varieties, and choricero and Gernika pepper. Seeds are non-GMO and organic. Secret Seed Cartel ships throughout the US.

secretseedcartel.com

Book by Lauded Barcelona Chefs on Cooking Sea Vegetables

Research shows that sea vegetables, rich in iodine, therapeutic sulfated polysaccharides, vitamins, carotenoids, and antioxidants, may protect against cancer. Chefs Eduard Xatruch and Oriol Castro, both from the Mediterranean-inspired, Michelin-starred Disfrutar in Barcelona, wrote *Cooking with Sea Vegetables* or *Cocina con Algas*. (Available in Spanish.)

Naturespirit Herbs: Sea Vegetables and Bath Therapy

Did you know that the use of seaweed to promote health goes back to the time of Aristotle? Or that iodine in seaweed helps fight infection? In Aristotle's day, when someone was injured, seaweed was used on wounds. Naturespirit Herbs harvests premier sea vegetables for supplementation and culinary usage. And for the bath, just ¾ cup of bladderwrack seaweed powder added to the water, softens skin and relieves headaches—home thalassotherapy like health spas of old Europe. In addition, bladderwrack reduces inflammation and rids the body of toxins. For cooking, Naturespirit's sea vegetables are added to miso soups. Their Wild Mushroom Mix, a blend of four Polypore fungi with immune-enhancing and antiviral properties, can be sipped or cooked with other foods as a base for soup. Naturespirit also produces herbal extracts, such as St. John's Wort tincture, effective in alleviating anxiety/depression while strengthening the heart. This liquid can be added to water or tea.

naturespiritherbs.com
@naturespiritherbs

Kettle & Fire Organic Bone Broths

Kettle & Fire simmers bone broths for more than twenty hours, ensuring high levels of collagen. Artisan-grade chicken, chicken/mushroom, and beef broths are basic soups, but a full line is offered. Packaging is environmentally friendly.

kettleandfire.com
@kettleandfire

Dr. Hauschka: Certified Natural and Organic Skin, Body Care and Cosmetics

Did you know that most skin care products contain additives of concern to breast cancer advocacy groups? Since 1967, Dr. Hauschka has been making skin and body care products free from toxic substances. Dedicated to purity, Hauschka bio-dynamically grows and wild-crafts most herbs and flowers for their products. Offering skin care programs geared toward different skin types of every age, Hauschka also makes body care, natural cosmetics, and a full line of fragrant, natural bath oils. Hauschka skin and body care is a daily routine for me. I especially love Rose Day Cream and Moor Lavender Calming Body Oil. Dr. Hauschka is opposed to animal testing and uses eco-friendly packaging.

drhauschka.com
@drhauschkausa

Flora Health

Flora has evolved into one of North America's premier natural health products companies. The U.S. and Canadian production plants employ sophisticated equipment for processing quality herbal teas and liquid tonics, encapsulating herbal extracts and cold-pressing certified organic seeds into health-benefitting oils. This includes Udo's 3-6-9 Blend oil and capsules.

florahealth.com
1-800-498-3610

More Health Resources, Books, Etc.

Brigitte Mars, A.H.G., Author and Aromatherapy Master

Brigitte Mars, founding member of the American Herbalists Guild, has written many books on aromatherapy and herbs, including *Herbs for Healthy Hair, Skin and Nails* and *Healing Herbal Teas: A Complete Guide to Making Delicious, Healthful Beverages.*

> brigittemars.com
> @brigitte.mars

Food for Breast Cancer Newsletter

In her June 16, 2021 digital newsletter, G. Sarah Charles writes: "The Mediterranean diet is a good starting point for breast cancer." Charles, a breast cancer survivor who writes the articles and compiles/presents research for her *Food for Breast Cancer* newsletter, has a science degree from UCLA and an MBA from Harvard.

> Foodforbreastcancer.com

Elena Pollard, MA

Elena Pollard, a clinical homeopath focusing on healing toxic damage is dedicated to educating families through classes and client consultation.

> SoleLunaBotanicals.com

Susun Weed: The Wise Woman Way

Herbalist Susun Weed's Wise Woman Center in Woodstock, NY offers seminars and work-study apprenticeships. Topics include "Identifying Wild Plants in Your Own Backyard" and "How to Make Simple Home Remedies." Weed's books, available at wisewomanbookshop.com and Amazon, are homey compendiums. Discover herbal teas, decoctions, compresses, and more. Weed, available for consultations, has a healing energy all her own.

> susunweed.com
> @susunsweed

Reflexology

The ages-old healing modality known as reflexology stimulates pressure points in the feet improving, for example, digestive and kidney function and other bodily systems. *Relax into Feeling Better*, a book by reflexologist Amon Sherriff, co-authored with his wife, Cina, explains classic reflexology pressure points. Amon, also a master flutist, offers his CD, *The Peace-Filled Journey*, featuring both percussion and flute.

awarehousehealth.net

More Reflexology

Barbara and Kevin Kunz are internationally recognized authorities in reflexology and best-selling authors of 24 books about reflexology. The Kunzes published in 24 languages with 60 foreign editions. Currently they are working with neuroscientists in an MRI reflexology research project conducted at the University of Minnesota School of Medicine. Look for their web presence via newsletter, Facebook, blog forums and Twitter.

Life Extension Magazine

This leading health publication reports advances in nutrition, including the latest research.

Lifeextension.com/magazine
@lifeextension

Culture and a Little History

Paradores

Paradores are Spanish government-owned, high-end, yet affordable hotels in converted monasteries, fortresses, and castles, usually in areas of striking natural beauty. Compared to top hotels across Europe, service at paradores is among the best, and values highly competitive. Most paradores have excellent restaurants featuring breakfast buffets and local dinner specialties with recipes of historic implication. Spain's oldest hotel, Parador de Santiago, in Galicia, is known for dramatic public rooms and spectacular local seafood. Some paradores, such as the one in the Pyrenees town of Vielha, offer swimming pools and spas. Many paradores carry legends that go back before they were hotels. At Parador de Hondarribia, housed in a converted 980 AD fortress in the Basque region, guests report creaking passageways from ghosts. Sophia Lauren, who stayed there, said this was true. In addition to ghosts, Parador de Hondarribia offers magnificent views from the wide stone terrace of coastal France.

Paradoresofspain.com

> Javier Marías (1951-2023) lauded at the time of his death as the best Spanish writer of the day, was a perennial contender for The Nobel prize. Author of 15 novels, published in 50 languages including *A Heart So White*, Marías was educated in Madrid, and taught Spanish literature at Oxford University. Called "a great philosopher of everyday absurdity," he was known as a keen observer of the games people play.

A Total Work of Art: Casa Milà, Barcelona (1906–1912)

Declared by UNESCO as a world heritage site, Casa Mila, known as "La Pedrera" or "rock quarry," was created by the architect Antoni Gaudí. Upon completion, his futuristic building with its rocky façade caused civic meltdown. Access to La Pedrera is through the lobby, designed with bronze hardware and ceramic tiles created by the most talented artisans of the day, making them art nouveau classics. Explore Casa Milà's rooftop terrace with its views of Barcelona. La Pedrera's preserved period apartment, detailing early nineteenth-century life with a fully outfitted kitchen, galvanizes. Fees to tour this historic structure contribute to environmental, educational, and cultural projects.

lapedrera.com
@lapedrera_barcelona

La Pedrera's Museum Shop: Architecture, Gastronomy, Furniture, etc.

The museum shop offers books on contemporary furnishings and design; magazines and books on gastronomy, architecture, and more. Solid bronze art nouveau-style ergonomic casts made from Casa Milà hardware are small enough to carry home.

store.lapedrera.com

The Basque Sculptor Eduardo Chillida, and Museo Chillida Leku

Eduardo Chillida (1924–2020), born in Donostia/San Sebastián, lived and worked close by in Hernani. Today, Museo Chillida Leku displays the master's work indoors in his studio, and outdoors on parklike grounds. Chillida's *The Comb of the Wind*, a massive installation of three primordial-looking forged iron sculptures embedded into gigantic shore boulders sited in the western end of La Concha Bay, is so majestic that the installation seems placed there on the day earth began. The Basque architect Luis Peña Ganchegui, who sited the work, knew that the frequently moody, windy bay adds even more power to the installation. The completed project is the ultimate expression of both the sculptor's and the architect's lifeworks. Chillida's *Elogio de Horizonte* sculpture in the coastal city, Gijón, in Asturias, also haunts. The heroic works of Chillida can be found throughout the world, including the UNESCO headquarters in Paris and the courtyard of the World Bank in Washington, DC.

museochillidaleku.com

Fundació Museu Picasso in Barcelona; and Picasso's Kitchen Exhibition

Museu Picasso, in the El Born neighborhood, displays many of Picasso's early works providing insight into the genius's formative years. The force of this collection in its entirety exceeds imagination. The 2018 exhibit *Picasso's Kitchen* paid tribute to the culinary motifs present in every genre of his work. An anecdote: Picasso created a rabbit cutout from the top of a cake box. When finished, the master held the cardboard rabbit forth to evaluate, but his dachshund, Lump, had another idea. Immediately snatching the cutout from the great artist's hands, the dog raced into the garden to eat it. Picasso found this extremely funny. The catalog, *Picasso's Kitchen*, published by Fundació Museu Picasso de Barcelona is available in English.

> museupicasso.bcn.cat
> @museupicasso

Guggenheim Bilbao and a Chef's Rooftop Garden in the Basque Country

This modernist structure houses the Guggenheim's collection. The building itself is so innovative it draws visitors from across the globe. The titanium structure, designed by Frank Gehry, was described by Philip Johnson as "the greatest building of our time." Guggenheim Bilbao exhibits large-scale modern and contemporary works by sculptors and offers nineteen galleries of exhibition space. Works by Willem de Kooning, David Hockney, Francisco Clemente, and others draw. Book reservations at Bilbao's Azurmendi, a three Michelin-starred delight. Chef Eneko Atxa features produce grown on its rooftop garden.

> guggenheim-bilbao.eus/en/
> @museoguggenheim

San Sebastián Jazz Festival

Known throughout the world by jazz lovers, this historic mid-July festival features jazz greats of the times.

> sansebastianturismo.com
> Instagram: @sansebastiantourism
> jazzaldia.com
> @heinekenjazzaldia

For more jazz in the Basque country, don't miss:

> basquecountrymagazine.com/en/festivals

Sitges Film Festival

A short drive south from Barcelona, one encounters the bohemian Mediterranean seaside town of Sitges, which hosts the annual Sitges Film Festival drawing worldwide directors and actors. Horror/fantasy genre rules. While in Sitges, check out the Cau Ferrat Museum in the former home-studio of the Catalan painter, dramatist and writer, Santiago Rusiñol (1861-1993).

sitgesfestival.com
@sitgesfestival

Galicia: Festival of the Celtic World in the Region A Coruña

This annual mid-July event in the seaside town of Ortigueira, near the northern most point of Iberia, features seaside concerts with established Celtic stars and new artists. The event is free. Nearby, one finds the highest cliffs in Europe in the fishing village of Cedeira.

festivaldeortigueira.com
@festivaldeortigueira

Gran Teatre del Liceu

Gran Teatre del Liceu, which opened in Barcelona in 1847, is the oldest opera house in Spain and one of the most respected in Europe. The Liceu hosts visiting opera companies and produces its own operas 2-3 times a year. In addition, programs featuring ballet and jazz are presented.

liceubarcelona.cat
@liceu_opera_barcelona

The famed diva, Montserrat Caballé (1933–2018), born in Barcelona, received her education at the Liceu. Caballé's international breakthrough occurred in 1965 at Carnegie Hall when she replaced Marilyn Horne with a performance of Donizetti's *Lucrezia Borgia* so astonishing that it earned Caballé a twenty-five-minute standing ovation. See YouTube, Montserrat Caballé, 50 anys al Liceu.

Barcelona's Club Apolo

Since its 1935 opening, this Barcelona nightspot has been one of Europe's most celebrated dance clubs. In 2000, Coldplay performed their first album there. See below for the book chronicling the history of the Apolo, including the club's many (noted) performers.

sala-apolo.com
@sala_apolo

Apolo, 75 Años Sin Parar de Bailar (Apolo, 75 Years with Nonstop Dance) by Eva Espinet (Comanegra, 2018), is available in Spanish and in Catalan. It contains hundreds of interviews.

El Born Centre de Cultura i Memòria

The El Born CCM stands as a testament to Barcelona's rich history, housed in one of the city's earliest iron architecture masterpieces designed by Josep Fontserè in 1876. Once the city's central market, its walls now reveal the remnants of the city from 1714, a poignant reminder of the fierce resistance against Philip V's final assault and the subsequent fall on September 11th. Today, this historic site serves as a vibrant center commemorating the enduring spirit of the struggle for freedom.

elbornculturaimemoria.barcelona.cat
@elbornccm

STREAMING TIPS: Catalan director Jordi Frades, described as "one of the highest profile creators of television drama series" by *Variety*, gives us *Cathedral of the Sea* bringing fourteenth century Barcelona to life. Viewers are transported to the time when the cathedral of Santa María del Mar was constructed by local guild craftsmen.

Basque Culinary Center

The Basque Culinary Center, spearheaded by the region's chefs, remains dedicated to training, research, and innovation. Events are aimed at development, management, science, and all disciplines related to gastronomy.

bculinary.com
@bculinary

The Picasso of Fashion: Cristóbal Balenciaga, and His Museum

The Basque seacoast village, Getaria, birthplace of Cristóbal Balenciaga (1895-1972), boasts the first museum in the world dedicated exclusively to a fashion designer. Committed to the relevance of Cristóbal Balenciaga, described by Christian Dior as "the master of us all," the museum exhibits more than three thousand items related to Balenciaga and remains involved in the education and forefront of fashion design. It is interesting that Balenciaga, said to be "the Picasso of fashion," opened his first boutique in San Sebastián in 1917 and then in Barcelona and Madrid. The Spanish Civil War forced Balenciaga to close his boutiques, and move to Paris, to open shop. It is said that during WWII, women risked their lives to shop there. Customers included the Duchess of Windsor and later, Jackie Onassis.

cristobalbalenciagamuseoa.com/en/
@cbmuseoa

Slow Food Spain

This group features a global network of chefs who embrace culinary tradition.

slowfood.es
@slowfood_international

Department of Basque Studies, Boise State University

The Basque Studies Program at Boise State offers a multidisciplinary course of advanced study overviewing varied aspects of language, history, politics, economics, and more. The mission is to empower students to generate self-directed lifelong learning into Basque culture and history.

basquestudies.boisestate.edu

The William A. Douglass Center for Basque Studies, University of Nevada

This organization is dedicated to Basque research, history, language, and literature. The founder, William A. Douglass, did more than any person in the United States to inspire understanding of the Basque people, one of the Western world's most advanced cultures. Douglass has authored or edited more than a dozen books about Basque history and culture. The William A. Douglass Center shares findings about the Basques through publications, conferences, lectures, and activities and offers a broad range of books including biographies, fiction, and children's books.

basque.unr.edu

Buber's Basque Page

Blas Pedro Uberuaga created this resource in 1994 covering Basque history, culture, and gastronomy. The site also publishes recipes.

buber.net

Catalan Literature, Translated into English

Springing from Catalunya's own energetic heritage, a deep-rooted inquisitiveness into other literary traditions is reflected in its qualities, further supported by an outstanding publishing industry. The illustrious publishing house Lletra presents Catalan writers/poets translated into English. Works by Mercè Rodoreda and Josep Pla are revealed. Links to literary organizations, such as an online library that catalogs the complete works of all noted Catalan authors, are offered through this site. YouTube presentations can also be discovered.

lletra.net

Discover Josep Pla

Joan Resina condenses and presents forty-seven volumes of Pla's work, including narrative fiction and history, organizing them into themes such as time, memory, religion, life, and metaphysics. Don't miss *Josep Pla: Seeing the World in the Form of Articles*.

Catalan Culture: Institut Ramon Llull

Institut Ramon Llull, with offices in New York City, Paris, London, Berlin, and Barcelona, promotes Catalan language, curriculum, and education. The Institute facilitates translation of Catalan literature into other languages and promotes Catalan art, architecture, science, films/television, literature, gastronomy, and music. Workshops and events are held, giving insight into how Catalans utilize culture to sustain their people during changing times. Llull headquarters in Barcelona, located in a remarkable Josep Puig 1900 building, can be toured.

llull.cat
@irllull

STREAMING TIPS: Ramon Salazar's *Sunday's Illness* is a gripping drama. The sophisticated comedic series, *Welcome to the Family*, directed by Pau Freixas, leaves you laughing. If you are into gross-out horror, the Basque *Witching and Bitching* will make you laugh so hard your sides will ache. *Bomb Scared*, a dark Basque comedy starring Javier Cámara, keeps humor moving fast and bright.

Etxepare Foundation, and a Food Writer You Should Not Miss

The first recorded book in the Basque language was written in 1545 by Bernart Etxepare. The Etxepare Institute, established to honor their genesis author, disseminates Basque language, culture, and gastronomy worldwide. The institute's teaching resources, available to universities, include translation services. Providing insight into the evolution of Basque gastronomy, Etxepare offers the free PDF English download "On Basque Cuisine" by the late Hasier Etxeberria. Etxeberria has focused on the New Basque Cuisine since the beginning of this world-shaping movement.

etxepare.eus/en

World Literature Today

One of the oldest, continuously published literary periodicals in the United States, *WLT* is an international magazine that has been presenting the best contemporary fiction, book reviews, poetry, essays, and interviews by authors from throughout the world for over 90 years. In addition to its articles, editorials from the editor, Daniel S. Simon, absorb. Graphics and art contribute to the publication's literary edge. The September 2009 issue was devoted to Catalan literature.

worldliteraturetoday.org
@worldlittoday

Cantabria: Botín Arts Center, Designed by Architect Renzo Piano

The Botín Arts Center, a daring structure nautical in spirit, is set in Santander's lovely Pereda Gardens. The boldly contemporary building is formed by two sections that seem randomly split in the middle, with walls of glass revealing the sparkling Bay. The Arts Center features exhibitions of modern art, workshops, classes, and offers a concert hall.

fundacionbotin.org

Galician Writers, Inspired by the Beauty of Their Land

Travel writer Annette M.B. Meakin (1867–1959) and author of *Galicia, The Switzerland of Spain*, understood the passion Galician writers and poets have for their "mountains, vales, and rivers." Based on this tradition, Galicia's leading Romantic poet, Rosalía de Castro, was the pen, guided by the land and waters of Galicia. Today, as with the work of de Castro, Galician writers continue to be moved by this beauty. Discover anthologies, single titles, dramas, essays, novels, poetry, and stories from these authors through the site below.

Galicianliterature.gal

STREAMING TIP: *All Is Silence*, a film based on the book by the Galician writer Manuel Rivas, captures the spirit of Rosalía de Castro's poetry, which inspired Rivas to write his own book and then make this powerful film. Footage in *All Is Silence* transmits longing from both de Castro and Rivas that somehow becomes your own.

Bold, Expressionistic Mural Art Adorns the Walls of Medieval Church in the Pyrenees

A fall road trip through the Pyrenees should include the hamlet, Saurí, in Lleida. The walls of the medieval church there are covered in contemporary mural art of mixed figuration with abstraction, making the experience mother nature's rave. The artist, Santi Moix, used expressionistic colors and style to depict the flora, animals, and birds of the surrounding valley. Moix, who has lived in New York since 1986, works in painting, sculpture, mural art, ceramics, prints, and illustration.

www.santimoix.com

PlayStation 4: Legends of Catalonia, Land of Barcelona

The PlayStation *Legends of Catalonia* throws one into dramatic locales that feel real. Action unfolds. Consider the rugged coastal town Cadaqués, a geological wonder so potent it draws people from across the globe. PlayStation 4 immerses you in this rugged splendour. YouTube offers a look.

isyourhome.catalunya.com/legendsofcatalonia/en/

Cantabria: Altamira Cave

Cantabria's Museo de Altamira's permanent exhibition, *The Times of Altamira*, is a presentation depicting prehistoric customs and traditions of the Iberian peninsula. Realistically represented, this exhibit takes one back to the dawn of civilization. Authentic archaeological artifacts from prehistory compose displays, creating a faithful replica of Altamira cave.

culturaydeporte.gob.es/mnaltamira
turismodecantabria.com

TIP: About 2 hours south of Altamira, near Burgos in Northern Spain, is Atapuerca, site of several limestone caves where one can find the earliest evidence of humans in Western Europe dating back 1.2 million years ago.

La Rioja: One of the Most Valuable Dinosaur Sites in Europe and Cutting Edge Architecture

Around 120 million years ago, during the Jurassic and Cretaceous periods, megasized dinosaurs crept throughout marshlands of La Rioja, with legs bigger than grand pianos, leaving fossilized footprints for us to marvel about today. Against a backdrop of tawny earth, one can imagine these giant creatures that weighed as much as seven elephants and were around 125 feet in length, plodding along.

dinosaurios-igea.com

Springing Forward to Present Day

Nestled in the heart of the wine country, the town of Elciego boasts approximately 275 thriving winegrowing farms. This picturesque locale is also home to the illustrious Bodegas Marqués de Riscal, where the landscape is graced by the iconic "Riojan Guggenheim." This architectural marvel, envisioned by the renowned Canadian architect Frank Gehry, stands as a symbol of innovation and elegance amidst the vineyards.

Tour Navarra: A Contemporary Hotel, Famed Produce, and Charlemagne's Only Defeat

Most associate Navarra with Pamplona's San Fermín Festival, but do not overlook Bardenas Reales Natural Park. Canyons, bizarre tower shapes of stone, and arid plateaus burst from desert plains. The area is so evocative that *Game of Thrones* was filmed there. To the north, the Camino de Santiago pilgrimage route starts in Roncesvalles where, in the 700s, an army of Basques successfully ambushed Charlemagne's troops, who were more numerous and better armed. This, the only major defeat Charlemagne suffered. In Tudela (the garden of Navarre), Aire de Bardenas Hotel, a modernist cube-like structure with generous windows brings the outdoors in, including fields of wheat. The minimalist restaurant inside serves the famed organic produce of Navarra. Tomatoes that taste like tomatoes. A promise fulfilled.

Airedebardenas.com

Asturias: Cave Paintings, and the Most Extensive Dinosaur Museum in Europe

Forty percent of Asturias is reserved undeveloped land. A trip to this region of natural wonder can include hikes in mountain valleys, explorations of Tito Bustillo Cave, which features prehistoric paintings, and a stop in Oviedo to view La Lluera Caves, housing even more spectacular cave art. As for dinosaurs that once roamed the beaches from Gijón to Ribadesella, fossilized footprints left by these massive creatures 150 million years ago are still visible today. Museo del Jurásico de Asturias, the most extensive dinosaur museum in Europe, fascinates.

turismoasturias.es/en

More Culture

Beebe Bahrami: Anthropologist, Writer, and Adventurer

By way of her blog and books written in memoir style, including *The Spiritual Traveler: Spain—A Guide to Sacred Sites and Pilgrim Routes* (Mahwah, NJ: Hidden Spring, 2009), Bahrami demonstrates knowledge of history and affinity for ancient spiritual customs.

beebebahrami.weebly.com

Piccavey, Travel Sherpa

Molly Piccavey began writing about Spain in 2011. Based in Andalusia, Piccavey reports on historic sites, gastronomy, travel tips, and more.

piccavey.com
@piccavey

A Few Favorite Cooking Blogs

Ruth Reichl

"My idea of good living is not about eating high on the hog. Rather, to me, good living means understanding how food connects us to the earth." A quote from Ruth Reichl, the last editor of *Gourmet* magazine. Ruth, the producer of *Gourmet's Diary of a Foodie* (PBS), wrote *My Kitchen Year: 136 Recipes That Saved My Life* (Random House, 2015). This book, along with Reichl's others, including *Delicious!*—an entertaining work of fiction—is available on Amazon.

> ruthreichl.com
> @ruth.reichl

Cara Eisenpress: Big Girls, Small Kitchen

Savvy New Yorker Cara Eisenpress offers tasty recipes. Don't miss her *Big Girls, Small Kitchen* blog or her book, *In the Small Kitchen: 100 Recipes from Our Year of Cooking in the Real World* (New York: William Morrow, 2011).

> biggirlssmallkitchen.com
> @bgsk

James Beard Foundation, and Its Book on Eliminating Food Waste

This organization honors and nurtures chefs who remain dedicated to making the food of America more sustainable, diverse, and delicious. For up-to-date food news and tasty recipes, don't miss the information below.

> jamesbeard.org
> @beardfoundation

Waste Not: How to Get the Most from Your Food, from the James Beard Foundation (*Rizzoli*, 2018), enlightens us on preventing food waste. One example: combine sautéed chard stems with garlicky pasta.

Janet Mendel: One of the First Cookbook Authors to Bring the Cooking of Spain to Light

An American cookbook writer, living in the south of Spain since 1966, Ms. Mendel has written six cookbooks filled with authentic recipes. Mendel's books, brimming with practical information, are rich in everyday experiences and traditions. Don't miss *My Kitchen in Spain: 235 Authentic Regional Recipes* (New York: HarperCollins, 2002).

> mykitcheninspain.blogspot.com

Marti Buckley, Cook, Writer, and YouTube Host: Why Spanish Food is So Underrated

Marti Buckley, a food/travel writer born in Alabama, lives in Donostia/San Sebastián and covers Basque cooking with the perspective of a native. Ms. Buckley's *Basque Country: A Culinary Journey through a Food Lover's Paradise* (Artisan, 2018) is packed with recipes. Don't miss the eloquent Ms. Buckley's April 17th, 2022, YouTube presentation on why she thinks Spanish food is underrated.

> Google YouTube, Marti Buckley
> travelcookeat.com
> @martibuckley

Maria Gilbert, The Mallorcan YouTube Grandmother Sensation

By way of her popular YouTube channel, *Recetas Mallorquinas*, the famous eighty-five-year-old grandmother demonstrates authentic Mallorcan recipes to almost 40,000 subscribers. Don't be left out.

> Recetas Mallorquinas YouTube

From the South of Spain: Nevenka's Organic Farm Blog

From her farm in Almeria, Nevenka—she likes just going by her first name—presents innovative farm-to-table vegan recipes. Nevenka is over the moon about her zero-miles produce and makes me want to start my own farm. Right now!

> fincafood.com

El Invitado de Invierno: *The Winter Guest* Blog and ...
Pies with Sneaky Eyes

Miriam García, chef and creator of *The Winter Guest*, loves spreading the word about the pleasures of Spain's Mediterranean diet. Visuals on the Winter Guest blog and García's vivid Instagram capture everyday life in her Madrid kitchen. Miriam's sense of play is apparent. One recipe features a picture of a couple of autumn stone fruit pies—eyes and mouths have been cut into crusts with sneaky, snarky expressions. Those pies are watching. You will not get away.

> invitadoinvierno.com
> @miriamelinvitado

Kanela y Limón; Some of The Hippest Food Styling Around

A party for the dessert lover's soul.

> kanelaylimon.blogspot.com

A Postscript Worthy of Your Consideration:
Does a Playful Approach Extend Life?

Investigating happiness, researcher Peter Dodds, from the University of Vermont, evaluated the ten most spoken languages in the world and found Spanish to include the most uplifting words such as laughter and love, and the fewest negative words, such as fighting or crying. We know that the Mediterranean diet helps the Spanish people to take their place among the longest living in the world. Could a positive attitude be a contributing factor as well? Epigenetics tells us that our mental state is as important to health as is eating a protective diet, by preventing the expression of genes programmed for disease. So the Spanish just might be on to something.

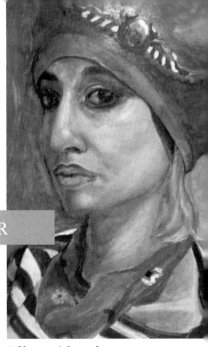

A NOTE ABOUT THE AUTHOR

Self-portrait by author

"And I got a strong feeling of the passage of time. Not the time of clouds and sun and rain and the moving stars that adorn the night, not spring when its time comes or fall, not the time that makes leaves bud on branches and then tears them off or folds and unfolds and colors the flowers, but the time inside me, the time you can't see but it molds us. The time that rolls on and on in people's hearts and makes them roll along with it and gradually changes us inside and out and makes us what we'll be on our dying day."

– Mercè Rodoreda, *The Time of the Doves*

Robin Keuneke, artist, writer, and natural foods cook, was born in Connecticut.

Drawing and painting since childhood, Keuneke studied classical drawing and anatomy at the Art Students League of New York with Robert Beverly Hale, curator for American paintings at the Metropolitan Museum of Art; and painting with Robert Beauchamp, a leading figure in the figurative expressionist movement; subsequently broadening her education at the Robert Blackburn Printmaking Workshop in Chelsea. Keuneke's oil paintings were featured in one-person shows in New York and in London at October Gallery, and her etchings in the permanent collection of the New York Public Library were exhibited with those of Sir Francis Bacon, Pablo Picasso, and others.

While pursuing her interest in fine art, she attended classes at the iconic but now closed Macrobiotic Center and Natural Gourmet Institute, which led to the development of a self-published, 100-page booklet featuring health research, tips, and original recipes. During the years that followed, she became a regular guest on national talk radio, advocating for women to make healthy food choices, especially regarding those rich in protective fats. She was interviewed by notables including Dr. Robert Atkins, and was profiled in Gary Null's *The Woman's Encyclopedia of Natural Healing.*

The author's pamphlet gave rise to her first book, with original recipes, *Total Breast Health: Power Foods for Protection and Wellness.* Released in hardcover by Kensington Books in 1998, it was distinguished by *Publisher's Weekly* in their Best Book of the Year List. The hardcover and two printings of the trade paperback sold a total of over 35,000 copies. Her second book, *The Detox Revolution: A Powerful Program for Boosting Your Body's Ability to Fight Cancer,* was published in 2003 with co-author Thomas J. Slaga, PhD., former Scientific Director of the AMC Cancer Research Center.

The Iberian Table is written with the observant eye of an artist, by someone who has devoted a lifetime to understanding natural health and cooking.

Keuneke is a member of the Culinary Historians of Southern California, the Independent Book Publishers Association, and the Florida Writers Association. With her husband, Thomas, the author divides her time between Atlanta and Delray Beach. Look for her next book project, a collection of short stories around the theme of Spanish gastronomy.

BIBLIOGRAPHY AND SUGGESTED READING

Benefits of the Mediterranean Diet

Shafqat, A. et al. "Mediterranean Diet Adherence and Risk of All-Cause Mortality in Women." *JAMA Network Open*, April 2024.

https://jamanetwork.com/journals/jamanetworkopen/fullarticle/2819335

Callahan, A. "The Magic of Olive Oil, Fish and Other Healthy Fats." *The New York Times*, January 2024.

www.nytimes.com/2024/01/19/well/eat/mediterranean-diet-oil-fish-healthy-fat.html

Pant, A. et al. "Mediterranean Diet and Risk of Cardiovascular Disease and Death in Women: A Systematic Review and Meta-Analysis." Prevention and Health Promotion: Nutrition and Lifestyle Digital Presentations, March 2023.

www.abstractsonline.com/pp8/#!/10674/presentation/20603

Bohn, K. "Mediterranean Diet with Lean Beef May Lower Risk Factors for Heart Disease." *Penn State University*, April 2021.

www.psu.edu/news/research/story/mediterranean-diet-lean-beef-may-lower-risk-factors-heart-disease/

Hinzey, E. "Mediterranean Diet...One of the Best Diets of 2023." *U.S. News & World Report*, January 2023.

http://health.usnews.com/best-diet/Mediterranean-diet

Segal, L. "The Mediterranean Diet Really is That Good for You. Here's Why." *The New York Times*, January 2023.

www.nytimes.com/2023/01/06/well/eat/mediterranean-diet-health.html

Delgado-Lista, J. et al. "Long-Term Secondary Prevention of Cardiovascular Disease with a Mediterranean Diet and a Low-Fat Diet (CORDIOPREV): A Randomized Controlled Trial." *The Lancet*, May 2022.

https://doi.org/10.1016/S0140-6736(22)00122-2

Calatayud-Saez, F. et al. "Effects of the Affinity to the Mediterranean Diet Pattern Together with Breastfeeding on the Incidence of Childhood Asthma and Other Inflammatory and Recurrent Diseases" *Allergologia et Immunopathologia, vol 9, number 6*, November 2021.

https://doi.org/10.15586/aei.v49i6338

Guasch-Ferré, M. et al. "Consumption of Olive Oil and Risk of Total and Cause-Specific Mortality Among U.S. Adults." *Journal of the American College of Cardiology*, January 2022.

Unattributed. "The Mediterranean Diet is a Good Starting Point for Breast Cancer." *foodforbreastcancer.com*, October 22, 2021

www.foodforbreastcancer.com/articles/the-mediterranean-diet-is-a-good-starting-point-for-breast-cancer

Shikany, J. et al. "Mediterranean Diet Score, Dietary Patterns and Risk of Sudden Cardiac Death in the REGARDS Study." *Journal of the American Heart Association*, June 2021.

https://doi.org/10.1161/120.019158

Meslier, V. et al. "Mediterranean Diet Intervention In Overweight And Obese Subjects Lowers Plasma Cholesterol and Causes Changes In The Gut Microbiome And Metabolome Independently of Energy Intake." *Gut*, April 2020.

https://doi.org/10.1136/gutjnl-2019-320438

Unattributed. "US News Reveals Best Diet Rankings for 2020," Jan. 2, 2020.

https://www.usnews.com/info/blogs/press-room/articles/2020-01-02/us-news-reveals-best-diets-rankings-for-2020

Papassotiriou, I. et al. "Adherence to Mediterranean Diet Is Associated With Lung Function in Older Adults: Data From the Health and Retirement Study." *Journal of the American College of Nutrition*, March 2020.

https://doi.org/10.1080/07315724.2020.1740114

LaMotte, S. "The Mediterranean Diet Scores Another Win for Longevity by Improving Gut Microbe," *CNN Health Online*, February 18, 2020.

www.cnn.com/2020/02/17/health/mediterranean-diet-microbiome-wellness/index.html

Ghosh, T. et al. "Mediterranean Diet Intervention Alters the Gut Microbiome in Older People Reducing Frailty and Improving Health Status: the NU-AGE 1-Year Dietary Intervention Across Five European Countries." *Gut*, April 2020.

https://doi.org/10.1136/gutjnl-2019-319654

Bolte, L. et al. "Towards Anti-Inflammatory Dietary Recommendations Based on the Relation Between Food and the Gut Microbione Composition in 1423 Individuals." Presented at UEG week, Barcelona October 21, 2019.

Unattributed. "2021 Best Diets Overall." *U.S. News & World Report*, 2021.

Al-Zoubi, J. "New Funding for Research on Dementia and Med Diet." *Olive Oil Times*, July 29, 2019.

www.oliveoiltimes.com/health-news/new-funding-for-research-on-dementia-and-meddiet/68798#:~:text=New%20Funding%20for%20Research%20on%20Dementia%20and%20MedDiet,Mediterranean%20diet%20and%20a%20reduced%20risk%20of%20dementia.

Al Wattar, B. et al. "Mediterranean-Style Diet in Pregnant Women with Metabolic Risk Factors (ESTEEM): A Pragmatic Multicentre Randomized Trial." *PLOS Medicine*, July 23, 2019.

https://doi.org/10.1371/journal.pmed.1002857

Argyropoulos, K. et al. "Adherence to Mediterranean Diet and Risk of Late-Life Depression." Presented at: APA Annual Meeting, SA Francisco, May 18-22, 2019.

https://doi.org/10.2478/gp-2019-0012

Afshin, A. et al. "Health Effects of Dietary Risks in 195 Countries, 1990-2017: A Systematic Analysis for the Global Burden of Disease Study 2017." *The Lancet*, April 3, 2019.

https://doi.org/10.1016/S0140-6736(19)30041-8

Huggins-Salomon, S. "8 Scientific Health Benefits of the Mediterranean Diet." *Everyday Health*, March 19, 2019.

https://www.everydayhealth.com/mediterranean-diet/scientific-health-benefits-mediterranean-diet/#:~:text=%208%20Scientific%20Health%20Benefits%20of%20the%20Mediterranean,May%20Prevent%20Cognitive%20Decline%20and%20Alzheimer's...%20More

Brancato, J. "Mediterranean Diet May Be Better for Diabetes Shows New Study." *Olive Tomato*, Spring 2019.

https://www.olivetomato.com/mediterranean-diet-better-diet-for-diabetes-shows-new-study/#:~:text=Mediterranean%20Diet%20May%20Be%20Better%20For%20Diabetes%20Shows,requirement%20for%20diabetes%20medications%20compared%20to%20other%20diets.

LaMotte, S. "Mediterranean Diet: How to Start (and Stay on) One of the World's Healthiest Diets." *CNN Health Online*, March 27. 2019.

Mediterranean Diet: How to Start (and Stay on) One of the World's Healthiest Diets

Foreman, K. et al. "Forecasting Life Expectancy, Years of Life Lost and All-Cause and Cause-Specific Mortality for 250 Causes of Death: Reference and Alternative Scenarios for 2016-40 for 195 Countries and Territories." *Global Health Metrics*, November 10, 2018.

https://doi.org/10.1016/S0140-6736(18)31694-5

Estruch, R. et al. "Primary Prevention of Cardiovascular Disease with a Mediterranean Diet Supplemented with Extra-Virgin Olive Oil or Nuts." *The New England Journal of Medicine*, June 13, 2018.

https://doi.org/10.1056/NEJMoa1800389

Kolata, G. "Mediterranean-Diet Study Is Retracted, Then Reissued With Same Findings." *The New York Times*, June 14, 2018.

https://www.nytimes.com/2018/06/13/health/mediterranean-diet-heart-disease.html

Bonaccio, M. et al. "Mediterranean Diet and Morality in the Elderly: A Prospective Cohort Study and a Meta-Analysis." *British Journal of Nutrition*, October 28, 2018.

https://doi.org/10.1017/s0007114518002179

Martínez-González, M. et al. "Design and Methods of the PREDIMED-Plus Randomized Trial." Epidemiology, April 2019.

doi.org/10.1093/ije/dyy225

Lazar, V. et al. "Aspects of Gut Microbiota and Immune System Interactions in Infectious Diseases, Immunopathology, and Cancer." *Frontiers in Immunology*, August 15, 2018.

https://doi.org/10.3389/fimmu.2018.01830

Pagliai, G. et al. "Mediterranean Diet, Food Consumption and Risk of Late-Life Depression: The Mugello Study." *The Journal of Nutrition, Health & Aging*, 2018.

https://doi.org/10.1007/s12603-018-1019-3

Bloomfield, H. et al. "Effects on Health Outcomes of a Mediterranean Diet With No Restriction on Fat Intake: A Systematic Review and Meta-analysis." *Annals of Internal Medicine*, October 4, 2016.

https://doi.org/10.7326/m16-0361

Yadav, H. et al. "Gut Microbiome Composition in Non-human Primates Consuming a Western or Mediterranean Diet." *Frontiers in Nutrition*, April 28, 2018.

https://doi.org/10.3389/fnut.2018.00028

Schwingshackl, L. et al. "A Network Meta-Analysis on the Comparative Efficacy of Different Dietary Approaches on Glycaemic Control in Patients with Type 2 Diabetes Mellitus." *European Journal of Epidemiology*, February 2018.

https://doi.org/10.1007/s10654-017-0352-x

Davis, C. et al. "A Mediterranean Diet Reduces F2-Isoprostanes and Triglycerides Among Older Australian Men and Women After 6 Months." *The Journal of Nutrition*, July 2017.

https://doi.org/10.3945/jn.117.248419

Toledo, E. et al. "Mediterranean Diet and Invasive Breast Cancer Risk Among Women at High Cardiovascular Risk in the PREDIMED Trial: A Randomized Clinical Trial." *JAMA Internal Medicine*, November 2015.

https://doi.org/10.1001/jamainternmed.2015.4838

Martínez-González, M. et al. "Benefits of the Mediterranean Diet: Insights from the PREDIMED Study." *Progress in Cardiovascular Disease*, July-August 2015.

https://doi.org/10.1016/j.pcad.2015.04.003

Delzo, J. "Following a Mediterranean Diet May Help Reduce the Health Harms of Air Pollution." *Everyday Health*, May 21, 2018.

Gunnars, K. "5 Studies on the Mediterranean Diet—Does it Really Work?" *healthline.com*, March 16, 2020.

www.healthline.com/nutrition/5-studies-on-the-mediterranean-diet

Campbell, Mi. "Newly Discovered Longevity Benefits of Mediterranean Diet." *Life Extension Institute Magazine*, April 2017.

Luciano, M. et al. "Mediterranean-Type Diet and Brain Structural Change from 73 to 76 Years in a Scottish Cohort." *Neurology*, January 4, 2017.

https://doi.org/10.1212/WNL.0000000000003559

Schwingshackl, L. et al. "Food Groups and Risk of All-Cause Mortality: A Systematic Review and Meta-Analysis of Prospective Studies." *American Journal of Clinical Nutrition*, June 2017.

https://doi.org/10.3945/ajcn.117.153148

Valls-Pedret, C. et al. "Mediterranean Diet and Age-Related Cognitive Decline: a Randomized Clinical Trial." *JAMA Intern Medicine*, July 2015.

https://doi.org/10.1001/jamainternmed.2015.1668

Bonaccio, M. et al. "High Adherence to the Mediterranean Diet is Associated with Lower Risk of Overall Mortality in Subjects with Cardiovascular Disease: Prospective Results from the MOLI-SANI Study." Paper presented 2016 at ESC Congress, Rome, Italy.

Martínez-González, M. "Benefits of the Mediterranean Diet Beyond the Mediterranean Sea and Beyond Food Patterns." *BMC Medicine*. October 14, 2016.

https://doi.org/10.1186/s12916-016-0714-3

Luciano, M. et al. "Mediterranean-Type Diet and Brain Structural Change from 73 to 76 Years in a Scottish Cohort." *Neurology*, January 2017.

https://doi.org/10.1212/wnl.0000000000003559

Widmer, R. et al. "The Mediterranean Diet, its Components, and Cardiovascular Disease." *American Journal of Medicine*, 2015.

https://doi.org/10.1016/j.amjmed.2014.10.014

Fundación Dieta Mediterránea. www.dietamediterranea.com

Blythmann, J. "The Secret of the Mediterranean Diet? There is No Secret." *The Guardian*, May 21, 2014.

www.theguardian.com/lifeandstyle/wordofmouth/2014/may/21/secret-mediterranean-diet-nitro-fatty-acids-healthy

Paravantes, E. "The Mediterranean Diet Can Save You Money." *Olive Tomato*, March 21, 2013.

https://www.olivetomato.com/new-study-the-mediterranean-diet-can-save-you-money/

Dosoff, A. et al. "The Compound in Mediterranean Diet that Makes Cancer Cells 'Mortal'." *Ohio State University*, May 13, 2013.

https://www.sciencedaily.com/releases/2013/05/130520154303.htm

Estruch, R. et al. "Primary Prevention of Cardiovascular Disease with a Mediterranean Diet." *New England Journal of Medicine*, 2013.

https://doi.org/10.1056/NEJMoa1200303

Bach-Faig, A. et al. "Mediterranean Diet Pyramid Today. Science and Cultural Updates." *Public Health Nutrition*. December 13, 2011.

https://doi.org/10.1017/S1368980011002515

Parvantes, E. "Mediterranean Diet Pyramid Gets a Makeover." *Olive Oil Times*, October 18, 2011.

https://www.oliveoiltimes.com/health-news/mediterranean-diet-pyramid-gets-a-makeover/21089#:~:text=Mediterranean%20Diet%20Pyramid%20Gets%20a%20Makeover.%20The%20Mediterranean,to%20rep%C2%ADre%C2%ADsent%20the%20Mediterranean%20lifestyle%20as%20a%20whole.

Vallverdú-Queralt, A. et al. "Bioactive Compounds Present in the Mediterranean Sofrito." *Food Chemistry*, December 15, 2013.

https://doi.org/10.1016/j.foodchem.2013.06.032

Sánchez, P. et al. "Adherence to the Mediterranean Diet and Quality of Life in the SUN Project." *European Journal of Clinical Nutrition*, March 2012.

https://doi.org/10.1038/ejcn.2011.146

Kok, F. et al. "Atherosclerosis—Epidemiological Studies on the Health Effects of the Mediterranean Diet." *European Journal of Nutrition*, March 2004.

https://doi.org/10.1007/s00394-004-1102-x

Koops, K. et al. "Mediterranean Diet, Lifestyle Factors, and 10-Year Mortality in Elderly European Men and Women: The HALE Project." *JAMA*, September 22, 2004.

https://doi.org/10.1001/jama.292.12.1433

Baker, J. "Golden Age. I'm the Oldest Woman in the World But I Have No Health Problems...Now Scientists Think I May Hold the Key to Immortality," *The Sun*, October 2023.

www.the-sun.com/health/9402264/oldest.woman.world-maria-branyas-key-immortality-spain/

Unattributed. "Spain, the Healthiest Country in the World." *Money UK*, March 2021.

http://goldenvisasinspain.com/blogs/spain-the-healthiest-country-in-the-world

Unattributed. "Bloomberg's Global Health Index for 2020." www.worldhealth.net, June 2020.

https://www.worldhealth.net/news/bloombergs-global-health-index-2020

Laliberte, M. "Why Spaniards are the Healthiest People in the World." *Reader's Digest*, 2019.

https://www.rd.com/list/spaniards-healthiest-in-world/

Thornton, A. et al. "These are the World's Healthiest Nations," *World Economic Forum*, February 24, 2019.

www.weforum.org/agenda/2019/02/these-are-the-world-s-healthiest-nations/

Foreman, K. et al. "Forecasting Life Expectancy, Years of Life Lost, and All-Cause and Cause-Specific Mortality for 250 Causes of Death: Reference and Alternative Scenarios for 2016-40 for 195 Countries and Territories." *The Lancet*, November 2018.

https://doi.org/10.1016/s0140-6736(18)31694-5

Taylor, E. "Why Spain is Set to Become the Country With the Longest Life Expectancy." *Vogue*, October 2018.

https://www.vogue.com/article/why-spain-is-set-to-become-the-country-with-the-longest-life-expectancy

Unattributed. "In Which Parts of Spain Do People Live Longest?" *National Statistics Institute*, June 2021.

www.thelocal.es/20210601/in-which-parts-of-spain-do-people-live-longest

Unattributed. "Healthy Food in Spain: The Basque Country, Aragón and Catalonia are the Communities that Spend Most on Fruit and Vegetables." *EAE Business School*, September 2017.

www.eae.es/en/news/eae-news/basque-country-aragon-and-catalonia-are-communities-spend-most-fruit-and-vegetables

Gómez-Rekondo, R. et al. "Emergence and Verification of Supercentenarians in Spain." In: Maier, H. et al. "Supercentenarians. Demographic Research Monographs." *Springer. Berlin. Heidelberg*. April 9, 2010.

https://doi.org/10.1007/978-3-642-11520-2_9

Comas, A. "Tips from Spain's Centenarians on How to Live to 100," *Reuter's News Service*, December 30, 2016.

https://www.reuters.com/article/us-spain-centenarians-idUSKBN14J128

World Health Statistics 2019. "Monitoring Health for SDGs, Sustainable Development Goals." *World Health Organization*, 2019.

www.who.int/gho/publications/world_health_statistics/2019/en/

Unattributed. "14 Places Where Life Expectancy is Unusually High." *Telegraph*, June 26, 2017.

www.telegraph.co.uk/travel/galleries/places-where-people-live-longest/

Whittaker, K. "Stay Young with Andorra's Secrets for a Longer Life." *Ezine Articles*, November 3, 2008.

www.ezinearticles.com/?Stay-Young-With-Andorras-Secrets-For-a-Longer-Life&id=1642596

Ribeiro, A. et al. "Where do People Live Longer and Shorter Lives? An Ecological Study of Old-Age Survival Across 4404 Small Areas from 18 European Countries." *Journal of Epidemiology & Community Health*, June 2016.

https://doi.org/10.1136/jech-2015-206827

Unattributed. "Large Gains in Life Expectancy." *World Health Organization, News Release Media Center*, May 2014.

www.who.int/mediacentre/news/releases/2014/world-health-statistics-2014/en/

Manesiotis, C. "Spain Lives Longest in Europe: Spanish Style Mediterranean Diet Explored." *Guardian Liberty Voice*, November 13, 2013.

www.guardianlv.com/2013/11/spain-lives-longest-in-europe-spanish-style-mediterranean-diet-explored/

Boseley, S. "Spanish Have Highest Healthy Life Expectancy in Europe." *The Guardian*, March 4, 2013.

www.theguardian.com/world/2013/mar/05/spanish-highest-life-expectancy-europe

Ribiero, A. et al. "Where Do People Live Longer and Shorter Lives? An Ecological Study of Old-Age Survival Across 4404 Small Areas From 18 European Countries." *BMJ of Epidemiology and Community Health*.

http://dx.doi.org/10.1136/jech-2015-206827

Buckland, Genevieve et al. "Olive Oil Intake and Mortality Within the Spanish Population (EPIC-Spain)." *American Journal of Clinical Nutrition*, July 2012.

https://doi.org/10.3945/ajcn.111.024216

Moreno, L. A. et al. "The Nutrition Transition in Spain: A European Mediterranean Country." *European Journal of Clinical Nutrition*, October 2002.

https://doi.org/10.1038/sj.ejcn.1601414

Zeinali, M. et al. "Immunoregulatory and Anti-Inflammatory Properties of Crocus Sativus (Saffron) and Its Main Activity Constituents: A Review." *Iranian Journal of Basic Medical Sciences*, December 11. 2018.

https://doi.org/10.22038/ijbms.2019.34365.8

Sofrito and Saffron

Black, J. "Love Saffron? How to Get Maximum Value From It in Your Kitchen." *Wall Street Journal*, March 16, 2022.

Alvarenga, J. et al. "Using Extra Virgin Olive Oil to Cook Vegetables Enhances Polyphenol and Carotenoid Extractability: A Study Applying the Sofrito Technique." *Molecules*, April 19, 2019.

https://doi.org/10.3390/molecules24081555

Reventiós, L. et al. "A Longer Cooking Time and Adding Onion to 'Sofrito' Makes it More Beneficial for Our Health." *Universitat de Barcelona*, May 2017.

http://www.ub.edu/web/ub/en/menu_eines/noticies/2017/05/044.html

Estruch, R. "Sofrito de Tomate, Dieta Mediterránea y Riesgo Cardiovascular." *Presentation, Hospital Clínic, Universidad de Barcelona & Instituto de Salud Carlos III, Madrid, Spain*, April 2014.

Vallverdú-Queralt, A. et al. "Bioactive Compounds Present in the Mediterranean Sofrito." *Food Chemistry*, December 2013.

https://doi.org/10.1016/j.foodchem.2013.06.032

Zeinala, M. et al. "Immunoregulatory and Anti-Inflammatory Properties of Crocus Sativus (Saffron) and Its Main Active Constituents: A Review." *Iran Journal of Basic Medical Science*, April 2019.

https://doi.org/10.22038/ijbms.2019.34365.8158

Shakiba, M. et al. "Saffron (Crocus Sativus) Versus Duloxetine for Treatment of Patients with Fibromyalgia: A Randomized Double-Blind Clinical Trial." *Avicenna Journal of Phytomedicine*, November-December 2018.

PMID: 30456199

Berezow, Alex. "Does Saffron Fight Cancer? A Plausible Biological Mechanism." *American Council on Science and Health*, July 20, 2017.

Granchi, C. et al. "Characterization of the Saffron Derivative Crocetin as an Inhibitor of Human Lactate Dehydrogenase 5 in the Antiglycolytic Approach Against Cancer." *Journal of Agricultural Food Chemistry*, June 23, 2017.

https://doi.org/10.1021/acs.jafc.7b01668

Amin, A. et al. "UAE Study Finds Cancer Fighting Properties in Saffron." *The National*, January 5, 2016.

https://www.thenational.ae/uae/health/uae-study-finds-cancer-fighting-properties-in-saffron1.205309#:~:text=AL%20AIN%20%2F%2F%20

Researchers%20at%20UAE%20University%20have,cancer%2C%20-
primarily%20the%20most%20common%20form%2C%20hepatocellular%20
carcinoma.

Tavakol-Afshari, J. et al. "Chapter 32—Anticancer Properties of Saffron." *Saffron: Science, Technology and Health*, 2020.

https://doi.org/10.1016/b978-0-12-818638-1.00033-2

Samarghandian, S. et al. "Anticarcinogenic Effect of Saffron (Crocus Sativus L.) and its Ingredients." *Pharmacognosy Research*, April 2014.

https://doi.org/10.4103/0974-8490.128963

Gutheil, W.G. et al. "Crocetin: An Agent Derived from Saffron for Prevention and Therapy for Cancer." *Current Pharmaceutical Biotechnology*, January 2012.

https://doi.org/10.2174/138920112798868566

Kamalipour, M. et al. "Cardiovascular Effects of Saffron: An Evidence-Based Review." *Journal Tehran Heart Center*, Spring 2011. PMID 2307406.

Bhargava, K. "Medicinal Uses and Pharmacological Properties of Crocus Sativus Linn (Saffron)." *International Journal of Pharmacy and Pharmaceutical Sciences*, April 2011. ISSN-0975-1491.

Falsani, B. et al. "Influence of Saffron Supplementation on Retinal Flicker Sensitivity in Early Age-Related Macular Degeneration." *Investigative Opthalmology & Visual Science*, December 2010.

https://doi.org/10.1167/iovs.09-4995

Blythman, J. et al. "Why Saffron is Good for You." *The Guardian*, August 2013.

www.theguardian.com/lifeandstyle/2013/aug/03/good-for-you-saffron-food-and-drink-health-and-wellbeing

Escribano, J. et al. "Crocin, Safranal and Picrocrocin from Saffron (Crocus sativus L.) Inhibit the Growth of Human Cancer Cells in Vitro." *Cancer Letter*, February 1996.

https://doi.org/10.1016/0304-3835(95)04067-6

Nutritional Dynamos: Extra-Virgin Olive Oil, Olives, Nuts and Fatty-Rich Fish

Tessier, A. J. et al. "Consumption of Olive Oil and Diet Quality and Risk of Dementia-Related Death." *JAMA Network Open*, March 2024.

https://jamanetwork.com/journals/jamanetworkopen/fullarticle/2818362

Craig, C. "Can Olive Oil Do All That?" *New York Times*, March 2023.

www.nytimes.com/2023/03/01/well/eat/olove-oil-health-benefits.html

Yassine, H. et al. "Good Cholesterol in Brain May Help Keep Alzheimer's at Bay." *Alzheimer's Association*, April 2022.

http://doi.org/10.1002/alz.12649

Unattributed. "Health Benefits of Nuts and Seeds." *Tufts Health & Newsletter*, June 2020.

www.nutritionletter.tufts.edu/healthy-eating/health-benefits-of-nuts-and-seeds/

Mellor, D "Fat: Why are We So Confused About Whether or Not We Should Include It in Our Diet?" *The Conversation*, July 2021.

https://theconversation.com/fat-why-are-we-so-confused-about-whether-or-not-we-should-include-it-in-our-diet-163462

Machek, D. et al. "Mediterranean Diet Ingredient May Extend Life; Olive Oil in the Diet, May also Help Mitigate Age-Related Diseases." *Science News*, University of Minnesota Medical School, February 21, 2020.

www.sciencedaily.com/releases/2020/02/200221125120.htm

Najt, C., Machek, D. et al. "Lipid Droplet-Derived Monounsaturated Fatty Acids Traffic via PLIN5 to Allosterically Activate SIRT1." *Molecular Cell*, December 31, 2019.

https://doi.org/10.1016/j.molcel.2019.12.003

Lozano-Castellón, J. et al. "Domestic Sautéing with EVOO: Change in the Phenolic Profile." *Antioxidants*, 2020.

https://doi.org/10.3390/antiox9010077

Unattributed. "Walnuts May be Good for the Gut and Help Promote Heart Health." *ScienceDaily*, January 16, 2020.

www.sciencedaily.com/releases/2020/01/200116112542.htm

Tindall, Alyssa et al. "Walnuts and Vegetable Oils Containing Oleic Acid Differentially Affect the Gut Microbiota and Associations with Cardiovascular Risk Factors: Follow-up of a Randomized, Controlled, Feeding Trial in Adults at Risk for Cardiovascular Disease." *The Journal of Nutrition*, December 18, 2019.

https://doi.org/10.1093/jn/nxz289

Canter, L. "Why You Still Need Omega-3 Fatty Acids." *Health Day News*, July 29, 2019.

https://consumer.healthday.com/vitamins-and-nutrition-information-27/food-and-nutrition-news-316/why-you-still-need-omega-3-fatty-acids-748012.html

Aglago, E. et al. "Consumption of Fish and Long-chain n-3 Polyunsaturated Fatty Acids Is Associated with Reduced Risk of Colorectal Cancer in a Large European Cohort." *Clinical Gastroenterology and Hepatology*, June 25, 2019.

https://doi.org/10.1016/j.cgh.2019.06.031

Noordermeer, T. "Olive Oil Research Takes Aim at Preventing Alzheimer's." *Opelika-Auburn News (oanow.com)*, July 29, 2019.

www.oanow.com/news/local/olive-oil-research-takes-aim-at-preventing-alzheimer-s/article_5002a0b0-b20a-11e9-afd0-179c14c236f7.html

Dawson, D. "Spain Sees Largest Olive Oil Consumption Increase in Nearly a Decade." *Olive Oil Times*, July 15, 2019.

www.oliveoiltimes.com/business/spain-sees-largest-olive-oil-consumption-increase-in-nearly-a-decade/68641

de Alvarenga, R. et al. "Using Extra Virgin Olive Oil to Cook Vegetables Enhances Polyphenol and Carotenoid Extractability: A Study Applying the *sofrito* Technique." *Molecules*, April 19, 2019.

https://doi.org/10.3390/molecules24081555

Friedman, G. et al. "Why the Low-Fat Diet Failed." *Tufts Health & Nutrition Update*, March 11, 2020.

www.nutritionletter.tufts.edu/healthy-eating/why-the-low-fat-diet-failed

Faloon, C. "Surprising Discoveries About Olive Oil." *Life Extension Magazine*, January 2018.

https://www.lifeextension.com/magazine/2018/1/olive-oil-markedly-extends-human-lifespan

Estruch, R. et al. "Primary Prevention of Cardiovascular Disease with a Mediterranean Diet Supplemented with Extra-Virgin Olive Oil or Nuts." *The New England Journal of Medicine*, June 13, 2018.

https://doi.org/10.1056/NEJMoa1800389

Keshavarz, S. et al. "Omega-3 Supplementation Effects on Body Weight and Depression Among Dieter Women with Co-Morbidity of Depression and Obesity Compared with the Placebo: A Randomized Clinical Trial." *Clinical Nutrition ESPEN*, June 2018.

https://doi.org/10.1016/j.clnesp.2018.03.001

Swanson, D. et al. "Omega-3 Fatty Acids EPA and DHA: Health Benefits Throughout Life." *Advances in Nutrition; An International Review Journal*, January 5, 2012.

https://doi.org/10.3945/an.111.000893

Rossman, S. "Extra Virgin Olive Oil Staves Off Alzheimer's, Preserves Memory, New Study Shows." *USA Today*, June 21, 2017.

www.usatoday.com/story/news/nation-now/2017/06/21/extra-virgin-olive-oil-staves-off-alzheimers-preserves-memory-new-study-shows/415279001/

Osborne, H. "Alzheimer's: How Extra Virgin Olive Oil Prevents Brain Plaques and Preserves Memory." *Newsweek*, June 21, 2017.

www.newsweek.com/extra-virgin-olive-oil-prevents-alzheimers-mediterranean-diet-627851

Casamenti, F., M. Stefani. "Olive Polyphenols: New Promising Agents to Combat Aging-Associated Neurodegeneration." *Expert Rev Neurother*, April 17, 2017.

https://doi.org/10.1080/14737175.2017.1245617

De la Torre, R. et al. "Protective Effect of Homovanillyl Alcohol on Cardiovascular Disease and Total Mortality: Virgin Olive Oil, Wine, and Catechol-

Methylanthion." *American Journal of Clinical Nutrition*, June 2017.

https://doi.org/10.3945/ajcn.116.145813

Cândido, F. et al. "Consumption of Extra Virgin Olive Oil Improves Body Composition and Blood Pressure in Women with Excess Body Fat: a Randomized Double-Blinded, Placebo-Controlled Clinical Trial." *European Journal of Nutrition*, October 2118.

https://doi.org/10.1007/s00394-017-1517-9

Lauretti, E. et al. "Extra-Virgin Olive Oil Ameliorates Cognition and Neuropathology of the 3xTg Mice: Role of Autophagy." *Ann Clin Transl Neurol*, July 21, 2017.

https://doi.org/10.1002/acn3.431

García-Gavilán, J. F. et al. "Extra Virgin Olive Oil Consumption Reduces the Risk of Osteoporotic Fractures in the PREDIMED Trial." *Clinical Nutrition*, February 2018.

https://doi.org/10.1016/j.clnu.2016.12.030

Dening, J. "Exclusive Olive Oil Consumption Protects Against Coronary Artery Disease." *Olive Oil Times*, February 2016.

https://www.oliveoiltimes.com/health-news/exclusive-olive-oil-consumption-protects-against-coronary-artery-disease/50537

Vanden Hueval, J. et al. "Mechanistic Examination of Walnuts in Prevention of Breast Cancer." *Nutr Cancer*, 2012.

https://doi.org/10.1080/01635581.2012.717679

Matthews, S. "Weak Bones? Eat a Mediterranean Diet! Fish, Olives and Oil Could Prevent Millions of at Risk Patients from Breaking Their Hips." *DailyMail.com*, July 11, 2018.

www.dailymail.co.uk/health/article-5938523/Millions-osteoporosis-patients-eat-Mediterranean-diet.html

Varela-López, A. et al. "Loss of Bone Mineral Density Associated with Age in Male Rats Fed on Sunflower Oil is Avoided by Virgin Olive Oil Intake or Coenzyme Q Supplementation." *Int J Mol Sci*. June 29, 2017.

https://doi.org/10.3390/ijms18071397

Unattributed. "Official Advice on Low-Fat Diet and Cholesterol is Wrong, Says Health Charity Press Association." *The Guardian*, May 23, 2016.

www.theguardian.com/society/2016/may/22/official-advice-to-eat-low-fat-diet-is-wrong-says-health-charity

Rigacci, S. et al. "Nutraceutical Properties of Olive Oil Polyphenols. An Itinerary from Cultured Cells Through Animal Models to Humans." *Int J Mol Sci*, May 31, 2016.

https://doi.org/10.3390/ijms17060843

Tejada, S. et al. "Cardioprotective Effects of the Polyphenol Hydroxytyrosol from Olive Oil." *Curr Drug Targets*, 2017.

https://doi.org/10.2174/1389450117666161005150650

Alice, R.D., "Trans Fats Banned; What That Could Mean for Your Cancer Risk."
  AICR Blog, June 16, 2015.

  www.aicr.org/resources/blog/trans-fats-banned-how-that-could-lower-your-
  cancer-risk/

Luu, H. N. et al. "Prospective Evaluation of the Association of Nut/Peanut
  Consumption with Total and Cause-Specific Mortality." *JAMA Intern Med*,
  August 1, 2016.

  https://doi.org/10.1001/jamainternmed.2014.8347

Brody, J. "Nuts are a Nutritional Powerhouse." *The New York Times*,
  March 30, 2015.

  https://well.blogs.nytimes.com/2015/03/30/nuts-are-a-nutritional-
  powerhouse-for-rich-and-poor/

Virruso, C. et. al. "Nutraceutical Properties of Extra-Virgin Olive Oil: A Natural
  Remedy for Age-Related Disease?" *Rejuvenation Res*, April 2014.

  https://doi.org/10.1089/rej.2013.1532

Yee, L.D. "Dietary Fish and Omega-3 Fatty Acids for Breast Cancer Prevention."
  The Ohio State University Comprehensive Cancer Center, August 2014.

  https://www.clinicaltrials.gov/ct2/show/NCT01282580

Chung, H. et al. "Omega-3 Fatty Acids Reduce Obesity-Induced Tumor Progression
  Independent of GPR120 in a Mouse Model of Postmenopausal Breast Cancer."
  Oncogene, July 2015.

  https://doi.org/10.1038/onc.2014.283

Gárcia-Arenzana, N. et al. "Calorie Intake, Olive Oil Consumption and
  Mammographic Density Among Spanish Women." *International Journal of
  Cancer*, April 15, 2014.

  http://doi.org/10.1002/ijc.28513

Chew, E. et al. "Lutein + Zeaxanthin and Omega-3 Fatty Acids for Age-Related
  Macular Degeneration: the Age-Related Eye Disease Study 2 (AREDS2)
  Randomized Clinical Trial." *JAMA*, May 15, 2013.

  https://doi.org/10.1001/jama.2013.4997

Puel, C., A. Quintin, et. al. "Olive Oil and Its Main Phenolic Micronutrient
  (Oleuropein) Prevent Inflammation-Induced Bone Loss in the Ovariectomised
  Rat." *Br J Nutr*, July 2014.

  https://doi.org/10.1079/bjn20041181

Solanas, M. et al. "Effects of a High Olive Oil Diet on the Clinical Behavior and
  Histopathological Features of Rat DMBA-Induced Mammary Tumors
  Compared with a High Corn Oil Diet." *Int J Oncol.* 2002 Oct;21(4):745-53

Unattributed. "LOVE THAT OLIVE: Why Olive Oil Lowers Blood Pressure."
  New York Daily News, May 20, 2014.

www.nydailynews.com/life-style/health/olive-oil-lowers-blood-pressure-article-1.1799073

Charles, R. et al. "Protection from Hypertension in Mice by the Mediterranean Diet is Mediated by Nitro Fatty Acid Inhibition of Soluble Epoxide Hydrolase." *Proceedings of the National Academy of Sciences of the United States of America*, June 2014.

https://doi.org/10.1073/pnas.1402965111

Schwingshackl, L., G. Hoffmann. "Monounsaturated Fatty Acids, Olive Oil, and Health Status: a Systematic Review and Meta-Analysis of Cohort Studies." *Lipids Health Dis*, October 1, 2014.

https://doi.org/10.1186/1476-511x-13-154

Khaw, K. "Dietary Fats and Breast Cancer Risk." *BMJ*, July 16, 2013.

https://doi.org/10.1136/bmj.f4518

Zheng, J. et al. "Intake of Fish and Marine n-3 Polyunsaturated Fatty Acids and Risk of Breast Cancer: Meta-Analysis of Data from 21 Independent Prospective Cohort Studies." *BMJ*, June 27, 2013.

https://doi.org/10.1136/bmj.f3706

Abuznait, A.H., et al. "Olive-Oil-Derived Oleocanthal Enhances β-Amyloid Clearance as a Potential Neuroprotective Mechanism Against Alzheimer's Disease: In Vitro and in Vivo Studies." *ACS Chem Neurosc*, June 19, 2013.

https://doi.org/10.1021/cn400024q

Elamin, M. et al. "Olive Oil Oleuropein has Anti-Breast Cancer Properties with Higher Efficiency on ER-Negative Cells." *Food Chem Toxicol*, March 2013.

https://doi.org/10.1016/j.fct.2012.12.009

Lucas L., A. Russell, R. Keast. "Molecular Mechanisms of Inflammation: Anti-Inflammatory Benefits of Virgin Olive Oil and the Phenolic Compound Oleocanthal." *Curt Phrm Des*, 2011.

https://doi.org/10.2174/138161211795428911

Solanas, M. et al. "Dietary Olive Oil and Corn Oil Differentially Affect Experimental Breast Cancer Through Distinct Modulation of the p21Ras Signaling and the Proliferation-Apoptosis Balance." *Carcinogenesis*, May 2010.

https://doi.org/10.1093/carcin/bgp243

Camargo, A. et al. "Gene Expression Changes in Mononuclear Cells in Patients with Metabolic Syndrome After Acute Intake of Phenol-Rich Virgin Olive Oil." *BMC Genomics*, April 20, 2010.

https://doi.org/10.1186/1471-2164-11-253

Macrae, F. "Olive Oil Protects Against Breast Cancer by Launching Multiple Attacks Against Tumors." *DailyMail.com*, July 2, 2010.

www.dailymail.co.uk/health/article-1291215/Olive-oil-protects-breast-cancer-launching-multiple-attack-tumours.html

Kim, J. et al. "Fatty Fish and Fish Omega-3 Fatty Acid Intakes Decrease the Breast Cancer Risk; A Case Control Study." *BMC Cancer*, June 30, 2009.

https://doi.org/10.1186/1471-2407-9-216

Ménendez, J. et al. "Extra-Virgin Olive Oil Polyphenols Inhibit HER2 (erbB-2)-Induced Malignant Transformation in Human Breast Epithelial Cells: Relationship Between the Chemical Structures of Extra-Virgin Olive Oil Secoiridoids and Lignans and their Inhibitory Activities on the Tyrosine Kinase Activity of HER2." *International Journal of Oncology*, 2009 Jan;34(1):43-51.

Cândido, F. et al. "Consumption of Extra Virgin Olive Oil Improves Body Composition and Blood Pressure in Women with Excess Body Fat: a Randomized, Double-Blinded, Placebo-Controlled Clinical Trial." *European Journal of Nutrition*, August 14, 2007.

https://doi.org/10.1007/s00394-017-1517-9

Goodrow, E. et al. "Consumption of One Egg Per Day Increases Serum Lutein and Zeaxanthin Concentration in Older Adults Without Altering Serum Lipid and Lipoprotein Cholesterol Concentrations." *J Nutr*, October 2006.

https://doi.org/10.1093/jn/136.10.2519

Bosetti, C. et al. "Olive Oil, Seed Oils, and Other Added Fats in Relation to Ovarian Cancer (Italy)." *Canc Causes Ctrl*, June 2002.

https://doi.org/10.1023/a:1015760004130

Erasmus, U. *Fats That Heal Fats That Kill: The Complete Guide to Fats, Oils, Cholesterol and Human Health*. Alive Books, 1993.

Olive Oil Fraud

Robbins, O. "Uncovering Food Fraud in the Olive and Avocado Oil Industry." *Food Revolution Network*, August 2020.

https://foodrevolution.org/blog/food-fraud-olive-oil-and-avocado-oil/

Downey, M. "Is Your Olive Oil Counterfeit?" *Life Extension Magazine*, September 2017.

www.lifeextension.com/magazine/2016/9/is-your-olive-oil-counterfeit

Rodriguez, C. "The Olive Oil Scam: If 80% is Fake, Why do You Keep Buying It?" *Forbes Online*, February 10, 2016.

www.forbes.com/sites/ceciliarodriguez/2016/02/10/the-olive-oil-scam-if-80-is-fake-why-do-you-keep-buying-it/#fe485af639d7

Protective Foods and Compounds: Spanish Mediterranean Diet

Mellor, D. "Six Reasons Potatoes are Good for You." *Metropolitan Barcelona*, July 2022.

www.barcelona-metropolitan.com/eating-and-drinking/six-reasons-potatoes-are-good

Ba, D. et al. "Higher Mushroom Consumption is Associated with Lower Risk of Cancer: A Systematic Review and Meta-Analysis of Observational Studies." *Advances in Nutrition*, April 2021.

http://doi.org/10.1093/advances/nmab015

Simes, D. et al. "Vitamin K as a Diet Supplement with Impact in Human Health: Current Evidence in Age-Related Diseases." *Nutrients*, January 3, 2020.

https://doi.org/10.3390/nu12010138

Li, Y. et al. "Prebiotic-Induced Anti-tumor Immunity Attenuates Tumor Growth." *Cell Rep*, February 11, 2020.

https://doi.org/10.1016/j.celrep.2020.01.035

Dehghan, M. et al. "Association of Egg Intake with Blood Lipids, Cardiovascular Disease, and Mortality in 177,000 people in 50 Countries." *American Journal of Clinical Nutrition*, January 2020.

https://doi.org/10.1093/ajcn/nqz348

DiSalvo, D. "Eating More Nuts to Improve Your Sex Life: What The Science Really Says." *Forbes*, July 29, 2019.

www.forbes.com/sites/daviddisalvo/2019/07/29/eating-nuts-to-improve-your-sex-life-what-the-science-really-says/#548455077265

Salas-Huetos, A. et al. "Effect of Nut Consumption on Erectile and Sexual Function in Healthy Males: A Secondary Outcome Analysis of the FERTINUTS Randomized Controlled Trial." *Nutrients*, June 2019.

http://doi.org/10.3390/nu11061372

Fletcher, J. "A Guide to Antioxidant Foods." *Medical News Today*, July 26, 2019.

www.medicalnewstoday.com/articles/325873

Unattributed. "What Happens When You Eat Raw Garlic Daily," *Times of India*, July 11, 2019.

https://timesofindia.indiatimes.com/life-style/food-news/what-happens-when-you-eat-raw-garlic-daily/photostory/70173905.cms

Ducharme, J. "Are Onions and Garlic Healthy? Here's What Experts Say," *TIME*, May 15, 2019.

https://time.com/5566916/are-garlic-and-onions-healthy/

Behera, J. et al. "Could Eating Garlic Reduce Aging-Related Memory Problems?" *Experimental Biology*, Apr 8, 2019.

www.sciencedaily.com/releases/2019/04/190408091259.htm

Osmond Cook, A. "5 Reasons Legumes Should be a Regular Part of Your Diet." *The Orange County Register*, July 10, 2019.

www.ocregister.com/2019/07/10/5-reasons-legumes-should-be-a-regular-part-of-your-diet/

Nelson, A. "4 Health Benefits of Figs." *Treehugger*, July 2, 2019.

www.treehugger.com/health-benefits-figs-4858765

Aglago, E. et al. "Consumption of Fish and Long-chain n-3 Polyunsaturated Fatty Acids Is Associated with Reduced Risk of Colorectal Cancer in a Large European Cohort." *Clinical Gastroenterology and Hepatology*, June 25, 2019.

https://doi.org/10.1016/j.cgh.2019.06.031

Powell, D. "Health Effects of Eggs: Where Do We Stand?" *CNN Health Online*, March 27, 2019.

www.cnn.com/2019/03/27/health/eggs-good-or-bad-where-do-we-stand/index.html

Li, W. *Eat to Beat Disease: the New Science of How Your Body Can Heal Itself.* Grand Central Publishing, March 19, 2019

Bharanidharan, S. "5 Health Benefits of Grapes." *Medical Daily*, February 21, 2019.

www.medicaldaily.com/5-health-benefits-grapes-430126

Wu, X. et al. "Allium Vegetables are Associated with Reduced Risk of Colorectal Cancer: A Hospital-Based Matched Case-Control Study in China." *Asia-Pacific Journal of Clinical Oncology*, February 20, 2019.

https://doi.org/10.1111/ajco.13133

Quartz, "The Health Benefits of Red Peppers." *The New Times*, February 3, 2019.

Vermeer, C. et al. "Menaquinone Content of Cheese." *Nutrients*, April 4, 2018.

https://doi.org/10.3390/nu10040446

Rabin, R. "Do Cruciferous Vegetables Really Fight Cancer?" *The New York Times*, December 7, 2018.

www.nytimes.com/2018/12/07/well/eat/do-cruciferous-vegetables-really-fight-cancer.html

Link, R. "The 13 Healthiest Root Vegetables." *Healthline*, December 6, 2018.

www.healthline.com/nutrition/root-vegetables

Liu, C. "Healthy Dietary Pattern with Daily Egg Consumption Might be the True Factor Associated with Decreased Risks of Cardiovascular Diseases and Mortality." *Heart*. November 2018.

doi.org/10.1136/heartjnl-2018-313774

Ghorbanian, D. et al. "Spatial Memory and Antioxidant Protective Effects of Raisin (Currant) in Aged Rats." *Preventive Nutrition & Food Science*, September 30, 2018.

https://doi.org/10.3746/pnf.2018.23.3.196

Unattributed. "Thyme Tea: A Potentially Beneficial Beverage Worth Your Time." *Mercola*, June 23, 2018.

https://articles.mercola.com/teas/thyme-tea.aspx

Sass, C. "6 Health Benefits of Onions." *Health*, June 22, 2018.

www.health.com/nutrition/health-benefits-onions

Fangping, L. et al. "A Potential Adjuvant Agent of Chemotherapy: Sepia Ink Polysaccharides," *Marine Drugs*, March 28, 2018.

https://doi.org/10.3390/md16040106

Chaker, A. "Beans: The Superfood You've Always Known." *The Wall Street Journal*, March 19, 2018.

www.wsj.com/articles/beans-the-superfood-you-ve-always-known-1521284401

Knott, S. et al. "Asparagine Bioavailability Governs Metastasis in a Model of Breast Cancer." *Nature*, February 7, 2018.

https://doi.org/10.1038.nature25465

Galenone, C. et al. "Onion and Garlic Use and Human Cancer." *American Journal of Clinical Nutrition*, November 2016.

https://doi.org/10.1093/ajcn/84.5.1027

Pasupuleti, V. et al. "Honey, Propolis, and Royal Jelly: A Comprehensive Review of Their Biological Actions and Health Benefits." *Oxidative Medicine and Cellular Longevity*, July 26, 2017.

https://doi.org/10.1155/2017/1259510

Valerio, L. "Setas, Cuidado Con Coger Lo Que Comes." *El Mundo*, November 2, 2015.

www.elmundo.es/vida-sana/2015/11/02/5631f8e346163f682f8b4632.html

Lahoz, A. "El Consume de Borraja Ayuda a Prevenir el Cáncer de Estómago." *El Periódico de Aragón*, December 22, 2013.

www.elperiodicodearagon.com/noticias/aragon/consumo-borraja-ayuda-prevenir-cancer-estomago_908434.html

Zheng, N. et al. "ERα Down-regulation Plays a Key Role in Silibinin-induced Autophagy and Apoptosis in Human Breast Cancer MCF-7 Cells." *Journal of Pharmacological Sciences*, July 2015.

https://doi.org/10.1016/j.phs.2015.05.001

Sanchez-Gonzalez, C. et al. "Health Benefits of Walnut Polyphenols: An Exploration Beyond Their Lipid Profile." *Critical Reviews in Food Science and Nutrition*, May 25, 2015.

https://doi.org/10.1080/10408398.2015.1126218

Atwood, M. "Fish Broth and Your Thyroid!" *Tips from the Traditional Cook*, Selene River Press. July 2015.

Gayot Editors. "Health Benefits of Figs." *Gayot.com*, 2015

Burnett, J. et al. "Natural Product Sulforaphane Selectively Inhibits Breast Cancer Stem Cells in Basal and Trastuzumab Resistant Her2+ Breast Cancer." *Cancer Research*, April 2013.

https://doi.org/10.1158/1538-7445.AM2013-913

Ramezanpour, M. et al. "Marine Bioactive Products as Anti-Cancer Agents: Effects of Sea Anemone Venom on Breast and Lung Cancer Cells." *Cancer Cell Microenviron*, January 15, 2014; 1: e29. doi: 10.14800/ccm.29.

Li, F. et al. "A Potential Adjuvant Agent of Chemotherapy: Sepia Ink Polysaccharides." *Mar. Drugs*, March 2018.

https://doi.org/10.3390/md16040106

Yancey, J. "Red Bell Peppers' Nutrition Beats Its Colorful Cousins." *Farm Flavor*, June 7, 2012.

www.farmflavor.com/lifestyle/red-bell-peppers-nutrition-beats-its-colorful-cousins/

Turrini, E. et al. "Potential Effects of Pomegranate Polyphenols in Cancer Prevention and Therapy." *Oxidative Medicine and Cellular Longevity*, 2015.

https://pubmed.ncbi.nim.nih.gov/26180600/

Jenkin, M. "Could Mushrooms be the Cure for Cancer?" *The Guardian*, March 2, 2014.

www.theguardian.com/lifeandstyle/2014/mar/02/could-mushrooms-cure-cancer

Juanola-Falgarona, M. et al. "Dietary Intake of Vitamin K is Inversely Associated with Mortality Risk." *The Journal of Nutrition*, May 2014.

https://doi.org/10.3945/jn.113.187740

Constantini, S. et al. "Potential Anti-Inflammatory Effects of the Hydrophilic Fraction of Pomegranate (Punica Granatum L) Seed Oil on Breast Cancer Cell Lines." *Molecules*, June 2014.

https://doi.org/10.3390/molecules19068644

Vallverdú-Queralt, A. et al. "Bioactive Compounds Present in the Mediterranean Sofrito." *Food Chemistry*, November 2013.

https://doi.org/10.1016/j.foodchem.2013.06.032

Enos, D. "4 Foods that are Good Sources of Resveratrol." *Live Science, Healthy Bites Column*, August 2013.

www.livescience.com/39125-foods-good-sources-resveratrol.html

Boggs, D. et al. "Fruit and Vegetable Intake is Associated with Lower Risk of ER-Breast Cancer." *American Journal of Epidemiology*, October 11, 2010.

https://doi.org/10.1093/aje/kwq293

Wang, L. et al. "Specific Carotenoid Intake is Inversely Associated with the Risk of Breast Cancer in Chinese Women." *British Journal of Nutrition*, February 2014.

https://doi.org/10.1017/s000711451300411x

Vadodkar, A. et al. "Chemoprevention of Breast Cancer by Dietary Compounds." *Anti-cancer Agents in Medicinal Chemistry*, December 2012.

https://doi.org/10.2174/187152012803833008

Coban, J. et al. "Olive Leaf Extract Decreases Age-Induced Oxidative Stress in Major Organs of Aged Rats." *Geriatrics Gerontology International*, May 23, 2014.

https://doi.org/10.1111/ggi.12192

Liu, X. et al. "Cruciferous Vegetables Intake is Inversely Associated with Risk of Breast Cancer: A Meta-Analysis." *The Breast*, August 9, 2012.

https://doi.org/10.1016/j.breast.2012.07.013

Gamaro, G. et al. "Effect of Rosmarinic and Caffeic Acids on Inflammatory and Nociception Process in Rats." *ISRN Pharmacology*, 2011.

https://pubmed.ncbi.nim.nih.gov/22084714/

Guciardi, A. "Study on How Eggs Prevent Cancer Shows Vast Healing Power of Foods." *Natural News*, August 2, 2011.

https://www.naturalnews.com/033199_eggs_cancer.html

Sharifiyan, F. et al. "Study of Pomegranate (Punica Granatum L.) Peel Extract Containing Anthocyanins on Fatty Streak Formation in the Renal Arteries in Hypercholesterolemic Rabbits." *Advanced Biomedical Research*, January 2016.

https://www.ncbi.nlm.nih.gov/pmc/articles/pmc4770606/

Bao, S. et al. "Inhibitory Effect of Luteolin on the Proliferation of Human Breast Cancer Cell Lines Induced by Epidermal Growth Factor." *PubMed,* February 25, 2016.

https://pubmed.ncbi.nlm.nih.gov/26915319/

Llanos, A. et al. "Diet Rich in Tomatoes May Lower Breast Cancer Risk." *Journal of Clinical Endocrinology & Metabolism*, December 2013.

www.sciencedaily.com/releases/2013/12/131218133543.htm

Bozkurt, E. et al. "Effects of Thymus Serpyllum Extract on Cell Proliferation." *Nutrition and Cancer*, 2012.

https://doi.org/10.1080/01635581.2012.719658

Li, Y. et al. "Sulforaphane, a Dietary Component of Broccoli/Broccoli Sprouts, Inhibits Breast Cancer Stem Cells." *Clinical Cancer Research*, May 1, 2010.

https://doi.org/10.1158/1078-0432.ccr-09-2937

Reagan-Shaw, S. et al. "Anti-proliferative Effects of Apple Peel Extract Against Cancer Cells." *Nutrition and Cancer*, July 2009.

https://doi.org/10.1080/01635580903441253

Ilow, R. et al. "Assessment of Dietary Flavonoid Intake Among 50-Year-Old Inhabitants of Wroclaw in 2008." *Adv Clin Exp Med*, May-June 2012.

https://pubmed.ncbi.nlm.nih.gov/23214199

Galeone, C. et al. "Onion and Garlic Use and Human Cancer." *American Journal of Clinical Nutrition*, November 2006.

https://doi.org/10.1093/ajcn/84.5.1027

Daniel, K. "Why Broth is Beautiful: Essential Roles for Proline, Glycerine, and Gelatin." *Weston A Price Foundation*, June 18, 2003.

www.westonprice.org/health-topics/why-broth-is-beautiful-essential-roles-for-proline-glycine-and-gelatin/

Bagchi, D. et al. "Cellular Protection with Proanthocyanidins Derived from Grape Seeds." *Annals of the New York Academy of Sciences*, January 24, 2006.

https://doi.org/10.1111/j.1749-6632.2002.tb02922.x

She, Q. et al. "Resveratrol-Induced Activation of p53 and Apoptosis is Mediated by Extracellular-Signal-Regulated Protein Kinases and p38 Kinase." *Cancer Research*, February 15, 2001.

https://pubmed.ncbi.nim.nih.gov/11245472/

Jorge, P. et al. "Effect of Eggplant on Plasma Lipid Levels, Lipidic Peroxidation, and Reversion of Endothial Dysfunction in Experimental Hypercholesterolemia." *Arquivos Brasileiros de Cardiologia*, February, 1998.

https://doi.org/10.1590/s0066-782x1998000200004

Ibérico De Bellota Pork Protective Effects on Cholesterol and Rich Source of Vitamins B1, B6, B12, E, and (Anti-Cancer) Selenium

Unattributed. "Ibérico 101: What Makes Jamón Ibérico the Best Ham in the World…" *Meat N' Bone*, Inc. November 2019.

www.meatnbone.com/blogs/the-clever-cleaver/the-best-ham-in-the-world

Unattributed. "About Jamón." *www.jamon.com*

Jiménez-Colmenero, F. et al. "Nutritional Composition of Dry-Cured Ham and its Role in a Healthy Diet." *Meat Science*, April 2010.

https://doi.org/10.1016/j.meatsci.2009.10.029

High Antioxidant Activity in Ibérico and Ewes Milk Cheese

Timó, M. et al. "Bioactive Low Molecular Weight Compounds in Two Traditional Spanish Products." *Food and Nutrition Sciences*, September 2013.

https://doi.org/10.4236/fns.2013.49a2003

Is Pork a Healthy Food?

Rajan, N. "BBC Future Releases List of Top Nutritional Foods and Pig's Fat is One of Them." *BBC Future*, January 31, 2018.

Xtalks.com/bbc-future-releases-list-of-top-nutritional-foods-and-pigs-fat-is-one-of-them-1136/

Health Enhancing Herbs and Spices
in the Spanish Pantry

Tweed, V. "Boost Your Mood with Saffron." *Better Nutrition*, July 15, 2021.

    www.betternutrition.com/conditions-and-wellness/mood-stress/saffron-mood/

Unattributed. "London-Based Spanish Chef José Pizarro, the King of Pimentón de la Vera. *Foods and Wines from Spain*. February 2020.

    www.foodswinesfromspain.com/spanishfoodwine/global/food/features/feature-detail/jose-pizarro-pimenton.html

Jiang. T. "Health Benefits of Culinary Herbs and Spices." *Journal of AOAC International*, March 2019

    http://doi.org/10.5740/jaoacint.18-0418

de Oliveira, J. et al. "Thymus Vulgaris L. Extract has Antimicrobial and Anti-Inflammatory Effects in the Absence of Cytotoxicity and Genotoxicity." *Archives of Oral Biology*, October 2017.

    https://doi.org/10.1016/j.archoralbio.2017.06.031

Caputo, L. et al. "Laurus Nobilis: Composition of Essential Oil and its Biological Activities." *Molecules*, May 2017.

    https://doi.org/10.3390/molecules22060930

Casamassima, D. et al. "The Effect of Laurus Nobilis on the Blood and Lenses Antioxidant Activity in Rabbit Under Fat-Enriched Diet." *Physiology Research*, June 2016.

    https://doi.org/10.33549/physiolres.933409

Chmit, M. et al. "Antibacterial and Antibiofilm Activities of Polysaccharides, Essential Oil, and Fatty Oil Extracted from Laurus Nobilis Growing in Lebanon." *Asian Pacific Journal of Tropical Medicine*, September 2014.

    https://doi.org/10.1016/s1995-7645(14)60288-1

Opara, E. et al. "Culinary Herbs and Spices: Their Bioactive Properties, the Contribution of Polyphenols and the Challenges in Deducing Their True Health Benefits." *International Journal of Molecular Sciences*, July 2014.

    https://doi.org/10.3390/ijms151019183

Dias, M. et al. "Nutritional and Antioxidant Contributions of Laurus Nobilis L. Leaves: Would be More Suitable a Wild or Cultivated Sample?" *Food Chemistry*, August 2014.

    https://doi.org/10.1016/j.foodchem.2014.01.122

Patrakar, R. et al. "Phytochemical and Pharmacological Review on Laurus Nobilis." *Int. J. Pharm. Chem. Sci.,* 2012.

    https://www.semanticscholar.org/paper/Phytochemical-and-Pharmacological-Review-on-Laurus-Patrakar-Mansuriya/1cd15010e12589a567edbcbde59a203502689794#citing-papers

Hyder, S. et al. "Breast Cancer Effectively Treated with Chemical Found in Parsley, Mouse Study Suggests." *University of Missouri-Columbia*, May 2012.

www.sciencedaily.com/releases/2012/05/120516093834.htm

Lu, T. et al. "Cinnamon Extract Improves Fasting Blood Glucose and Glycosylated Hemoglobin Level in Chinese Patients with Type 2 Diabetes." *Nutrition Research*, June 2012.

https://doi.org/10.1016/j.nutres.2012.05.003

Jaganathan, S. et al. "Molecules: Antiproliferative and Molecular Mechanism of Eugenol-Induced Apoptosis in Cancer Cells." *Molecules*, March 2012.

https://doi.org/10.3390/molecules17066290

Arreola, R. et al. "Immunomodulation and Anti-Inflammatory Effects of Garlic Compounds." *Journal of Immunology Research*, January 2015.

https://doi.org/10.1155/2015/401630

Lee, K. et al. "Effects of Macelignan Isolated from Myristica Fragrans (Nutmeg) on Expression of Matrix Metalloproteinase-1 and Type I Procollagen in UVB-Irradiated Human Skin Fibroblasts." *Biological and Pharmaceutical Bulletin*, June 2012.

https://doi.org/10.1248/bpb.b12-00037

Kaefer, C. et al. "Herbs and Spices in Cancer Prevention and Treatment." *Herbal Medicine: Biomolecular and Clinical Aspects, 2nd Edition, Boca Raton, CRC Press/Taylor & Francis*, 2011.

https://www.ncbi.nlm.nih.gov/books/nbk92774/

Martinez-Tome, M. et al. "Antioxidant Properties of Mediterranean Spices Compared with Common Food Additives." *Journal of Food Protection*, September 2001.

https://doi.org/10.4315/0362-028x-64.9.1412

Willoughby, J. "Pimentón: It's Spanish for 'Better Than Paprika." *New York Times*, April 13, 2010.

O'Shea, T. "Hip, Hip Ole for the Fresh Flavors of Spain: Thyme Soup; Sopa de Tomillo." *Mother Earth Living*, February/March 2009.

García, M. et al. "Agronomic Characteristics and Carotenoid Content of Five Bola-Type Paprika Red Pepper (*Capsicum annuum* L.) Cultivars." *Scientia Horticulturae*, June 26, 2007.

https://doi.org/10.1016/j.scienta.2007.02.003

Yance, D. *Herbal Medicine, Healing, & Cancer: A Comprehensive Program for Prevention and Treatment*. New Canaan, CT: Keats Publishing, 1st Edition, 1999.

Singletary, K. et al. "Inhibition by Rosemary and Carnosol of 7,12-Dimethylbenz[a] anthracene (DMBA)-Induced Rat Mammary Tumorigenesis and in Vivo DMBA-DNA Adduct Formation." *Cancer Letters*, June 24, 1996.

https://doi.org/10.1016/0304-3835(96)04227-9

Zargari, A. "Medicinal Plants." *Tehran University Press*, Tehran, 1990.

Yance, D. "Rosemary (Rosmarinus Officinalis)." *Rosemary Monograph* (V 2.9).

Mediterranean Diet/Lifestyle Protects Against Heart Disease, Breast, Lung, Prostate, and Colorectal Cancers; Childhood Asthma, Cognitive Decline, Alzheimer's, Osteoporosis, Fractures, Geriatric Fraility, Macular Degeneration, Psoriasis, Depression and Stroke

Tessier, A. "Olive Oil Intake and Fatal Dementia Risk in Two Large Prospective U.S. Cohort Studies." *Nutrition 2023*, July 24, 2023.

Tchounwu, P. et al, "Olives and Bone: A Green Osteoporosis Prevention Option." *International Journal of Environmental Research and Public Health*, August 2016.

http://doi.org/10.3390/ijerph13080755

Farvid, M. et al. "Post Diagnostic Fruit and Vegetable Consumption and Breast Cancer Survival: Prospective Analyses in the Nurse' Health Studies" *Cancer Research*, November 2020.

www.doi.org/10.1158 /0008-5472.CAN-18-3515

Farvid, M. et al. "Postdiagnostic Dietary Glycemic Index, Glycemic Load, Dietary Insulin Index, and Insulin Load and Breast Cancer", *Cancer Epidemiol Biomarkers Prevention*, February 2021.

www.doi.org/10.1158/1055-9965.EPl-20-0764

Zhong, Y. et al. "Association Between Mediterranean Diet Adherence and Colorectal Cancer: A Dose-Response Meta-Analysis." *The American Journal of Clinical Nutrition*, June 2020.

https://doi.org/10.1093/ajcn/nqaa083

Kindelan, K. "Mediterranean Diet Tops List of Best Diets For 2020. What to Know About This Plant-Based Way of Eating," *Good Morning America Online*, January 2, 2020.

Bolte, L. et al. "Towards Anti-Inflammatory Dietary Recommendations Based on the Relation Between Food and the Gut Microbiome Composition in 1423 Individuals." Abstract OP052. Presented at UEG Week Barcelona October 21, 2019.

Kim, H. et al. "Plant-Based Diets are Associated with a Lower Risk of Incident Cardiovascular Disease, Cardiovascular Disease Mortality, and All-Cause Mortality in a General Population of Middle-Aged Adults." *Journal of the American Heart Association*, August 7, 2019.

https://doi.org/10.1161/jaha.119.012865

Unattributed. "FDA Issues Revised 'Advice about Eating Fish for Women Who Are or Might Become Pregnant, Breastfeeding Mothers, and Young Children.'" *U.S. Food & Drug Administration*, July 2, 2019.
www.fda.gov/food/cfsan-constituent-updates/fda-issues-revised-advice-about-eating-fish-women-who-are-or-might-become-pregnant-breastfeeding

Unattributed. "Cholesterol Does Not Cause Heart Disease." *Mercola*, July 24, 2019.
www.articles.mercola.com/sites/articles/archive/2019/07/24/cholesterol-myth-what-really-causes-heart-disease.aspx

Racey Gleeson, J. "Fish, Fruit, Healthy Fats: What Should Heart Disease Patients Eat?" *Michigan Health*, May 2019.
https://healthblog.uofmhealth.org/heart-health/fish-fruit-healthy-fats-what-should-heart-disease-patients-eat

Reynolds, A. et al, "Carbohydrate Quality and Human Health: a Series of Systematic Reviews and Meta-Analyses." *The Lancet*, January 10, 2019.
https://doi.org/10.1016/s0140-6736(18)31809-9

Buckingham, C. "8 Reasons Why Spain is Skinny." *Eat This, Not That!*, August 2016.
www.eatthis.com/why-spain-is-skinny/

Phan, C. et al. "Association Between Mediterranean Anti-inflammatory Dietary Profile and Severity of Psoriasis." *JAMA Dermatology*, September 2018.
http://doi.org/10.1001/jamadermatol.2018.2127

"Diet, Nutrition, Physical Activity, and Cancer: A Global Perspective. Landmark Cancer Prevention Report Shows Consensus Among Global Experts on 10 Steps to Reduce Risk." *American Institute for Cancer Research*, Continuous Update Project Expert Report 2018. www.dietandcancerreport.org

Zheng, J. et al., "Association Between Post-Cancer Diagnosis Dietary Inflammatory Potential and Mortality Among Invasive Breast Cancer Survivors in the Women's Health Initiative." *Cancer Epidemiology, Biomarkers & Prevention*, April 2018.
https://doi.org/10.1158/1055-9965.epi-17-0569

MacMillian, A. "What Can You Eat On the Mediterranean Diet?" *TIME*, January 16, 2018.
www.time.com/5101886/what-can-you-eat-on-the-mediterranean-diet/

Castelló, A. et al. "Mediterranean Dietary Pattern is Associated with Low Risk of Aggressive Prostate Cancer: MCC-Spain Study." *The Journal of Urology*, February 1, 2018.
https://doi.org/10.1016/j.juro.2017.08.087

Aridi, Y. et al. "The Association Between the Mediterranean Dietary Pattern and Cognitive Health: A Systematic Review." *Nutrients*, June 2017.
https://doi.org/10.3390/nu9070674

Medina-Remón A. et al. "Polyphenol Intake from a Mediterranean Diet Decreases Inflammatory Bio-Markers Related to Atherosclerosis: a Sub-study of the PREDIMED Randomized Trial." *British Journal of Clinical Pharmacology.* April 2016

https://doi.org/10.1111/bcp.12986

Biasini, C. "Mediterranean Diet Influences Breast Cancer Relapse: Preliminary Results of the SETA PROJECT." *Journal of Clinical Oncoloty*, 2016.

https://doi.org/10.1200/jco.2016.34.15_suppl.e13039

Veronese, N. et al. "Adherence to the Mediterranean Diet is Associated with Better Quality of Life: Data from the Osteoarthritis Initiative." *The American Journal of Clinical Nutrition.* September 2016.

https://doi.org/10.3945/ajcn.116.136390

Nelson, Mya. "Vast Majority of Cancers Caused by Lifestyle, Not 'Bad Luck.'" *American Institute of Cancer Research Blog*, December 2015

Martínez-González, M. "Mediterranean Diet Plus Olive Oil Associated with Reduced Breast Cancer Risk." *JAMA Internal Medicine*, September 2015.

www.sciencedaily.com/releases/2015/09/150914092837.html

Ramírez-Anaya, J. et al. "Phenols and the Antioxidant Capacity of Mediterranean Vegetables Prepared with Extra Virgin Olive Oil Using Different Domestic Cooking Techniques." *Food Chemistry*, December 2015.

https://doi.org/10.1016/j.foodchem.2015.04.124

Castelló A., et al, "Spanish Mediterranean Diet and Other Dietary Patterns and Breast Cancer Risk: Case-Control EpiGEICAM Study." *British Journal of Cancer*, August 2014.

https://doi.org/10.1038/bjc.2014.434

Pérez-Jiménez, J. et al. "Contribution of Macromolecular Antioxidants to Dietary Antioxidant Capacity: A Study in the Spanish Mediterranean Diet." *Plant Foods for Human Nutrition*, October 2015.

https://doi.org/10.1007/s11130-015-0513-6

Dernini, S. "Mediterranean Diet: From a Healthy Diet to a Sustainable Dietary Pattern." *Frontiers in Nutrition*, May 2015.

https://doi.org/10.3389/fnut.2015.00015

Malmir, H. et al. "Adherence to Mediterranean Diet in Relation to Bone Mineral Density and Risk of Fracture: a Systematic Review and Meta-Analysis of Observational Studies." *European Journal of Nutrition*, June 2017.

https://doi.org/10.1007/s00394-017-1490-3

Savanelli, M. et al. "Preliminary Results Demonstrating the Impact of Mediterranean Diet on Bone Health." *Journal of Translational Medicine*, April 2017.

https://doi.org/10.1186/s12967-017-1184-x

Link, L.B. et al. "Dietary Patterns and Breast Cancer Risk in the California Teachers Study Cohort." *American Journal of Clinical Nutrition*, December 2013.

https://doi.org/10.3945/ajcn.113.061184

Estruch, R. et al. "Towards an Even Healthier Mediterranean Diet." *Nutrition, Metabolism and Cardiovascular Diseases*. December 2013.

https://doi.org/10.1016/j.numecd.2013.09.003

Abuznait, A.H. et al. "Olive-Oil-Derived Oleocanthal Enhances β-Amyloid Clearance as a Potential Neuroprotective Mechanism Against Alzheimer's Disease: In Vitro and in Vivo Studies." *ACS Chemical Neuroscience*. June 2013.

https://doi.org/10.1221/cn400024q

Eliassen, A.H. et al. "Circulating Carotenoids and Risk of Breast Cancer: Pooled Analysis of Eight Prospective Studies." *Journal of the National Cancer Institute*, December 2012.

https://doi.org/10.1093/jnci/djs461

Rodríguez-Hernández, M. et al. "Natural Antioxidants in Purple Sprouting Broccoli Under Mediterranean Climate." *Journal of Food Science*, August 2012.

https://doi.org/10.1111/j.1750-3841.2012.02886.x

Yao, F. et al. "Lentil Polyphenol Extract Prevents Angiotensin II-Induced Hypertension, Vascular Remodeling, and Perivascular Fibrosis." *Food Function*, February 2012.

https://doi.org/10.1039/c1fo10142k

Davis, A. et al. "Metabolic Syndrome and Triple-Negative Breast Cancer: A New Paradigm." *International Journal of Breast Cancer*, 2012.

https://doi.org/10.1155/2012/809291

Ismail, T. et al. "Pomegranate Peel and Fruit Extracts: a Review of Potential Anti-Inflammatory and Anti-Infective Effects." *Journal of Ethmopharmacology*, September 2012.

https://doi.org/10.1016/j.jep.2012.07.004

Baglietto, L. et. al. "Dietary Patterns and Risk of Breast Cancer." *British Journal of Cancer*, December 2010.

https://doi.org/10.1038/sj.bjc.6606044

Pollán, M. et al. "Recent Changes in Breast Cancer Incidence in Spain 1980-2004." *Journal of the National Cancer Institute*, November 2009.

https://doi.org/10.1093/jnci/djp358

Touillaud, M. et al. "Dietary Lignan Intake Postmenopausal Breast Cancer Risk by Estrogen and Progesterone Receptor Status." *Journal of the National Cancer Institute*, March 2007.

https://doi.org/10.1093/jnci/djk096

Menédez J. et al. "HER2 (erbB-2) -Targeted Effects of the Omega-3 Polyunsaturated Fatty Acid, Alpha-Linolenic Acid (ALA; 18:3n-3), in Breast Cancer Cells: The 'Fat Features' of the 'Mediterranean Diet' as an 'Anti-HER2 Cocktail.'" *Clinical and Transactional Oncology*, November 2006.

https://doi.org/10.1007/s12094-006-0137-2

Fernandez San Juan, P. "Dietary Habits and Nutrition Status of School Aged Children in Spain." *Nutrición Hospitalaria*, May-Jun 2006;21(3):374-8

Willett, W. "The Mediterranean Diet: Science and Practice." *Public Health Nutrition*, February 2006.

https://doi.org/10.1079/phn2005931

Nkondjock, A. et al. "Diet, Lifestyle and BRCA-Related Breast Cancer Risk Among French-Canadians." *Epidemiology*, March 2006.

https://doi.org/10.1007/s10549-006-9161-8

Kode, A. et al. "Effect of Ethanol and Thermally Oxidized Sunflower Oil Ingestion on Phospholipid Fatty Acid Composition of Rat Liver: Protective Role of Cuminum Cyminum L." *Annals of Nutrition and Metabolism*. September-October 2005.

https://doi.org/10.1159/000087333

Shedding Light on Cancer Screening/ Prevention Is Key

Bretthauser, M. et al, "Effect of Colonoscopy Screening on Risks of Colorectal Cancer and Related Death" *The New England Journal of Medicine*, October 9, 2022.

https://doi.org/10.1056/NEJMoa2208375

Excess Body Weight

Sanz, J. et al. "Eating a Diet Rich in Fruit and Vegetables Could Cut Obesity Risk." *European Association for the Study of Obesity*, May 2017.

www.sciencedaily.com/releases/2017/05/170518220955.htm

Estruch R. et al. "Effect of High-Fat Mediterranean Diet on Bodyweight and Waist Circumference: a Prespecified Secondary Outcomes Analysis of the PREDIMED Randomized Controlled Trial." *The Lancet Diabetes & Endocrinology*, May 2019.

https://doi.org/10.1016/s2213-8587(19)30074-9

Martínez-González, M. et al. "Yogurt Consumption, Weight Change and Risk of Overweight/Obesity: The SUN Cohort Study." *Nutrition, Metabolism and Cardiovascular Diseases*, November 2014.

https://doi.org/10.1016/j.numecd.2014.05.015

Adams, J. "Obesity, Epigenetics and Gene Regulation." *Nature*, 2008.

http://www.nature.com/scitable/topicpage/obesity-epigenetics-and-gene-regulation-927

Health Destructive Effects
of Various Diets, Including Keto

Napoli, N. "'Keto-Like' Diet May be Linked to Higher Risk of Heart Disease, Cardiac Events." *American College of Cardiology*, March 2023.

www.acc.org/About-ACC/Press-Releases/2023/03/05/15/07/Keto-Like-Diet-May-Be-Linked-to-Higher-Risk

Hoffman, R. "Ultra-Processed Foods: It's Not Just Their Low Nutritional Value that's a Concern," September 12, 2022

www.theconversation.com/ultra-processed-foods-it-not-just-their-low-nutritional-value-thats-a-concern-189918

Wang, Lu et al. "Association of Ultra-Processed Food Consumption with Colorectal Cancer Risk Among Men and Women: Results from Three Prospective US Cohort Studies." *The British Journal of Medicine*, August 2022.

https://doi.org/10.1136/bmj-2021-068921

Papier, Keren et al. "Meat Consumption and Risk of Ischemic Heart Disease: A Systematic Review and Meta-analysis." *Critical Reviews in Food Science and Nutrition*, July 2021.

https://doi.org/10.1080/10408398.2021.1949575

Safford, M. et al. "The Southern Diet—Fried Foods and Sugary Drinks—May Raise Risk of Sudden Cardiac Death." *Journal of the American Heart Association*, June 2021.

www.sciencedaily.com/releases/2021/06/210630091407.htm

Chazelas, E. et al. "Sugary Drinks, Artificially-Sweetened Beverages, and Cardiovascular Disease in the NutriNet-Santé Cohort." *Journal of the American College of Cardiology*, November 2020

http://doi.org/10.1061/j.jacc.2020.08.075

Stevenson, R. et al. "Hippocampal-Dependent Appetitive Control is Impaired by Experimental Exposure to a Western-Style Diet." *Royal Society Open Science*, Febuary 2020.

https://doi.org/10.1098/rsos.191338

Junxiu, L. et al. "Quality of Meals Consumed by Adults at Full-service and Fast-Food Restaurants, 2003-2016:

Persistent Low Quality and Widening Disparities". *The Journal of Nutrition*, January 2020.

https://doi.org/10.1093/jn/nxz299

Goldberg, E. et al. "Ketogenesis Activates Metabolically Protective γδT Cells in Visceral Adipose Tissues" *Nature Metabolism*, January 2020.

https://doi.org/10.1038/s42255-019-0160-6

Zen, D. et al, "Association of Sulfur Amino Acid Consumption with Cardiometabolic Risk Factors: Cross-sectional Findings from NHANES III." *EClinicalMedicine*, 2020.

https://doi.org/10.1016/j.eclinm.2019.100248

Junxiu Liu, et al, "Quality of Meals Consumed by US Adults at Full-Service and Fast-Food Restaurants, 2003-2016: Persistent Low Quality and Widening Disparities." *The Journal of Nutrition*, 2020.

Yance, D. "Glyphosate, Not Gluten, Is the True Villain." *Donnie Yance*, October 3, 2019.
www.donnieyance.com/glyphosate-not-gluten-is-the-true-villain/

Beckett, E. "Stop Hating on Pasta, It Actually has a Healthy Ratio of Carbs, Protein and Fat." *Barcelona-Metropolitan*, April 2023.
www.barcelona-metropolitan.com/eating-and-drinking/stop-hating-on-pasta/

Johnston, B. et al. "Unprocessed Red Meat and Processed Meat Consumption: Dietary Guideline Recommendations From the Nutritional Recommendations (NutriRECS) Consortium." *Annals of Internal Medicine*, October 2019.
https://doi.org/10.7326/m19-1621

Baldridge, A, et al. "The Healthfulness of the US Packaged Food and Beverage Supply: A Cross-Sectional Study." *Nutrients*, July 2019.
https://doi.org/10.3390/nu11081704

Rico-Campà, A. et al. "Association Between Consumption of Ultra-Processed Foods and All Cause Mortality: SUN Prospective Cohort Study." *British Medical Journal*, May 2019.
https://doi.org/10.1136/bmj.l1949

Gupta, S. et al. "Characterizing Ultra-processed Foods by Energy Density and Cost," *Frontiers in Nutrition*, May 2019
www.doi.org/10.3389/fnut.2009.00070

Davies, M. et al. "Management of Hyperglycemia in Type 2 Diabetes, 2018. A Consensus Report by the American Diabetes Association (ADA) and the European Association for the Study of Diabetes (EASD)." *Diabetes Care*, December 2018.
https://doi.org/10.2337/dci18-0033

Gómez-Donoso, C. et al. "Ultra-Processed Food Consumption and the Incidence of Depression in a Mediterranean Cohort: the SUN Project." *The European Journal of Nutrition*, May 2019.
https://doi.org/10.1007/s00394-019-01970-1

Afshin, A. et al. "Health Effects of Dietary Risks in 195 Countries, 1990-2017: A Systematic Analysis for the Global Burden of Disease Study 2017." *The Lancet*, April 2019.
https://doi.org/10.1016/s0140-6736(19)30041-8

The Editorial Board. "The World Doesn't Need Trans Fats." *The New York Times*, May 14, 2018.
www.nytimes.com/2018/05/14/opinion/eliminate-trans-fats.html

Unattributed. "HDL Cholesterol Could Have Brain Benefits." *Tufts Health & Nutrition Letter*, March 2018.

www.nutritionletter.tufts.edu/healthy-eating/hdl-cholesterol-could-have-brain-benefits#:~:text=The%20researchers%20speculated%20that%20HDL%20cholesterol%20might%20protect,to%20prevent%20the%-20degeneration%20of%20the%20brain's%20neurons.

Micha, R. et al. "Association Between Dietary Factors and Mortality from Heart Disease, Stroke, and Type 2 Diabetes in the United States." *Journal of the American Medical Association*, March 2017.

https://doi.org/10.1001/jama.2017.0947

Lauretti, E. et al. "Effect of Canola Oil Consumption on Memory, Synapse and Neuropathology in the Triple Transgenic Mouse Model of Alzheimer's Disease." *Scientific Reports*, December 2017.

https://doi.org/10.1038/s41598-017-17373-3

Viennois, E. et al. "Dietary Emulsifier-Induced Low-Grade Inflammation Promotes Colon Carcinogenesis." *Cancer Research*, January 2017.

https://doi.org/10.1158/0008-5472.can-16-1359

Unattributed "Spanish Towns and Regions Agree to Ban Glyphosate in Public Areas." *gmwatch.org*, March 2016.

www.gmwatch.org/en/news/archive/2016/16820-spanish-towns-and-regions-agree-to-ban-glyphosate-in-public-areas

Guallar-Castillón, P. et. al. "Consumption of Fried Foods and Risk of Coronary Heart Disease: Spanish Cohort of the European Prospective Investigation into Cancer and Nutrition Study. *British Medical Journal*, January 2012.

https://doi.org/10.1136/bmj.e363

Jiang, Y, et al. "Dietary Sugar Induces Tumorigenesis in Mammary Gland Partially Through 12 Lipoxygenase Pathway." *Cancer Research*, August 2015.

https://doi.org/10.1158/1538-7445.am2015-3735

Vlassara, H. "What are Advanced Glycation End Products? The A.G.E. Less Diet." *Life Extension*, 2018.

https://blog.lifeextension.com/2018/11/what-are-advanced-glycation-end.html

Luo, S. et al. "Differential Effects of Fructose Versus Glucose on Brain and Appetitive Responses to Food Cues and Decisions for Food Rewards." *Proceedings of the National Academy of Sciences*, May 2015.

https://doi.org/10.1073/pnas.1503358112

Guo, J. et al. "Red and Processed Meat Intake and Risk of Breast Cancer: A Meta-Analysis of Prospective Studies." *Breast Cancer Research and Treatment*, April 2015.

https://doi.org/10.1007/s10549-015-3380-9

Papaioannou, M. et al., "The Cooked Meat Derived-Mammary Carcinogenic 2-Amino-1-Methl-6-Phenylimidazo [4.5-b] Pyridine (PhIP) Elicits Estrogenic-Like MicroRNA Responses in Breast Cancer Cells." *Toxicology Letters*, August 2014.

https://doi.org/10.1016/j.toxlet.2014.05.021

Yang, B. et al. "Ratio of n-3/n-6 PUFAs and Risk of Breast Cancer; a Meta-Analysis of 274,135 Adult Females from 11 Independent Prospective Studies." *BMC Cancer*, February 2014.

https://doi.org/10.1186/1471-2407-14-105

Farvid, M. et al., "Dietary Protein Sources in Early Adulthood and Breast Cancer Incidence: Prospective Cohort Study." *BMJ*, June 2014.

https://doi.org/10.1136/bmj.g3437

Chang, N. et al. "High Levels of Arachidonic Acid and Peroxisome Proliferation-Activated Receptor-Alpha in Breast Cancer Tissues are Associated with Promoting Cancer Cell Proliferation." *The Journal of Nutritional Biochemistry*, January 2013.

https://doi.org/10.1016/j.jnutbio.2012.06.005

Guallar-Castillón, P. et al. "Consumption of Fried Foods and Risk of Coronary Heart Disease: Spanish Cohort of the European Prospective Investigation into Cancer and Nutrition Study." *BMJ*, January 24, 2012.

https://doi.org/10.1136/bmj.e363

Kris-Etherton, P. "Trans-Fats and Coronary Heart Disease." *Critical Reviews in Food Science and Nutrition*, December 2010.

https://doi.org/10.1080/10408398.2010.526872

Tappel, A. "Heme of Consumed Red Meat Can Act as a Catalyst of Oxidative Damage and Could Initiate Colon, Breast, and Prostate Cancers, Heart Disease, and Other Diseases." *Medical Hypotheses*, October 2006.

https://doi.org/10.1016/j.mehy.2006.08.025

Heaney, R. et al. "Carbonated Beverages and Urinary Tract Calcium Excretion." *American Journal of Clinical Nutrition*, September 2001.

https://doi.org/10.1093/ajcn/74.3.343

Sinha, R. et al. "Dietary Intake of Heterocyclic Amines, Meat-Derived Mutagenic Activity, and Risk of Colorectal Adenomas." *Cancer Epidemiology, Biomarkers & Prevention*, May 2001.

https://cebp.aacrjournals.org/content/10/5/559

Zeng, W. et al. "Well-Done Meat Intake and the Risk of Breast Cancer." *Journal of the National Cancer Institute,* November 1998.

https://doi.org/10.1093/jnci/90.22.1724

Erasmus, Udo. "Fats That Heal Fats That Kill," *Alive Books*, 1993.

Iberia's Singular Place in European Botany and Archaeology

Unattributed, "Over 100 Prehistoric Engravings Found in a Cave in Northeastern Spain, *El País*, March 2023.

http://english.elpais.com/culture/2023-03-17/over-100-prehistoric-engravings-found-in-a-cave-in-northeastern-spain.html

Pietroni, D. "A New Monumental City Discovered in Northern Spain." *The Art Insider*, July 2022.

http://art-insider.com/a-new-monumental-city-discovered-in-northern-spain/3947

Olaya, V. "Archaeologists Find Previously Unknown Roman City at the Foothills of the Pyrenees." *El Pais English Edition*, July 2022.

http://english.elpais.com/culture/2022-07-13

Unattributed. "Jawbone Found in Spain Could be Oldest European Human Fossil." *The Guardian*, July 2022.

http://www.theguardian.com/science/2022/jul/08/jawbone-found-in-spain-could-be-oldest-human-fossil

Alvarez, C. "Two Generations of Botanists End Titanic Task: Describing the 6,120 plants of Spain and Portugal." *El Pais*, October 14, 2021

www.english.elpais.com/science-tech/2021-10-14/two-generations-of-botanists-end-titanic-task-decribing-the-6120-plants-of-spain-and-portugal.html

Barrat, John. "Beetle and Pollen Trapped in 105 Million-Year-Old Amber Reveal Fourth Major Pollination Mode in Mid-Mesozoic." *Smithsonian Insider*, March 2, 2017.

https://insider.si.edu/2017/03/beetle-and-pollen-trapped-in-105-million-year-old-amber-confirm-fourth-major-pollination-mode-during-mid-mesozoic/

Barras, Colin. "Meet a Lamprey. Your Ancestors Looked Just Like It." *BBC.com*, November 2, 2015.

www.bbc.com/earth/story/20151102-meet-a-lamprey-your-ancestors-looked-just-like-it

Environment

Planelles, M. "Spain to Ban Sale of Fruit and Vegetables in Plastic Wrapping From 2023." *El País*, September 22, 2021

www.english.elpais.com/society/2021-09-22/spain-to-ban-sale-of-fruit-and-vegetables-in-plastic-from-2023.html

Pennino, M. et al. "Ingestion of Microplastics and Occurrence of Parasite Association in Mediterranean Anchovy and Sardine." *Marine Pollution Bulletin*, September 2020.

https://doi.org/10.1016/j.marpolbul.2020.111399

Cohut, M. "Harmful Hospital Bacteria Evolved in Response to Modern Diets.'" *Medical News Today*, August 13, 2019.

www.medicalnewstoday.com/articles/326029

Chen, F. et al. "Lower Concentrations of Phthalates Induce Proliferation in Human Breast Cancer Cells." *Climacteric*, August 2014.

https://doi.org/10.3109/13697137.2013.865720

Are Saturated Fats and Eggs Really Linked to Heart Disease?

Astrup, A. et al. "Saturated Fats and Health: A Reassessment and Proposal for Food-Based Recommendations." *Journal of the American College of Cardiology: JACC State of the Art Review*, June 2020.

https://doi.org/10.1016/j.jacc.2020.05.077

Dehghan, M. et al. "Association of Egg Intake with Blood Lipids, Cardiovascular Disease, and Mortality in 177,000 People in 50 Countries." *The American Journal of Clinical Nutrition*, April 2020.

https://doi.org/10.1093/ajcn/nqz348

Johnston, B. et al. "Unprocessed Red Meat and Processed Meat Consumption: Dietary Guideline Recommendations from the Nutritional Recommendations (NutriRECS) Consortium." November 2019.

https://doi.org/10.7326/m19-1621

Otto, M. et al. "Serial Measures of Circulating Biomarkers of Dairy Fat and Total and Cause-Specific Mortality in Older Adults: the Cardiovascular Health Study." *The American Journal of Clinical Nutrition*, July 2018.

https://doi.org/10.1093/ajcn/nqy117

Lordan, R. et al. "Dairy Fats and Cardiovascular Disease: Do We Really Need to be Concerned?" Foods, March 2018.

www.doi.org/10.3390/foods7030024

Chen, G. et al. "Cheese Consumption and Risk of Cardiovascular Disease: A Meta-Analysis of Prospective Studies. *European Journal of Nutrition*, January 2019.

https://doi.org/10.1007/s00394-016-1292-z

Nimalaratne, C. et al. "Free Aromatic Amino Acids in Egg Yolks Show Antioxidant Properties" *Journal of Food Chemistry*, July 2011.

https://doi.org/10.1016/j.foodchem.2011.04.058

Unattributed, "7 Myths About Cholesterol Debunked" *Yahoo*, June 2023.

> https://www.yahoo.com/lifestyle/7-myths-about-cholesterol-debunked-120030351.html

Mercola, J. "New Scientific Analysis Confirms Fats Have No Links to Heart Disease." *Mercola*, August 31, 2015.

> https://articles.mercola.com/sites/articles/archive/2015/08/31/saturated-fats-heart-disease.aspx

White, J. "Is Full-Fat Milk Best? The Skinny on the Dairy Paradox." *New Scientist*, February 21, 2014.

> www.newscientist.com/article/dn25102-is-full-fat-milk-best-the-skinny-on-the-dairy-paradox/

Reiser, R. "Saturated Fat in the Diet and Serum Cholesterol Concentration: A Critical Examination of the Literature." *The American Journal of Clinical Nutrition*, May 1973.

> https://doi.org/10.1093/ajcn/26.5.524

Teicholz, N. *The Big Fat Surprise: Why Butter, Meat, and Cheese Belong in a Healthy Diet*. New York: Simon & Schuster, 2014.

Benefits of Artisan Cheese

Donnelly, Catherine W. *Cheese and Microbes*. Washington DC: ASM Press, April 2014.

Benefits of Organic Foods, Grass-Fed Beef

Grandjean, P. "Human Health Implications of Organic Food and Organic Agriculture," *Directorate-General for Parliamentary Research Services (DG EPRS) of the European Parliament*. December 2016.

> doi: 978-92-846-0395-4

Daley, C. et al. "A Review of Fatty Acid Profiles and Antioxidant Content in Grass-Fed and Grain-Fed Beef." *Nutrition Journal*, March 2010.

> https://doi.org/10.1186/1475-2891-9-10

Robinson, J. "Breeding the Nutrition out of Food." *New York Times*, May 26, 2013.

> www.nytimes.com/2013/5/26/opinion/sunday/breeding-the-nutrition-out-of-our-food.html

Hallmann, E. et al. "The Seasonal Variation in Bioactive Compounds Content in Juice from Organic and Non-Organic Tomatoes." *Plant Foods for Human Nutrition*, April 2013.

> https://doi.org/10.1007/s11130-013-0352-2

McAfee, A. et al. "Red Meat From Animals Offered a Grass Diet Increases Plasma and Platelet n-3 PUFA in Healthy Consumers." *British Journal of Nutrition*, January 2011.

https://doi.org/10.1017/s0007114510003090

Tsiplakou, E. et al. "Differences in Sheep and Goat's Milk Fatty Acid Profile Between Conventional and Organic Farming Systems." *Journal of Dairy Research*, August 2010.

https://doi.org/10.1017/s0022029910000270

Long, C. "Industrially Farmed Foods Have Lower Nutritional Content." *Mother Earth News*, June-July 2020.

www.motherearthnews.com/nature-and-environment/nutritional-content-zmaz09jjzraw#:~:text=Industrially%20Farmed%20Foods%20Have%20Lower%20Nutritional%20Content.%20A,as%20the%20use%20of%20high-yield%20industrial%20farming%20

Davies, D. "Declining Fruit and Vegetable Nutrient Composition: What is the Evidence?" *HortScience*, February 2009.

https://doi.org/10.21273/hortsci.44.1.15

Benbrook, C. et al. "New Evidence Confirms the Nutritional Superiority of Plant-Based Organic Foods." *State of Science Review*, The Organic Center. March 2008.

www.plantnutritiontech.com/wp-content/uploads/2019/12/NutrientContentReport.pdf

Mercola, J. "What Are the Best Type of Eggs to Get?" *Mercola*, November 8, 2007.

Staff of Life: Bread and Whole Grains

Miller, K. et al. "Nutrition Economics: Four Analyses Supporting the Case for Whole Grain Consumption." *Journal of Cereal Science*, May 2022.

http://doi.org/10.1016/j.jcs.2022103455

Shivakoti, R. et al. "Intake and Sources of Dietary Fiber, Inflammation, and Cardiovascular Disease in Older US Adults." *JAMA Network Open Conversations*, March 2022.

http://doi.org/10.1001/jamanetworkopen.2022.5012

Yance, D. "Bread as Sustenance for Body and Soul." *Donnie Yance*, May 2015.

www.donnieyance.com/bread-as-sustenance-for-body-and-soul/

Unattributed. "Bread in Europe." *Wikipedia*, October 2015,

https://en.wikipedia.org/Bread_in_Europe

Vanegas, S. et al. "Substituting Whole Grains for Refined Grains in a 6-wk Randomized Trial has a Modest Effect on Gut Microbiota and Immune and Inflammatory Markers of Healthy Adults." *American Journal of Clinical Nutrition*, October 2017.

http://doi.org/10.3945/ajcn.117.155424

Aune, D. et al. "Whole Grain Consumption and Risk of Cardiovascular Disease, Cancer, and All Cause and Cause Specific Mortality: Systematic Review and Dose-Response Meta-Analysis of Prospective Studies." *British Journal of Medicine*, June 2016.

https://doi.org/10.1136/bmj.i2716

Jannalagadda, S. et al. "Putting the Whole Grain Puzzle Together: Health Benefits Associated with Whole Grains—Summary of American Society for Nutrition 2010 Satellite Symposium." *Journal of Nutrition*, May 2011.

https://doi.org/10.3945/jn.110.132944

Harris, D. "The Quest for Organic Artisan Bread." *La Tienda*, October 2009.

www.tienda.com/learn-about-spain/the-quest-for-organic-artisan-bread.html

Shultz, A. et al. "The Thiamin Content of Wheat Flour Milled by the Stone Milling Process." *Cereal Chemistry*. 1942. Volume 19 pp.529-531

www.cabdirect.org/cabdirect/abstract19421402074

Red Wine and Coffee

Mezue, K. et al. "Reduced Stress-related Neural Activity Mediates the Effect of Alcohol on Cardiovascular Risk." *Journal of the American College of Cardiology*, June 2023.

www.doi.org/10.1016/j.jaee.2023.04.015

Roeder, A. "Should Red Wine be Removed from the Mediterranean Diet." *Harvard School of Public Health*, February 2024.

www.hsph.harvard.edu/news/features/red-wine-mediterranean-diet/

White, A. et al. "Using Death Certificates to Explore Changes in Alcohol-Related Mortality In the United States, 1999-2017," *Alcoholism Clinical & Experimental Research*, January 2020.

https://doi.org/10.1111/acer.14239

Unattributed. "Alcohol Facts and Statistics." *National Institute on Alcohol Abuse and Alcoholism*, February 24, 2020.

www.niaaa.nih.gov/brochures-and-fact-sheets/alcohol-facts-and-statistics

Zhu, X. et al. "The Antidepressant- and Anxiolytic-Like Effects of Resveratrol: Involvement of Phosphodiesterase-4D Inhibition." *Neuropharmacology*, July 2019.

https://doi.org/10.1016/j.neuropharm.2019.04.022

Prysyazhna, O. et al. "Blood Pressure-Lowering by the Antioxidant Resveratrol is Counter-Intuitively Mediated by Oxidation of cGMP-Dependant Protein Kinase." *Circulation*, May 2019.

https://doi.org/10.1161/circulationaha.118.037398

Lichtenstein, A. et al. "Drinking in Moderation: What That Means and Why It's Recommended." *Tufts University Health & Nutrition Newsletter*, September 2019.

www.nutritionletter.tufts.edu/ask-experts/drinking-in-moderation-what-that-means-and-why-its-recommended

Huang, S. et al. "Longitudinal Study of Alcohol Consumption and HDL Concentrations: A Community-Based Study." *American Journal of Clinical Nutrition*, March 13, 2017.

https://doi.org/10.3945/ajcn.116.144832

Gunter, M. et. al. "Coffee Drinking and Mortality in 10 European Countries: A Multinational Cohort Study." *Annals of Internal Medicine*, July 2017.

https://doi.org/10.7326/m16-2945

Carroll, A. "More Consensus on Coffee's Benefits Than You Might Think." *The New York Times*, May 2015.

www.nytimes.com/2015/05/11/upshot/more-consensus-on-coffees-effect-on-health-than-you-might-think.html

Shay, N. et al. "Another Reason to Drink Wine: It Could Help You Burn Fat." *Sciencedaily.com/releases/2015/02/150206111702.htm.* Study: *Journal of Nutritional Biochemistry*, February 2015.

https://doi.org/10.1016/j.jnutbio.2014.09.010

Ornstrup, M. et al. "Resveratrol Increases Bone Mineral Density and Bone Alkaline Phosphatase in Obese Men: A Randomized Placebo-Controlled Trial." *Journal of Clinical Endocrinology & Metabolism*, December 2014.

https://doi.org/10.1210/jc.2014-2799

Underwood, A. "9 Superfoods for Your Heart." *Prevention*, January 18, 2012.

www.prevention.com/food-nutrition/a20437827

Freedman, N. et al. "Association of Coffee Drinking with Total and Cause-Specific Mortality." *The New England Journal of Medicine*, May 2012.

https://doi.org/10.1056/nejmoa1112010

Soohan, J. et al. "Cellular Antioxidant and Anti-Inflammatory Effects of Coffee Extracts with Different Roasting Levels." *Journal of Medicinal Food*, June 2017.

https://doi.org/10.1089/jmf.2017.3935

Bagchi, D. et al. "Cellular Protection with Proanthocyanidins Derived from Grape Seeds." *Annals of the New York Academy of Sciences*, January 2006.

https://doi.org/10.1111/j.1749-6632.2002.tb02922.x

Genetics, DNA, and Diet

Zierath, J. et al. "Acute Exercise Remodels Promoter Methylation in Human Skeletal Muscle." *Cell Metabolism*, March 2012.

https://doi.org/10.1016/j.cmet.2012.01.001

Reynolds, G. "How Exercise Can Change Our DNA." *The New York Times*, December 17, 2014.

Brown, W. "Exercise-Associated DNA Methylation Change in Skeletal Muscle and the Importance of Imprinting Genes: A Bioinformatics Meta-Analysis." *British Journal of Sports Medicine*, March 2015.

https://doi.org/10.1136/bjsports-2014-094073

Peikoff, K. "I Had my DNA Picture Taken with Varying Results." *The New York Times*, December 2013.

www.nytimes.com/2013/12/31/science/i-had-my-dna-picture-taken-with-varying-results.html

Stefanaska, B. et al. "Epigenetic Mechanisms in Anti-Cancer Actions of Bioactive Food Components – The Implications in Cancer Prevention." *British Journal of Pharmacology*, September 2012.

https://doi.org/10.1111/j.1476-5381.2012.02002.x

Shi, Y.Y. et al. "Diet and Cell Size Both Affect Queen-Worker Differentiation Through DNA Methylation in Honey Bees (Apis Mellifera, Apidae)." *PLOS One*, April 2011.

https://doi.org/10.1371/journal.pone.0018808

Kolodziejski, Kevin. "Epigenetic Diet Shows Good Food Negates Bad Genes." *Times News Online*, (September 3, 2011).

Hodge, Anne-Marie C., "Food We Eat Might Control Our Genes." *Scientific American*, November 25, 2011.

Berner C. et al. "Epigenetic Control of Estrogen Receptor Expression and Tumor Suppressor Genes is Modulated by Bioactive Food Compounds." *Annals of Nutrition and Metabolism*, March 2010.

https://doi.org/10.1159/000321514

Adams, J. "Obesity, Epigenetics, and Gene Regulation." *Nature*, 2008.

www.nature.com/scitable/topicpage/obesity-epigenetics-and-gene-regulation 927

Nikondjock, A. et al. "Diet, Lifestyle, and BRCA-Related Breast Cancer Risk Among French-Canadians." *Breast Cancer Research & Treatment*, March 2006.

https://doi.org/10.1007/s10549-006-9161-8

Deckelbaum, R. et al. "n-3 Fatty Acids and Gene Expression." *The American Journal of Clinical Nutrition*, June 2006.

https://doi.org/10.1093/ajcn/83.6.1520s

Ferguson, L. "Nutrigenomics: Integrating Genomic Approaches into Nutrition Research." *Molecular Diagnosis & Therapy*, August 2012.

https://doi.org/10.1007/bf03256449

Affman, L. et al. "Nutrigenomics: From Molecular Nutrition to Prevention of Disease." *Journal of the Academy of Nutrition and Dietetics*, April 2006.

https://doi.org/10.1016/j.jada.2006.01.001

Slaga, T, R. Keuneke. "The Detox Revolution: A Powerful New Program for Boosting Your Body's Ability to Fight Cancer and Other Diseases." New York: McGraw-Hill, 2003

Additional Protective Foods/Compounds Not Limited to the Mediterranean Pantry

Ba, D. et al. "Mushroom Intake and Depression: A Population-based Study Using Data from the US National Health and Nutrition Examination Survey (NHANES), 2005-2016." *J. Affect Discord*. July 2021.

http://doi.org/10.1016/j.jad.2021.07.080

Fonseca, S. et al. "Association Between Consumption of Fermented Vegetables and COVID-19 Mortality at a Country Level in Europe." *MedRxiv*, July 2020.

https://doi.org/10.1101/2020.07.06.20147025

Unattributed. "A Word About Eggs and Dairy." *Tufts University Health & Nutrition Letter*, April 2018.

www.nutritionletter.tufts.edu/healthy-eating/a-word-about-eggs-and-dairy

Seidelmann, S. et al. "Dietary Carbohydrate Intake and Mortality: a Prospective Cohort Study and Meta-Analysis." *The Lancet*, September 2018.

https://doi.org/10.1016/s2468-2667(18)30135-x

Hare, H. "'Forbidden' Black Rice Is Instagram's Newest Superfood Obsession." *The Daily Meal*, June 2018.

www.thedailymeal.com/healthy-eating/forbidden-black-rice-instagram-superfood

Yance, D. "Kamut: An Ancient Grain with Many Health Benefits." *Donnie Yance*, October 2016.

www.donnieyance.com/kamut-an-ancient-grain-with-many-health-benefits/

Unattributed. "What's New and Beneficial about Watermelon." *The World's Healthiest Foods*, 2015

www.whfoods.com/genpage.php?tname=foodspice&dbid=31

Keenan, M. et al. "Role of Resistant Starch in Improving Gut Health, Adiposity, and Insulin Resistance." *Advances in Nutrition*, March 2015

http://doi.org/10.3945/an.114.007419

Conner, T. et al. "On Carrots and Curiosity; Eating Fruit and Vegetables is Associated with Greater Flourishing in Daily Life." *British Journal of Health Psychology*, July 2014.

https://doi.org/10.1111/bjhp.12113

Goodson, A. "Why Turmeric and Black Pepper is a Powerful Combination." July 2018.

www.healthline.com/nutrition/turmeric-and-black-pepper

Moyle, C. et al. "Potent Inhibition of VEGFR-2 Activation by Tight Binding of Green Tea Epigallocatechin Gallate and Apple Procyanidins to VEGF: Relevance to Angiogenesis." *Molecular Nutrition & Food Research*. December 2014.

https://doi.org/10.1002/mnfr.201400478

Yao, Y. et al. "Anti-Inflammatory Activity of Saponins from Quinoa (Chenopodium Quinoa Willd.) Seeds in Lipopolysaccharide-Stimulated RAW 264.7 Macrophages Cells." *Journal of Food Science*, May 2014.

https://doi.org/10.1111/1750-3841.12425

Lai, L. et al. "Piperine Suppresses Tumor Growth and Metastasis in Vitro and in Vivo in a 4T1 Murine Breast Cancer Model." *Acta Pharmacologica Sinica*, March 2012.

https://doi.org/10.1038/aps.2011.209

Douglas, C. et. al. "Soy and Its Isoflavones: The Truth Behind the Science in Breast Cancer." *Anti-Cancer Agents in Medicinal Chemistry*, 2013.

https://doi.org/10.2174/18715206113139990320

Weintraub, A. "The New Science of Living Longer: A Handful of Exotic and Familiar Foods Can Influence How Quickly Your Cells Age." *MORE Magazine*, November 2013.

Teas, J. et al. "Consumption of Seaweed as a Protective Factor in the Etiology of Breast Cancer: Proof of Principle." *Journal of Applied Phycology*, November 2012.

https://doi.org/10.1007/s10811-012-9931-0

Wien, M. et al. "A Randomized 3x3 Crossover Study to Evaluate the Effect of Hass Avocado Intake on Post-Ingestive Satiety, Glucose, and Insulin Levels, and Subsequent Energy Intake in Overweight Adults." *Nutrition Journal*, November 2013.

https://doi.org/10.1186/1475-2891-12-155

Jung, S. et al. "Fruit and Vegetable Intake is Associated with Lower Risk of ER-Breast Cancer." *Journal of the National Cancer Institute*, January 2013.

www.sciencedaily.com/releases/2013/01/130124163336

Lindahl, G. et al. 'Tamoxifen, Flaxseed, and the Lignan Enterolactone Increase Stroma-and Cancer Cell-Derived IL-1Ra and Decrease Tumor Angiogenesis in Estrogen-Dependent Breast Cancer." *Cancer Research*, January 2011.

https://doi.org/10.1158/0008-5472.can-10-2289

Roizman, T. "Health Benefits of Cloves, Allspice, Nutmeg, Cinnamon, & Ginger." *AZ Central*.

https://healthyliving.azcentral.com/health-benefits-cloves-allspice-nutmeg-cinnamon-ginger-17114.html

Kakarala, M. et al. "Targeting Breast Stem Cells with the Cancer Preventive Compounds, Curcumin and Piperine." *Breast Cancer Research and Treatment*, November 2009.

https://doi.org/10.1007/s10549-009-0612-x

Unattributed. "What is Raw Honey Good For?" *Mercola*, May 2017.

https://foodfacts.mercola.com/raw-honey.html

Hui, C. et al. "Anticancer Activities of an Anthocyanin-Rich Extract from Black Rice Against Breast Cancer Cells in Vitro and in Vivo." *Nutrition and Cancer*, November 2010.

https://doi.org/10.1080/01635581.2010.494821

Angulo, L. et al. "Microflora Present in Kefir Grains of the Galician Region (Northwest of Spain)." *Journal of Dairy Research*, June 2009.

http://dio.org/10.1017/s002202990002759x

Story, E. et al. "An Update on the Health Effects of Tomato Lycopene." *Annual Review of Food Science & Technology*, November 2009.

https://doi.org/10.1146/annurev.food.102308.124120

Liu, J. et al. "Fresh Apples Suppress Mammary Carcinogenesis and Proliferative Activity and Induce Apoptosis in Mammary Tumors of the Sprague-Dawley Rat." *Journal of Agricultural and Food Chemistry*, January 2009.

https://doi.org/10.1021/jf801826w

Eberhardt, M. et al. "Antioxidant Activity of Fresh Apples." *Nature*, June 2000.

https://doi.org/10.1038/35016151

Kawashima H. et al., "Effects of Vitamin K2 (Menatetrenone) on Atherosclerosis and Blood Coagulation in Hypercholesterolemic Rabbits." *The Japanese Journal of Pharmacology*, October 1997.

https://doi.org/10.1254/jjp.75.135

The Seven Countries Study

Keys PhD, Dr. Ancel. "The Seven Countries Study. Countries and Cohorts: USA, Finland, Former Yugoslavia, Netherlands, Italy, Greece, Japan." 1947.

www.sevencountriesstudy.com

Kahn, J. "The Posthumous Assassination of Dr. Ancel Keys." *The Huffington Post*, December 19, 2016.

www.huffpost.com/entry/the-posthumous-assassination-of-dr-ancel-keys_b_58581561e4b0d5f48e165198

Allbaugh, L. "CRETE: A Case Study of an Undeveloped Area, *Princeton University Press*, 1953.

Carbohydrates and Breast Cancer

Kaaks, R. et al. "Insulin-like Growth Factor I and Risk of Breast Cancer by Age and Hormone Receptor Status—A Prospective Study Within the EPIC Cohort." *International Journal of Cancer*, June 2014.

https://doi.org/10.1002/ijc.28589

Romieu, I. et al. "Dietary Glycemic Index and Glycemic Load and Breast Cancer Risk in the European Prospective Investigation into Cancer and Nutrition (EPIC)." *The American Journal of Clinical Nutrition*, August 2012.

https://doi.org/10.3945/ajcn.111.026724

Fung, T. et al. "Low-Carbohydrate Diets, Dietary Approaches to Stop Hypertension-Style Diets, and the Risk of Postmenopausal Breast Cancer." *American Journal of Epidemology*, September 2011.

https://doi.org/10.1093/aje/kwr148

Wu, M. et al. "Relationships Between Critical Period of Estrogen Exposure and Circulating Levels of Insulin-Like Growth Factor-I (IGF-I) in Breast Cancer: Evidence from a Case-Control Study." *International Journal of Cancer*, January 2010.

https://doi.org/10.1002/ijc.24722

Yun, S. et al. "The Association of Carbohydrate Intake, Glycemic Load, Glycemic Intake, and Selected Rice Foods with Breast Cancer Risk: A Case-Control Study in South Korea." *Asian Pacific Journal of Clinical Nutrition*, 2010.

https://pubmed.ncbi.nlm.nih.gov/20805083

Suggested Reading

Kliger, I. "These are Spain's Newest Michelin-Starred Restaurants." *Forbes*. November 2023.

forbes.com/sites/isabellekliger/2023/11/29.

Álvarez, P. "Ferran Adrià: If elBulli Had Stayed Open, I Could Have Hit Rock Bottom," *El País English*, April 2023.

http://English.elpais.com/culture/2023-04-08/ferran-adria-if-elbulli-had-stayed-open-i-could-have-hit-rock-bottom.html

Berrill, A. "Tinned Fish: Your Easy Meal Fix." *The Guardian*, January 2022.

http://theguardian.com/food/2022/jan/18/tinned-fish-recipes-your-easy-meal-fix-kitchen-aide

Unattributed. "Six of the Top 100 Restaurants in the World are Basque." *Euskal Kazeta*, October 5, 2021.

www.euskalkazeta.com/seven-of-2018-top-restaurants-in-the-world-are-basque/

Unattributed. "The Best Chef Awards 2021 Winners Announcement: Chef Dabiz Muñoz Wins the Top 100." *The Best Chef*, September 2021 www.thebestchefawards.com/amsterdam2021/

Lakhani, N. et al. "Revealed: The True Extent of America's Food Monopolies and Who Pays the Price." July 14, 2021.

www.theguardian.com/environment/ng-interactive/2021/food-monopoly-meals-profits-data-investigations

Editorial Staff. "Chef Xanty Elías Wins Basque Culinary World Prize 2021." *Basque Culinary Center*, July 2021.

www.basqueculinaryworldprize.com

Whitelocks, Sadie. "The Best Restaurants for 2021 are named by Tripadvisor." *Daily Mail Online*, July 21, 2021.

www.dailymail.co.uk/travel/travel_news/article-9805701/The-best-restaurants-2021-named-Tripadvisor-eatery-LAKE-DISTRICT-No1.html

Woolever, Laurie. "Five of Anthony Bourdain's Favorite Food Destinations." *The Guardian*, May 19, 2021

https://www.theguardian.com/travel/2021/may/19/five-of-anthony-bourdains-favourite-food-destinations

Sevilla, María José. *Delicioso*. London: Reaktion Books Ltd, January 2020.

Tish, Ben. *Moorish: Vibrant Recipes from the Mediterranean*. Bath, England: Bloomsbury Absolute, October 22, 2019.

Mohacho, Nieves Barragan. *Sabor: Flavours from a Spanish Kitchen*. London: Fig Tree, May 1, 2019.

Spector, N. "What the 'Blue Zone' Island of Sardinia Can Teach Us About Living Longer." *NBC News*, June 2019.

https://www.nbcnews.com/better/lifestyle/what-blue-zone-island-sardinia-can-teach-us-about-living-ncnc1011051

Eckhardt, R. "On the Costa Brava, a Sea Urchin Quest." *The New York Times*, March 6, 2016.

Linton, Monika. *Brindisa: The True Food of Spain*. New York: Harper Collins, 2016.

Clark, Samantha. *Morito*. London, England: Ebury Press, September 15, 2015.

Harmon Jenkins, Nancy. *Virgin Territory, Exploring the World of Olive Oil*. New York: Houghton Mifflin Harcourt, 2015.

Casas, Penelope. *1000 Spanish Recipes*. New York: Houghton Mifflin Harcourt, 2014.

Jenkins, Debbie. *Spanish Village Cooking: Recetas del Campo*. www.nativespain.com, 2014

loren24250. "Variations on the Theme of Lamb Shoulder." *Radio Free Dagan*, September 12, 2013

www.loren24250.wordpress.com/2013/09/12/variations-on-the-theme-of-lamb-shoulder

Allibhoy, Omar. *Tapas Revolution*. London: Ebury Press, August 1, 2013.

Koehler, Jeff. *Spain: Recipes and Traditions from the Verdant Hills of the Basque County to the Coastal Waters of the Andalusia*. San Francisco: Chronicle Books, 2013.

Stewart, Chris. *Driving Over Lemons*. New York: Vintage Books, 1999.

Roden, Claudia. *The Food of Spain*. New York: Penguin Group, 2012.

Stein, Rick. *Rick Stein's Spain: 140 New Recipes Inspired by My Journey Off the Beaten Track*. London: BBC Books; 1st Edition, September 1, 2012.

Adrià, Ferran. *The Family Meal; Home Cooking with Ferran Adrià*. New York: Phaidon Press, 2011.

Berga, M. *50 Años del Hotel Empordà HISTORIAS DEL MOTEL, Con 50 Recetas de la Casa*. Ara Llibres, 2011.

Monné, Tonni, Oriol Alue (Photographer), Ana Torróntegui (Contributor). *Barcelona, Gastronomy, and Cuisine*. Saint Lluis (Menorca): Triangle Postals, 2011.

Casas, Penelope. *One Pot Spanish; More Than 80 Easy, Authentic Recipes*. Portland, ME: Sellers Publishing, 2009.

Ruscalleda, Carme. *CR20: 20 Years of the Sant Pau*. Mont-Ferrant, 2009.

Andrés, José. *Made in Spain; Spanish Dishes for American Kitchens*. Danvers, MA: Clarkson Potter Publishers, 2008.

Barlow, John. *Everything but the Squeal: Eating the Whole Hog in Northern Spain*. New York: Farrar, Straus and Giroux, 2008.

Batali, Mario, w/ Gwyneth Paltrow. *Spain*. New York: Harper-Collins Publishers, 2008.

Andrews, Colman. *Ferran: The Inside Story of El Bulli and the Man Who Reinvented Food*. New York: Gotham Books, 2010.

Casas, P. *Tapas: The Little Dishes of Spain*. New York: Knopf, 2007.

Chandler, Jenny, Jean Cazals (Photographer). *The Food of Northern Spain: Recipes from the Gastronomic Heartland of Spain*. London, England: Pavilion Books, 2006.

Casas, Penelope. *La Cocina de Mama: The Great Home Cooking of Spain*. New York: Clarkson Potter, 2005.

von Bremzen, Anya. *The New Spanish Table*. New York: Workman Publishing Company, 2005.

Harmon Jenkins, Nancy. *The Essential Mediterranean: How Regional Cooks Transform Key Ingredients into the World's Favorite Cuisines*. New York: Harper Collins Publishers, 2003.

Kurlansky, Mark. *Choice Cuts, a Savory Selection of Food Writing from Around the World and Throughout History*. New York: Ballantine Books, 2002.

Casas, Penelope. *Paella! Spectacular Rice Dishes from Spain*. New York: Henry Holt and Co., 1999.

Barrenechea, Teresa. *The Basque Table; Passionate Home Cooking from One of Europe's Great Regional Cuisines*. Cambridge, MA: Harvard Common Press, 1998.

Andrews, Colman. *Catalan Cuisine; Europe's Last Great Culinary Secret*. Atheneum, 1988.

Casas, Penelope. *Delicioso! The Regional Cooking of Spain*. New York: Knopf, 1996.

Busca Isusi, Jose Maria, Nancy Peppin. *Traditional Basque Cooking: History and Preparation* (Basque Series). Reno, NV: University of Nevada Press, 1993.

Torres, Marimar. *The Catalan Country Kitchen: Food and Wine from the Pyrenees to the Mediterranean Seacoast of Barcelona*. Cambridge, MA: De Capo Press, 1992.

Torres, Marimar. *The Spanish Table: The Cuisines and Wines of Spain*. New York: Doubleday & Co, 1986.

Wolfert, Paula. *The Cooking of Southwest France: A Collection of Traditional and New Recipes from France's Most Rustic Cuisine*. New York: Doubleday & Co, 1983.

Casas, Penelope. *The Foods and Wines of Spain*. New York: Knopf, 1982.

Robert, Mestre, *Libre del Coch*. Edited by Veronika Leimgruber. 2nd ed. Barcelona: Bibliotheca Torres Amat/Curial Edicions Catalanes,1982 (C). Definitive edition of book published in Barcelona in 1520 by Robert de Nola.

Crewe, Rudolfe, Editor. *Libre de Sent Sovi/Receptari de Cuina*. Barcelona: Editorial Barcino, 1979. Modern edition of the 1324 manuscript.

Ruscalleda, Carme. *Carme Ruscalleda's Meditteranean Cuisine: 100 Recipes to Cook at Home*. Salsa Books.

Spanish Culture

Hunter, M "The World's 50 Best Restaurants for 2023 Revealed" *CNN*, June 2023.

https:// www.cnn.com/travel/worlds-50-best-restaurants-2-23/index.html

Nabais, M. et al. "The Exploitation of Crabs by Last Interglacial Iberian Neanderthals: Evidence from Gruta da Figueira Brava (Portugal)." *Frontiers in Environmental Archaeology*, February 2023.

https://doi.org/10.3389/fearc.2023.1097815

Olaya, V. "Researchers Claim to Have Found Earliest Document Written in Basque 2,100 Years Ago." *El Pais*, November 2022.

https://english.elpais.com/culture/2022-11-14

Arranz, J. "Gourmet Neanderthals Cooked Seafood and Joined Forces with Other Clans to Hunt Giant Elephants." *El Pais*, February 2023.

https://english.elpais.com/science-tech/2023-02-12

Gracián, Baltasar. "The Pocket Oracle and Art of Prudence." *Penguin Classics*

Gracián, Baltasar. "A Pocket Mirror for Heroes." *Doubleday*, 1996

Avalle, Nico "Controversial 'World's 50 Best Restaurants' Group Announces 2022 Winners," July 18, 2022

www.bonappetit.com/story/worlds-50-best-restaurants-2022-winners

Moran, C. "Calais of the Costa Brava: Part 2." *Metropolitan Barcelona Magazine*, August 10, 2021.

www.barcelona-metropolitan.com/travel/calais-of-the-costa-brava-part-2

Bennett, Annie. "The Spectacular Spanish Region That the British Haven't Discovered." *The Telegraph*, July 22, 2019.

www.telegraph.co.uk/travel/destinations/europe/spain/articles/galicia-travel-guide-where-to-go/

Walker, Kira. "The Mediterranean Diet that Benefits from the Food of the Moors." *The Nation, Lifestyle*, May 27, 2019.

www.thenational.ae/lifestyle/food/the-mediterranean-diet-that-benefits-from-the-food-of-the-moors-1.866812#:~:text=The%20Mediterranean%20diet%20that%20benefits%20from%20the%20food,Vibrant%20Recipes%20from%20the%20Mediterranean'%20by%20Ben%20Tish

Hargitai, Q. "Is this the Home of the Holy Grail?", *BBC Travel*, May 2018.

www.bbc.com/travel/article/20180528-is-this-the-home-of-the-holy-grail

Sconzo, John. "The Legacy of el Bulli." *DocSconz; Musings on Food and Life*, July 9, 2018.

http://docsconz.com/2018/07/the-legacy-of-elbulli/

ACN Barcelona. "Three Michelin Star Restaurant Sant Pau to Close Down After 30 Years." *Catalan News*, July 6, 2018.

https://www.catalannews.com/life-style/item/three-michelin-star-restaurant-sant-pau-to-close-down-after-30-years

León, Pablo. "How Spanish Chefs are Still Revolutionizing the Global Food Scene." *EL PAÍS*, June 29, 2018.

https://english.elpais.com/elpais/2018/06/27/inenglish/1530100747_679502.html#:~:text=How%20Spanish%20chefs%20are%20still%20revolutionizing%20the%20global,dessert%20served%20at%20El%20celler%20de%20Can%20Roca.

Unattributed. "Taking the Kids to Basque Country." *Goop*, 2018.

https://goop.com/travel/experiences/taking-the-kids-to-basque-country/

Unattributed. "Healthy Living at This Year's *BioCultura* Fair in Barcelona." *Catalan News*, May 6, 2018.

www.catalannews.com/life-style/item/healthy-living-at-this-year-s-biocultura-fair-in-barcelona

Unattributed. "Catalonia; Tradition and Creativity from the Mediterranean." *Smithsonian Folk Life Festival*, 2018.

https://festival.si.edu/2018/catalonia

Unattributed. "Chef Ruscalleda to Open Restaurant for Two Months Abroad." *Catalan News*, April 18, 2018.

https://www.catalannews.com/life-style/item/chef-ruscalleda-to-open-restaurant-for-two-months-abroad

Uberauga, Blas Pedro. "Buber's Basque Page."

https://buber.net/Basque/

Unattributed. "Wooden Remains of Roman Shipwreck Discovered." *Catalan News*, March 20, 2018.

https://www.catalannews.com/culture/item/wooden-remains-of-roman-shipwreck-discovered#:~:text=Wooden%20remains%20of%20Roman%20shipwreck%20discovered%20Off%20the,structure%20was%20also%20-protected%20by%20over%20100%20amphoras

Unattributed. "Rioja Launches New Global Message." *Foods & Wines From Spain*, March 12, 2018.

https://www.foodswinesfromspain.com/spanishfoodwine/global/whats-new/news/new-detail/rioja-launches-new-global-message.html

Barrena, Pepe. "Playing with Fire at Etxebarri Restaurant." *Foods & Wines from Spain*, March 15, 2018.

https://www.foodswinesfromspain.com/spanishfoodwine/global/whats-new/features/feature-detail/etxebarri-restaurant.html

Hotz, Robert Lee. "Neanderthals Had a Creative Side, New Cave Art Studies Suggest." *The Wall Street Journal*, February 22, 2018.

Unattributed. "The Roca Brothers Prepare Menu for Elton John's Oscars Night Dinner." *Catalan News*, February 10, 2018.

https://www.catalannews.com/life-style/item/the-roca-brothers-prepare-menu-for-elton-john-s-oscars-night-dinner

Fernández, Rodrigo García. "12 Months of Gourmet Jewels from Spain." *Foods & Wines from Spain*, January 1, 2018.

https://www.foodswinesfromspain.com/spanishfoodwine/global/food/features/feature-detail/12-months-foodie-festivities-spain.html

Rey, Manuel. "Confirman o Avistamento 'Histórico' da Balea Azul na Ría de Muros e Noia." *GCiencia*, September 13, 2017.

www.gciencia.com/medioambiental/balea-azul-avistamento/

Mourenza, Paula. "Catalan Cheese, Part 1: Reviving Old Traditions." *Culinary Backstreets*, April 14, 2015.

www.culinarybackstreets.com/cities-category/barcelona/2015/catalan-cheese-part-1/

Andrei, M. "Spanish is the Happiest Language in the World, New Study Reveals." *ZME Science*, February 2015.

www.zmescience.com/research/language-happiness-02102015

Foster, Kirsten. "Wild Things: Foraging for Wild Food in the Catalan Countryside." *Metropoitan Barcelona*, 2014.

www.barcelona-metropolitan.com/eating-and-drinking/wild-things/

Mourenza, Paula. "Catalonia's Magic Mushroom Season." *Culinary Backstreets*, November 30, 2012.

www.culinarybackstreets.com/cities-category/barcelona/2012/catalonias-magic-mushrooms/

Besant, Alexander. "First Known Insect Pollen Carrier Found in Northern Spain." *Dadant*, May 15, 2012.

www.dadant.com/scientists-discover-first-ever-record-of-insect-pollination-from-100-million-years-ago/

Unattributed. "Spanish Olive Oil Triumphs at the New York International Olive Oil Competition." *Foods & Wine from Spain*, May 4, 2018.

www.foodswinesfromspain.com/spanishfoodwine/global/food/news/new-detail/new-york-olive-oil-competition.html

Dawes, Gerry. "God and Men (Godello and Menacía) in Ribeira Sacra: Winemaking in Spain's Most Exciting Wine Region for Terroir-Driven Wines." *Gerry Dawes's Spain: An Insider's Guide to Spanish Food, Wine, Culture, and Travel*, May 2012.

Finn, Maria. *The Whole Fish: How Adventurous Eating of Seafood Can Make You Healthier, Sexier, and Help Save the Ocean*. Ted Books, 2012.

Harris, Donald, B. *The Heart of Spain; Families and Food*. Portland, OR: Duende Press, 2011.

"*World Literature Today* Devotes a Monographic Dossier to Catalan Literature." *Institut Ramon Llull*, September 28, 2009.

Reguant-Aleix, J. et al. "Mediterranean Heritage: an Intangible Cultural Heritage." *Public Health Nutrition*, September 2009.

https://doi.org/10.1017/s1368980009990413

Bahrami, Beebe. *The Spiritual Traveler: Spain; A Guide to Scared Sites and Pilgrim Routes*. Hidden Springs, CA: Hidden Springs Publishing, 2009.

Williams, Mark. *The Story of Spain: The Dramatic History of Europe's Most Fascinating Country*. San Mateo, CA: Golden Era Books, 2009.

Xamar. *Orhipean; The Country of Basque* (2nd Edition). Navarre: Pamiela Publishing, 2009.

Young, Sue. *Antoni Gaudi 1852-1926*. *Sue Young Histories*. November 2008.

www.sueyounghistories.com/2008-11-22-antoni-gaudi-1852-1926/

Burnett, V. "Spain's Top Chefs Clash Over Ingredients and Culinary Innovations." *The New York Times*, June 1, 2008.

> https://www.nytimes.com/2008/06/01/world/europe

Santanach, Joan; Translated by Robin Vogelzang. *The Book of Sent Soví: Medieval Recipes from Catalonia*. Rochester, NY: Barcino-Tamesis, June 19, 2008.

Zubiri, Nancy. *A Travel Guide to Basque America: Families, Feasts, and Festivals*. Reno, NV: University of Nevada Press, 2006.

Kurlansky, Mark. *The Basque History of the World: The Story of a Nation*. New York: Penguin Books, 1999.

Casas, Penelope. *Discovering Spain: An Uncommon Guide*. New York: Knopf, 1996.

Andrews, Colman. "Ramon Cabau Gausch: A 'Poet of the Ovens.'" *The Los Angeles Times*, June 28, 1987.

> www.latimes.com/archives/la-xpm-1987-06-28-ca-70-story.html

Gray, Patience. *Honey from a Weed, Fasting and Feasting in Tuscany, Catalonia, The Cyclades and Apulia*. London: Prospect Books, 1986.

Markham, James M. "A Nouvelle Cuisine with a Catalan Flair." *New York Times*, October 25, 1981.

> www.nytimes.com/1981/10/25/travel/a-nouvelle-cuisine-with-a-catalan-flair.html

de Ugalde, Martin. "A Short History of Basque Country." *Buber.net*, 1980.

> www.buber.net/Basque/History/shorthist.php

Pla, Josep. *The Gray Notebook*. Edited & Translated by the heirs of Joseph Pla. New York: New York Review of Books. 1966.

Orwell, George. *Homage to Catalonia*. New York: Houghton Mifflin Harcourt, 1952.

Ford, Richard. *Gatherings from Spain*. London: *Clowes and Sons*, 1906. (Nabu Public Domain Reprints).

Additional Reading: Booklets, Articles, Blogs and More

Severson, K. "How Will We Eat in 2021? 11 Predictions to Chew On." *The New York Times*, December 22, 2020

> www.nytimes.com/2020/12/22/dining/food-trends-predictions-2021.html

Ann Abel, "Michelin Awards 18 Restaurants in Spain and Portugal Stars for 2020" *Forbes*, Nov 2019.

> www.forbes.com/sites/annabel/2019/11/21/2020-michelin-stars-in-spain-and-portugal-who-got-the-new-stars/#3cb963836124

Dunlop, Fiona. "Spain's Best Young Chefs and the Restaurants where You'll Discover Them." *The Guardian*, January 30, 2020.

> www.theguardian.com/travel/2020/jan/30/spain-best-young-chefs-restaurants-where-youll-discover-them

Number of Michelin 3-star Restaurants Goes up to Four in Catalonia." *Catalan News*, November 23, 2017.

www.catalannews.com/life-style/item/number-of-michelin-3-star-restaurants-goes-up-to-four-in-catalonia

Tanis, David. "You Say Tomato, I Say Tomato Toast." *The New York Times*, July 20, 2018.

www.nytimes.com/2018/07/20/dining/pan-con-tomate-recipe.html

Tanis, David. "Duck in Summertime, Spicy and Fruity." *The New York Times*, August 7, 2015.

www.nytimes.com/2015/08/12/dining/duck-in-summertime-spicy-and-fruity.html

Fernández, Rodrigo Garcia. "Balfegó, the Spanish Company that is Fighting to Save Bluefin Tuna." November 22, 2017.

www.foodswinesfromspain.com/spanishfoodwine/global/wine/features/feature-detail/balfego-bluefin-tuna.html

Kemper, Benjamin. "How a Chef with 8 Michelin Stars Cooks at Home." *The Wall Street Journal*, July 12, 2017.

www.wsj.com/articles/how-a-chef-with-8-michelin-stars-cooks-at-home-1499888140

Unattributed. "Study Reveals Neanderthals at El Sidrón in Northern Spain had Knowledge of Plants' Healing Qualities." *University of York*, 2012.

www.york.ac.uk/news-and-events/features/el-sidron/

Aparicio, S. "From Sea to Mountain in 5 Cheeses." *Spain Gourmet Travel Tour, Food & Wine*, 2008.

Harmon Jenkins, Nancy. "The New Spanish Mediterranean Diet." *Bantam*, 2008.

Perry, Charles, "The Oldest Mediterranean Noodle: A Cautionary Tale." *Petit Propos Culinaires* 9, October, 1981.

Dean, M. et al. "Longstanding Dental Pathology in Neanderthals from El Sidrón (Asturias, Spain) with a Probable Familial Basis." *Journal of Human Evolution*, June 2013.

https://doi.org/10.1016/j.jhevol.2013.03.004

Turismo de Aragón. *Food and Recipes from Aragón*. Departmento de Industria Comercio y Turismo de Aragón.

McHenry, H. "Atapuerca", *Britannica*.

www.britannica.com/place/atapuerca

black cumin, 134–135

black currants, 124–125, 129

black pepper, 133

black sausage, 174

bladderwrack, 335

Blanc, 302

blood cancer, 137

blood clotting, 97, 108, 140

blood pressure, 50, 59, 110, 128–129, 276

blood sausage, 174

blood sugar, 48–49, 95, 104, 136, 171. *See also* diabetes; insulin

blueberries, 124, 162

boars, wild, 110

bocadillos, 179

Bodega Torres, 316–317

body care, 336

bomba rice, 92, 164, 175

bone broth, 112, 166, 198, 335. *See also* stock

bone cancer, 137

bone health, 27, 67–68, 97, 106, 112, 120, 129, 198, 276, 299. *See also* osteoporosis

bones in cooking, 111–112

boquerones, 175

borage *(borraja),* 93

botanical medicine, 328. *See also* herbs: medicinal use

botifarra amb mongetes, 106

botifarra sausage, 24, 72, 174

Botín Arts Center, 347

bowel cancer. *See* colon cancer

BPA, 17

brain function, 115, 270–271, 276. *See also* Alzheimer's disease; cognitive decline; memory

bread, 24, 113, 161, 163, 166, 179–180

breadcrumbs, 247, 333

bread sticks, 179

breakfast, 281–286

breast cancer, 16, 23, 54, 109 prevention, 28–29

and essential oils, 336

and fruit, 123–126, 128

and herbs, 104

and legumes, 106–107, 229

and nuts, 85, 87

and olive oil or olives, 22, 47–52, 59, 68

and seafood, 71–73, 276

and vegetables, 78–79, 81–82, 96–98, 101, 105

resources, 314, 331, 337

Breast Cancer Prevention Partners, 314

broccoli, 80–81, 83, 97

broccoli sprouts, 94

bromelain, 129

broth. *See* bone broth; fish broth; seafood broth; stock

brussels sprouts, 81, 97

Buckley, Marti, 352

buckwheat, 164

burned meat, 54

butifarra sausage. *See* *botifarra* sausage

butter, 51, 119

Bye Bye Plastic Bags, 325

Cabau, Ramón, 68

cabbage, 24, 81–82, 162

Cabellé, Montserrat, 342

Cabrales cheese, 122, 163

Cadí cooperative, 119

café con leche, 172, 281–282

caffeic acid, 93

calabacín. See zucchini

calabaza. See pumpkins

calamar, 91

Calatrava, Santiago, 349

calciferol. *See* vitamin D

calcium, 48–49, 68, 93, 97, 106, 120, 125, 128, 276

calcium d-glucarate, 126

Cal Codina, 120

calçots, 66

Caldo de pescado, 172

cherries, 129
chestnuts, 85–86, 163
Chez Panisse, 311
chicken, 108, 164
chicken feet, 111
chickpeas, 106–107
Chillida, Eduardo, 339–340
chives, 164
chlorogenic acid, 99
chocolate, 115, 125, 131, 161,
    165–166, 299
chocos, 70
cholesterol, 49, 85, 101, 110, 114–115,
    123, 276
    LDL, 99, 107, 115, 120, 124
choline, 94, 114–115
choricero peppers, 163, 175, 177–178,
    240, 334
chorizo, 173–174
churches, 64, 140, 327, 347. *See also*
    cathedrals
cider, 44, 318
cigalas, 70
cinnamon, 136
citrus fruit, 123. *See also specific types*
CLA, 120
clams, 71, 106. *See also specific types*
clay pot cooking, 172–173
clementines, 123–124
cloves, 137
cobalamin. *See* vitamin B12
cocido lebaniego, 107
cocido montañés, 106
cocidos, 82
cocina de vanguardia, 18, 26. *See also*
    gastronomy: Spanish
cod, 72–73, 175
Codorníu Raventós, 317
coffee, 172, 281–282
cognitive decline, 124, 168, 276, 315.
    See also Alzheimer's disease;
    brain function; memory
cojones, 113
Colbin, Anne Marie, 4, 33

collagen, 111–112, 136, 198, 334–335
colon cancer, 17, 21–23, 75, 108,
    115, 128
conjugated linoleic acid, 120
cooking, 29–30, 33, 46, 52, 147, 152,
    167–168, 170. *See also under*
    gastronomy
    resources, 350–353
    training (*see* culinary education)
    with bones, 111–112
    with fish, 52, 72, 153
    with potatoes, 153–154
    with seafood, 52, 75, 145
    with spices, 132–136
    with vegetables, 154
    with vinegar, 138
coronary disease. *See* cardiovascular
    disease
Cortes de Navarra, 114
cortisol, 332
courgettes, 98, 162
couscous, 164
Covid-19, 3, 75
COX-2 enzyme, 78, 133
crabs, 70
cranberries, 124
crema catalana, 136
criadillas de toro, 113
CR20: 20 Years of Sant Pau
    (Ruscalleda), 219, 224
cruciferous vegetables, 81–82, 97
Cruz, Jordi, 290
Cua Ferrat Museum, 341
cucumbers, 98
CUICK, 150
Cuinar per ser feliç (Ruscalleda), 147
culinary education, 310–311, 313, 343
cumin, 133–134
cumin, black, 134–135
currants, black, 124–125, 129
cuttlefish, 70, 91
cuttlefish ink, 91, 175. *See also* squid ink
cysteine, 138

glycemic load, 95. *See also* blood sugar
glycine, 112
glyphosate, 181
goat milk, 119–120
Godello wine, 256
González-Solla, José (Pepe), 26
González Sotres, Ricardo, 25
Gordal olives, 67, 162
grains, 161, 164, 181. *See also*
    specific types
Gran Teatre del Liceu, 342
grapefruit, 123
grapes, 125–126, 140. *See also* raisins
greenmarkets, 27, 33, 46, 63–64,
    298–299. *See also la* Boqueria
green tea, 78
grelos. See turnip greens
Grupo Nove, 26
Guggenheim Bilbao, 340–341
guindilla peppers, 102, 166, 178
gut health. *See* gastrointestinal health
gut microbiome, 22, 49, 75, 85,
    106–107, 120, 299. *See also*
    gastrointestinal health

Hadid, Zaha, 349
hair, 112, 198
hake, 72, 242
ham, 110–111, 149, 164
hazelnuts, 163
HCAs, 54
health and diet. *See* diet: effect
    on health
health and wellness resources,
    328–332, 334–338. *See also*
    nutrition resources
heart disease. *See* cardiovascular
    disease
heavy metals, 137
Hemingway, Ernest, 140–141
hemoglobin, 112
herbs, 103–104, 163–164, 269–271.
    See also specific herbs

medicinal use, 270–271, 298,
    329–331, 335 (*see also*
    botanical medicine)
resources, 337
herpes simplex virus, 137
heterocyclic amines, 54
high blood pressure. *See* blood pressure
Hispània, 24
hogs, 110
homeopathy, 331, 337
homocysteine, 111
honey, 29, 138, 164
horchata de chufa, 304
Hudson, Tori, 331
Huesca, 39, 46, 172, 326
huevos revueltos con ajos tiernos, 76
hydroxytyrosol, 68
hypertension. *See* blood pressure

*Iberian Table, The (*Keuneke), xiii–xiv,
    3, 6–7, 9–10, 14–17, 19, 289,
    298, 356
Ibérico pig, 110
Idiazábal cheese, 122, 163
immunity and immune system, 30, 75,
    83, 93, 113, 185, 235, 333
    and bone broth, 112, 198
    and dairy products, 120, 299, 330
    and fruit, 125, 129
    and mushrooms, 78, 335
    and seafood, 91, 235, 276
indoles, 81–82
infertility, 17
inflammation, 17, 22, 104, 120, 133, 168,
    335. *See also* anti-inflammatory
    properties
ingredients in Spanish cooking. *See*
    Spanish pantry
Institute of Culinary Education, 310
Institut Ramon Llull, 345
insulin, 86. *See also* blood sugar;
    diabetes
Intangible Cultural Heritage of
    Humanity, xiii, 6

rabbit, 164
rabo de buey, 112
Racó de Can Fabes, 290
Rafa's, 76, 201
raisins, 126, 129. *See also* grapes
raspberries, 124, 162
ratatouille, 99
razor clams, 71
Recuit cheese. See *Mató* cheese
red meat, 54, 109. *See also* beef; meat
red wine. *See* wine: red
reflexology, 337–338
Reichl, Ruth, 350
reinetas, 126
Reixach, Lolita, 24
Reixach, Paquita, 24
Rekondo (restaurant), 126
Rekondo, Edurne, 126
Rekondo, Txomin, 126
Representative List of Intangible
    Cultural Heritage of Humanity,
    xiii, 6
resistant starch, 94, 106
respiratory problems, 104
Restaurant Indigo, 7, 271
restaurant meals, 168
restaurants, 290, 326, 338. *See also*
    specific restaurants
resveratrol, 125, 140
riboflavin, 110
rice, 92, 164, 175, 225
RNA, 112
Roca brothers (Joan, Josep, and Jordi),
    290, 298
rockfish, 70
Rodoreda, Mercè, 345
Román, María José San. *See* San
    Román, María José
romesco sauce, 66, 85, 102, 166, 259
Roncal cheese, 122, 163
rosemary, 8, 104, 164, 270–271
rosewater, 164
rosmarinic acid, 104
rouge de roussillons, 127

Rubia Gallega beef, 24
Rubio, Ana Vela. *See* Vela Rubio, Ana
Ruscalleda, Carme, 7, 16, 26, 82–83,
    89, 143, 150, 155, 224, 264,
    275, 290
    CR20: 20 Years of Sant Pau,
    219, 224
    Cuinar per ser feliç, 147
    interview with, 145–149
    recipes, 149–150
    restaurants, 144–148, 302
Ruscalleda, Raul, 144
Rusiñol, Santiago, 341
rutabagas, 162

saffron, 29, 132–133, 163, 175–176
Sage Mountain Retreat Center and
    Nature Preserve, 331
Sagrada Familia cathedral, 117, 343
St. James legend of scallop shells,
    74–75
St. John's wort, 335
salicylic acid, 98
salmorreta, 102
salsa gallega, 179
Salsa Para tu Coco (Berasategui), 18
salsa vizcaína, 177–178
salt, 162, 168, 170
salted cod, 72–73, 175
Salt Island (Connecticut), 13–14
samfaina, 99
San Román, María José, 7, 9, 199, 225,
    227, 290
San Sebastián. *See* Donostia
San Sebastián Jazz Festival, 341
Santamaría, Santi, 290
Santa María del Mar, 343
Sant Pau (Japan), 144, 147–148
Sant Pau (Spain), 144–147
sardines, 42, 166
saturated fat, 51, 109, 114, 120–121.
    See also fats, dietary
sausages, 173–174. *See also*
    specific types

Color Inserts

1   Mural cameo, La Senorita with Brick, Manu Manu. Photo, Lourdes Solana Carné.

2   Mural cameo, La Senora, Manu Manu. Photo, Lourdes Solana Carné.

3   Barcelona street art mural, *M'agraden* les mares I dones del món sencer, Manu Manu. Photo, Lourdes Solana Carné.

4   Monastrell grapes. Photo courtesy of Gerry Dawes.

5   Vegetable Menestra. Food styling and photo, Eva Espinet and Olga Moya.

6   Basque Piperrada Vasca. Food styling and photo, Eva Espinet and Olga Moya.

7   Cod on a Bed of Multi-Color Vegetables. Photo, author.

8   Dried Salt Cod Croquetas. Food styling and photo, Eva Espinet and Olga Moya.

9   Pa amb Tomáquet. Food styling and photo, Eva Espinet and Olga Moya.

10 Minced Leek and Tomato Salad with Queen Olives. Food styling and photo, Eva Espinet and Olga Moya.

11 Mediterranean Seafood Paella. Photo, author.

12 Migas and Grapes. Food styling and photo, Eva Espinet and Olga Moya.

13 Fabada Austuriana. Photo, author.

14 *A Private Country*, oil on canvas, by author.

Chapter Openings including Parts One and Two

Black and white cameos of Barcelona street art mural. Photos, Lourdes Solana Carné.

Author page. Self-Portrait, oil on canvas. Author's photo.

Front Cover Flap. Author's photo.

BASQUE TO BARCELONA!
... and Stories Along the Way

ROBIN KEUNEKE

The stories in this collection revealed themselves, as if waiting to be discovered—by me. Apparently my 'literary spring' that had bubbled before Spain had finally been freed. I began assuaging a thirst I did not know I had. Someone said that 'water teaches thirst'. Well, Spain is my water.

But how does the published author of three non-fiction books, including, *The Iberian Table*, suddenly change and write fiction? Perhaps, as Washington Irving experienced, after traveling to Spain, I discovered my Self.

Irving found himself in Spain expecting to make translations of documents relating to a biography of Christopher Columbus. Instead he found his artistic spirit "in poor, wild, legendary proud-spirited, romantic Spain where the old magnificent barbaric spirit still contends." After Spain, Irving produced his best work in four subsequent books he had no idea he would write."

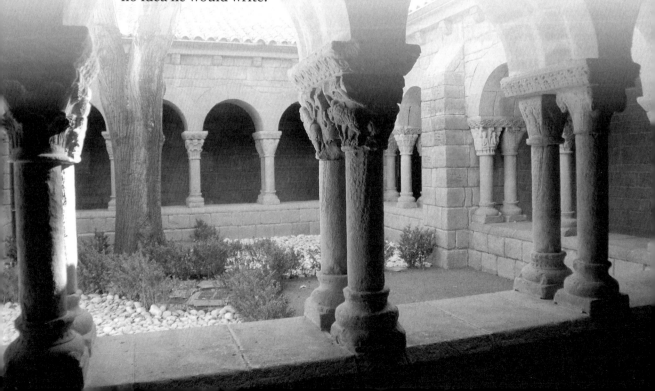